Recent Progress in Toxicity and Drug Testing

Recent Progress in Toxicity and Drug Testing

Edited by **Judith Baker**

New Jersey

Published by Foster Academics,
61 Van Reypen Street,
Jersey City, NJ 07306, USA
www.fosteracademics.com

Recent Progress in Toxicity and Drug Testing
Edited by Judith Baker

International Standard Book Number: 978-1-63242-351-1 (Hardback)

Printed in the United States of America.

Contents

Preface

This book was inspired by the evolution of our times; to answer the curiosity of inquisitive minds. Many developments have occurred across the globe in the recent past which has transformed the progress in the field.

Present-day drug design and testing includes experimental in-vitro and in-vivo measurements of the drug candidate's adsorption, distribution, metabolism, elimination and toxicity (ADMET) properties in the initial stages of drug discovery. Just a poor percentage of the recommended drug candidates get the authorization of government and reach the market place. Disadvantageous pharmacokinetic properties, bad bioavailability and efficiency, negative side effects, poor solubility and toxicity matters are responsible for most of the drug failures confronted in the pharmaceutical industry. Authors from across the globe have provided information elucidating pharmaceutical concerns, regulatory policies and clinical properties in their respective countries hoping that the open trade of scientific ideas and outcomes compiled in this book will result in enhanced pharmaceutical products. This book has a section on drug design covering several research chapters.

This book was developed from a mere concept to drafts to chapters and finally compiled together as a complete text to benefit the readers across all nations. To ensure the quality of the content we instilled two significant steps in our procedure. The first was to appoint an editorial team that would verify the data and statistics provided in the book and also select the most appropriate and valuable contributions from the plentiful contributions we received from authors worldwide. The next step was to appoint an expert of the topic as the Editor-in-Chief, who would head the project and finally make the necessary amendments and modifications to make the text reader-friendly. I was then commissioned to examine all the material to present the topics in the most comprehensible and productive format.

I would like to take this opportunity to thank all the contributing authors who were supportive enough to contribute their time and knowledge to this project. I also wish to convey my regards to my family who have been extremely supportive during the entire project.

Editor

Drug Design

Blood Brain Barrier Permeation

Abolghasem Jouyban[1] and Somaieh Soltani[2]
[1]Drug Applied Research Center and Faculty of Pharmacy,
[2]Liver and Gastrointestinal Diseases Research Center,
Tabriz University of Medical Sciences, Tabriz,
Iran

1. Introduction

The large surface area and the short diffusion distance from capillaries of the blood brain barrier (BBB) to the neurons facilitate the drugs and nutrients access to the brain. Penetration of chemicals to the BBB occurs using a combination of intra and intercellular passages. Tight junctions regulate the intracellular passage of molecules according to their physico- chemical properties (e.g. lipophilicity, ionisation and polarity), where inter cellular penetration is regulated by influx and efflux transporters, endocytosis and passive diffusion. Poor pharmacokinetic properties (absorption, distribution, metabolism and excretion) and toxicity are responsible for most of the failures in drug discovery projects. This problem is more evident for CNS drugs because of the restrict barrier function of blood brain barrier. The CNS drug discovery attracted more attentions since the diseases pattern has been changed during recent decades and aging disorders are one of the major health problems. Drug exposure is controlled by plasma pharmacokinetic properties of drug which are different from brain pharmacokinetic and can be studied using common pharmacokinetic studies, where BBB permeability depends on physicochemical properties of drug compound and physiologic function of the BBB (physical barrier, transport, metabolic, ...) and need special study techniques. In this chapter, fundamentals of BBB, permeation mechanisms, penetration measurement methods and penetration prediction methods are discussed.

2. Fundamentals of BBB

2.1 Cellular properties of Blood Brain Barrier

BBB consisted of a monolayer of brain micro vascular endothelial cells (BMVEC) joined together by much tighter junctions than peripheral vessels and formed a cellular membrane which known as the main physical barrier of BBB (Abbott, 2005; Cardoso et.al., 2010). The main characteristics of this cellular membrane are, uniform thickness, no fenestrae, low pinocytotic activity, continues basement membrane and negative surface charge. In addition to the BMVECs, the neurovascular unit consisted of the capillary basement membrane, pericytes, astrocytes and microglia. The BMVECs are surrounded by a basement membrane which composed of structural proteins (collagen and elastin), specialized proteins (fibronectin and laminin) and proteoglycans. This structural specificity gives the basement membrane a cell establishment role. Pericytes are cellular constituents of microvessels including capillaries and post capillary venules that covered about 22-32% of the capillaries and shared the same basement membrane. Pericytes are responsible for a wide variety of structural and non-structural tasks in BBB. In summary they synthesis some of structural and signalling proteins and they are involved in the BMVECs proliferation, migration and differentiation. More details and references about pericytes role in BBB can be found in the literature (Cardoso et al., 2010). Fine lamellae closely opposed to the outer surface of the capillary endothelium and respective basement membrane formed by astrocytes end feet. Like pericytes, astrocytes involve in various functional and structural properties of neurovascular unit.

Microglia is immunocompetent cells of the brain that continuously survey local micro environment with highly motile extensions and change the phenotype in response to the homeostatic disturbance of the CNS (Prinz & Mildner, 2011). The interactions of brain micro vascular endothelial cells with basement membrane, neighbouring glial cells (microglia and astrocytes), neurons and perivascular pericytes leads to specific brain micro vascular biology. Presence of matrix adhesion receptors and signalling proteins form an extensive and complex matrix which is essential for maintenance of the BBB (Cardoso et al., 2010). Figure 1 shows a schematic illustration of neurovascular unit and BBB cellular components.

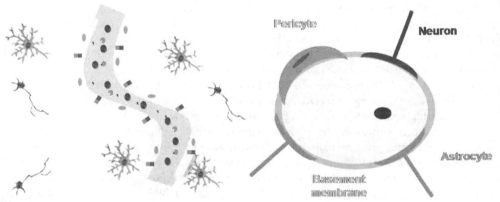

Fig. 1. Schematic illustration of the neurovascular unit and BBB cellular components adopted from (Cardoso et al., 2010).

2.2 Molecular properties of BBB

The BMVECs assembly are regulated by molecular constituents of tight junctions, adherence junctions and signalling pathways. Tight junctions are highly dynamic structures which are responsible for the barrier properties of BBB. Apical region of the endothelial cells sealed together by tight junctions and paracellular permeability of BMVECs are limited by them. Structurally tight junctions formed by interaction of integral transmembrane proteins with neighbouring plasma membrane. Among these proteins junction adhesion molecules, claudins and occludins (inter membrane) which bind to the cytoplasmic proteins (e.g. zonula occludens, cinguline, ...) are well studied and their role in tight junctions and BBB have been evaluated (Figure 2). Beyond the main role in physical restriction of BBB, other functions such as control of gene expression, cell proliferation and differentiation have been suggested for tight junctions. Below the tight junctions, actin filaments (including cadherins and catenins) linked together and form a belt of adherence junctions. In addition to the contribution in the barrier function some other events such as adhesion of BMVECs to each other, the contact inhibition during vascular growth, the initiation of cell polarity and the regulation of paracellular permeability have been suggested for adherence junctions. A dynamic interaction between tight junctions and adherence junctions through signalling pathways regulate the permeability of BBB. These signalling routes mainly involve protein kinases, members of mitogen – activated protein kinases, endothelial nitric oxide synthase and G-proteins. Dynamic interactions between these pathways control the opening and closing of the paracellular route for fluids, proteins and cells to move across the endothelial cells through two main types of signal transduction procedures (e.g. signals from cell interior to tight junctions to guide their assembly and regulate their permeability, signals transmitted from tight junctions to cell interior to modulate gene expression, proliferation and differentiation). The molecular mechanisms of these interactions can be found in the literature (Ballab et al., 2004; Abbott et al., 2006). In addition to the proteins with enzymatic activities, there are other specific proteins (drug efflux transporters, multi drug resistance proteins, organic anion transporting polypeptides) work as BBB transporters which are responsible for rapid efflux of xenobiotics from the CNS (Losscher & Potschka, 2005) and delivery of the essential nutrients and transmitters to the brain.

The combined effect of the special cellular and molecular properties of central nervous system result in the specific barrier functions of BBB which is important for preventing CNS from harmful xenobiotics. Because of these properties drug delivery to the CNS is among the most challenging drug development areas. In order to develop successful drug candidates for CNS disorders drug uptake mechanisms should be studied. In the next section, these mechanisms are briefly reviewed.

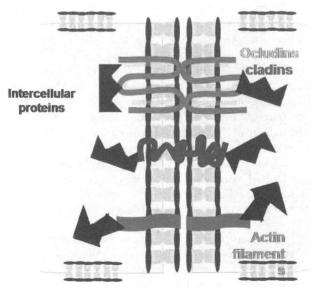

Fig. 2. Tight junctions and adherent junctions.

3. BBB permeation mechanisms

Like other cellular membranes in the body, permeation through BBB can occur by passive diffusion, endocytosis and active transport (Diagram 1). Combined effects of the mentioned mechanisms modulate the compound (e.g. Drugs) penetration to the brain.

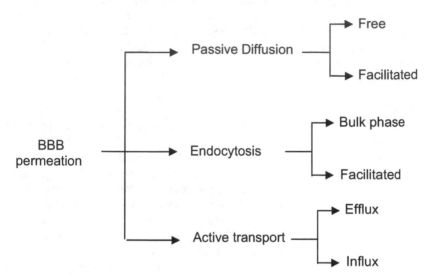

Diagram 1. Main permeation mechanisms in the brain.

3.1 Passive diffusion

A limited number of drugs and drug like compounds with high lipophilicity and low molecular size can penetrate to the brain mainly by passive diffusion. In order to overcome the surface tension difference between a compound and cellular membrane, physical work is needed and the smaller molecules will need less work. The uncharged forms of the weak acidic and basic compounds have higher permeability rate in comparison with charged molecules in physiologic pH of brain. The charged forms possess hydrophilic characteristics and hydrophilic drugs distribute within blood and cannot cross the endothelial cells and excreted from brain parenchyma. Therefore, the molecules with higher fraction of uncharged form in physiologic pH have higher permeability rate (Fischer et al., 1998).

Passive diffusion occurs via two mechanisms (Figure 3):

- Free diffusion in which some compounds move freely paracellularly (e.g. sucrose) between cells to a limited extent due to tight junctions or transcellularly (transcytosis) across the cells for lipophilic substances (e.g. ethanol) (Alam et al., 2010). These mechanisms are non-competitive, nonsaturable and occur in downhill concentration direction.
- Facilitated diffusion in which target compounds bind to a specific membrane protein and carry to the other side of the membrane through conformation change of the protein. This mechanism is a form of carrier mediated endocytosis which occurs from high to low concentration like free diffusion and contributes for transport of some amino acids, nucleosides, small peptides, mono-carboxylates and glutathione (Alam et al., 2010).

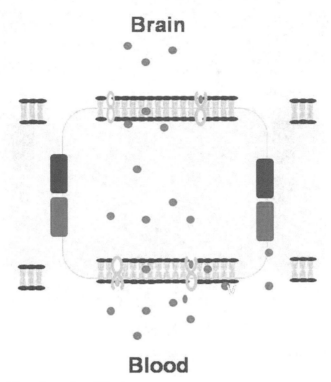

Fig. 3. Free and facilitated passive diffusion.

3.2 Endocytosis

In this method, substances (e.g. macromolecules) are engulfed by membrane and pass through the cell by vesicles and release in the other side (Kerns & Di, 2008). Endocytosis occurs via two main methods: bulk phase endocytosis (fluid phase or pinocytosis) and mediated or facilitated endocytosis (receptor and absorptive mediated). Fluid phase endocytosis is a nonsaturable, non-competitive and non-specific method for uptake of extra cellular fluids which is temperature and energy dependent.

Receptor mediated endocytosis facilitates the larger essential molecules uptake selectively using specific receptors present in luminal membrane. Hormones, growth factors, enzymes and plasma proteins are targets for specific receptors (Pardridge, 2007).

Absorptive mediated endocytosis is based on an electrostatic interaction between negatively charged plasma membrane luminal surfaces (glycocalyx which is a negatively charged proteoglycan or glycosaminoglycan) with cationic substances (e.g. peptides) and uptake it in a vesicle into the endothelial cell and release it on the other side (Figure 4) (Ueno, 2009).

This has lower affinity and higher capacity than receptor mediated endocytosis (Alam et al., 2010). Mechanism of vesicle formation (caveolin dependent, dynamin dependent and caveolin- dynamin independent) is not discussed in this chapter and more details could be found in the literature (Lajoie et al., 2010).

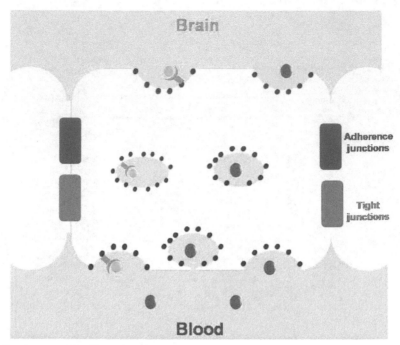

Fig. 4. Bulk phase and facilitated endocytosis.

3.3 Active transport

Hydrophilic drugs which cannot penetrate the brain through passive diffusion and lipophilic drugs which cannot penetrate the brain, in contrast of their suitable characteristics for BBB permeation are substrate for drug transporters of the BBB. Also some compounds are substrates for transporters and at the same time they are delivered by passive diffusion or endocytosis. Drug transporters are integral membrane proteins which is able to carry the drug usually against the concentration gradient into and out of the cell.

The overall exposure of xenobiotics to brain through these transporters depends on their location and expression level according to the normal and pathophysiologic conditions. Two types of drug transporters according to their driving forces (ATP dependent and ATP independent) are known. Active transporters broadly categorized as primary (ATP dependent), secondary or tertiary (ATP independent) (Murk et al., 2010).

There are two types of transporters:

1. Carrier mediated transporters which express on both the luminal and abluminal membranes and operates in both blood to brain and brain to blood directions.
2. Active efflux transporters which mediate extruding drugs and other compounds from brain (Alam et al., 2010). Although the main role of the drug transporters is carrying the drugs and other xenobiotics into and out of the brain but they are responsible for other cell processes such as inflammation, differentiation of immune cells, cell detoxification, lipid trafficking, hormone secretion and development of stem cells (Murk et al., 2010).

3.3.1 Influx transporters

Essential hydrophilic nutrients (e.g. glucose, amino acids, fatty acids, organic and inorganic ions) reach to brain through influx transporters and receptors. According to the structural similarity of the target drug to the biologic molecules; it can be delivered to the brain using appropriate transporter. Solute carrier family encodes most of the influx transporters which include facilitated, ion coupled and ion exchange transporters that do not need ATP (Eyal et al., 2009). These transporters are responsible for uptake of a broad range of substrates including glucose, amino acids, nucleosides, fatty acids, minerals and vitamins (Alam et al., 2010). The most well studied groups of these bidirectional transporters along with their properties and activities are summarized in Table 1.

3.3.2 Efflux transporters

Efflux occurs in BBB through both passive and active routes in order to detoxify the brain and prevent from drugs and xenobiotics exposures. There are several kinds of efflux transporters such as ATP binding cassette transporters (ABC), organic anion transport systems, amino acid transport systems and so on (Ueno, 2009). ABC transporters are primary active systems which are responsible for different efflux activities including P-glycoprotein (P-gp), multi-drug resistance proteins (MRPs), and breast cancer related protein (BCRP). P-gp (the most studied ABC transporter), located in luminal side of BBB, immediately pump most of the drugs and xenobiotics back to the blood and decrease the net penetration to the brain. A broad range of drugs, generally including un-conjugated and cationic substances (Table 1) are substrates for P-gp, where some of them are able to inhibit P-gp and lead to increased permeability of co-administered drugs. This fact can be used as a drug delivery strategy to the brain. Along with P-gp, MRPs and BCRP are responsible for main part of drug efflux in BBB and their effect are dependent to their localization and expression level in normal and pathologic conditions. Over expression of these transporters considered as one of the major reasons of pharmacoresistance of brain diseases and their inhibition, bypassing and regulating methods are important for CNS drug development (Loscher & Potschka, 2005).

3.4 Metabolism in BBB (Enzymatic barrier)

Existing enzymes in BBB can be regarded as second barrier after negative surface charge. These enzymes involve in disposition of drugs and xenobiotics before entering the endothelial cells of capillaries. Alkaline phosphatase, acid phosphatase, 5′-nucleotidase, adenosine tri-phosphatase and nucleoside di-phosphatase are among well studied enzymes distributed within BBB (Ueno, 2009).

4. BBB permeation measurement methods

The rate and the extent of drug transport to the brain are needed for drug discovery studies (both peripheral and CNS drugs) and different methods developed in order to study the pharmacokinetic profile of drug candidates. BBB permeability depends on physicochemical properties of drug compound and physiologic functions of the BBB (physical barrier, transport, metabolic pathways) and need special study techniques. These techniques include *in vivo*, *in vitro*, and *in silico* methods (Diagram 2) which are complement in most cases and researchers are able to define different aspects of drug passage to the brain using these methods.

Transporter name	Substrates	Sample drugs and nutrients	Influx/ Efflux
Organic anion transporting polypeptides	Anionic amphipathic molecules with molecular weight greater than 450 Daltons and a high degree of albumin binding	Fexofenadine, Digoxin, Methotrexate	Influx
Organic anion transporters	Anionic drugs and nucleotides	Benzylpenicillin, Valacyclovir, Zidovudine, Mercaptopurine, Methotrexate, Valproic acid	Influx
Organic cation transporters	Bidirectional transport of small hydrophilic positively charged compounds	Cimetidine , Desipramine, Metformin, Amantadine, Memantine, Cisplatine, Quinin	Influx / Efflux
System L.	Bidirectional transport of large neutral amino acids with branched or aromatic side chains	L-phenylalanine, L-tyrosine, L-tryptophan, L-lucine, Levodopa, α-Methyldopa, Baclofen, Melphalan, Gabapentin, Pregabalin	Influx / Efflux
Monocarboxylate transporters	HMG-CoA reductase inhibitors that contain a carboxylic acid moiety	Simvastatin, γ- Hydroxybutyrate	Influx
Nucleoside transporters	Purine and pyrimidine nucleosides	Adenosine	Influx
Hexose transporters	Hexose nucleosides	Glucose	Influx
Ion transporters	Bidirectional transport of small ions	Cl^-, Na^+, K^+, H^+, $HCO3^-$	Influx / Efflux
P-glycoproteins	A broad range of drugs and xenobiotics (normally un-conjugated, cationic substances)	Anti cancer drugs, corticoids	Efflux
Multi-drug resistance proteins	Drugs and xenobiotics (normally conjugated, anionic substances)	Anti cancer and anti HIV Drugs	Efflux
Breast cancer resistant proteins	Drugs and xenobiotics (overlap with P-glycoproteins and multi-drug resistance proteins)	Some anti cancer Drugs	Efflux

Table 1. Some of the well studied influx and efflux transporters of brain.

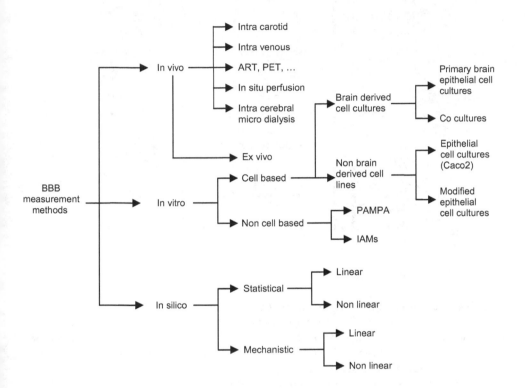

Diagram 2. Brain drug testing methods.

4.1 BBB permeation data
4.1.1 Bound and unbound drug concepts

The drug is available in blood in the free (unbound) and bounded (protein bounded, erythrocyte bounded, tissue bounded) forms. The unbound drug molecules equilibrate across the BBB and brain. The spaces that these equilibria occur are: blood, interstitial fluid, intercellular and intracellular fluids. Figure 5 shows these equilibria schematically. The speed of the equilibria to reach the steady state define the rate of drug distribution within brain, and the slowest one would be the rate limiting step. For poor CNS penetrantes, the BBB permeation or the diffusion of drug molecules within the brain tissue is the rate limiting step. Total brain concentration which allow us just to rank drug candidates according to their CNS total levels and general CNS penetrability can be measured using most of the *in vivo* methods, while there is just a few methods which are able to provide free fractions directly.

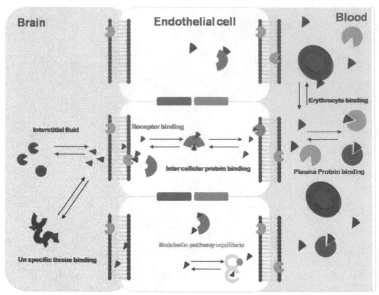

Fig. 5. Different equilibria in brain.

4.1.2 The importance of free drug measurement

The free drug is responsible for pharmacokinetic and pharmacodynamic properties of drugs and relation between dose and response is correct when free drug supplies in target tissue get into account. In this regard interstitial fluid and intra cellular fluid drug levels in brain are important data for drug discovery.

The traditional methods of brain homogenization destroy all compartments of brain (including brain tissue binding and plasma protein binding) and drug levels in specific compartments cannot be measured (Reichel, 2009). The plasma free fractions data cannot be used in CNS drug discovery studies, because of the different physiological properties, blood brain interstitial fluid free fractions. Some researchers used cerebrospinal drug levels (CSF sampling) as an estimate of the unbound drug levels in brain which is not so reliable because of lower tightness of cerebra-spinal blood barrier which leads to higher diffusion and overestimation of free drug concentration in brain (Read & Braggio, 2010). The microdialysis is the only *in vivo* method to provide such data directly, which is limited by its practicability.

4.1.3 The rate and extent of drug penetration to the brain

Neuropharmaceuticals should be able to permeate the BBB and enter the brain parenchyma in order to treat desired disorders whereas peripheral drugs should have limited entrance to the brain in order to decrease their neurological side effects. The drug entrance to the brain was evaluated and quantified using different methods, among them BUI, logBB, $K_{p,uu}$ etc, are well studied and frequently used to measure the rate and the extent of brain drug penetration (Jeffrey & Summerfield, 2010).

Brain uptake index (BUI%) is one of the earliest indicators of BBB permeability of compounds and is calculated by:

$$BUI\% = 100\frac{E}{E_{ref}} \tag{1}$$

where E denotes the first pass extraction and the E_{ref} referred to freely diffusible internal standard. This indicator provides information about the total concentration of the drug in the brain at early time point after administration (Lanevskij et al., 2010).

The logBB which describes the ratio between brain and blood (or plasma) concentrations and provide a measure of the extent of drug permeation is calculated using (Kerns & Di, 2008):

$$\log BB \text{ or } K_p = \frac{AUC_{tot.brain}}{AUC_{tot.blood}} \tag{2}$$

The only information provided by K_p is passive lipid partitioning of the drug which is affected by metabolism, relative binding affinity to proteins and lipid content of brain and blood or plasma and it is not a net measure of BBB permeability (Abbott, 2004; Mehdipour & Hamidi, 2009). It is highly time dependent and in order to get an overall estimation, usually is measured under steady-state conditions.

Another approach based on unbound drug fraction, for quantifying the extent of brain penetration is recommended, which is calculated by:

$$K_{p,uu} = \frac{AUC_{u,brain}}{AUC_{u,blood}} \tag{3}$$

$K_{p,uu}$ affected by both passive diffusion and active influx/efflux and can give information about the permeation mechanism, beyond these, it is not affected by plasma protein and brain tissue binding which interfere in logBB values (Mehdipour & Hamidi, 2009). For drugs delivered by passive diffusion, this index will be close to unity while for efflux and influx substrates it will be less than and more than unity respectively (Hammarlund- Udenaes et al., 2008).

To assess the brain drug permeability rate, the unidirectional influx constant from blood to the brain (K_{in}) and the product of the BBB permeability surface area (PS) which is a measure of the unidirectional clearance from blood to brain have been developed. Both parameters expressed as ml/min/g of brain (Rooy et al., 2010). PS is able to reflect the BBB permeation step more accurately (Abbott, 2004) and is valuable parameter for follow up permeation ability of drug candidates in the pharmaceutical industry and although in pathologic conditions. PS gives an estimation of unbound drug in brain but it is affected by the possible association of the drug with active influx or efflux transporters (Hammarlund- Udenaes et al., 2008).

According to the measurement method K_{in} and PS can be calculated from Crone-Renkin equation:

$$K_{in} = F\left(1 - e^{\frac{-PS}{F}}\right) \tag{4}$$

where F could be considered as perfusion flow rate, or cerebral blood flow rate and PS is computed using:

$$PS = -F \times \ln\left(1 - \frac{K_{in}}{F}\right) \tag{5}$$

Methods for measuring efflux of the drugs out of the brain (brain efflux index (BEI)) have been developed which represent the elimination rate constant of the drugs in brain. Using these parameters, scientists can provide information about the mechanism of BBB permeation in which for passive diffusion the efflux and influx constants will be similar.

To measure all of these data, the remained drug in brain microvascular should be calculated and subtracted from total brain concentration.

4.2 *In vivo*

The resulted data from *in vivo* experiments are valuable and regarded as gold standard in CNS drug discoveries. This value comprises from the experiment which uses anesthetized or cautious animals which represent full physiologic condition for study and the obtained data reflect different aspects of BBB permeation. Demanding skilled scientists and equipped laboratories are the main disadvantage of these techniques.

4.2.1 Intra venous injection

Intra venous injection methods have been developed during primary CNS studies in order to assess the BBB permeability and brain distribution of the CNS drug candidates. The radio-labelled compounds are injected intravenously and blood samples are obtained in different time intervals and a single brain tissue can be obtained at the designated time point. The measured compound concentrations in plasma and brain plotted against the time and after calculating AUC values the logBB computed using equation 2. For each time interval three animals are needed and in order to get a plot using 7 data points, 21 animals are required which is the main limitation of the method (Rooy et al., 2010). The logBB are interesting for pharmaceutical companies, because they can be easily used to rank the goals and other pharmacokinetic parameters such as C_{max} and time length that the compound remains above *in vitro* determined effective concentration can be calculated. Recently these data are questioned about their ability to reflect the permeability properties of studied compounds mainly because: 1) The obtained concentrations are total, while the free fraction of the compounds are responsible for most of their pharmacokinetic properties and 2) It is a brain distribution value and the permeation rate of compounds cannot be obtained (Kerns & Di, 2008). The other parameters which can be calculated using the obtained data are rate parameters (i.e. K_{in} and PS).

4.2.2 Single carotid injection

Single intra carotid injection is one of the earliest BBB permeation study methods and can be done by injection of a given concentration of a labelled compound through common carotid artery of an animal along with a reference standard and experiment stopped after 5 - 15 seconds. Then the brain sampling is done and the brain uptake index (BUI%) can be calculated using the concentration of the compound and the reference standard (Pardridge, 2007). Because of the low sensitivity of the method (limited sampling time), this method has been replaced by *in situ* brain perfusion which provide higher control on experimental condition (Kerns & Di, 2008).

4.2.3 *In situ* brain perfusion
The desired concentration of the studied drug was prepared using the perfusion fluid and the resulted solution is perfused directly to the brain through common artery of an anesthetized animal (commonly rat) for the suitable time and the brain sampling carry out on the predefined time intervals after stopping the perfusion (Amith & Allen, 2003). Similar to the intravenous injection method the remained intravascular perfusion fluid should be removed by brain flashing or calculated using an impermeable compound injection (Rooy et al., 2010). Direct perfusion enables scientists to study the BBB drug permeation in the absence of the first pass metabolism or drug elimination methods. Using this method, the mechanism of drug permeation can be studied using co-administered transporter inhibitors. But such as intravenous injection high resource demanding is a limitation for this method. The K_{in} and PS can be calculated using the obtained data from this method.

4.2.4 Quantitative auto radiography
Another method for CNS drug partitioning study is quantitative auto radiography which can be used for regional study of total drug exposure. Using this method, the amount of radio labelled compound is measured in desired regions (e.g. stroke affected areas, brain tumours) following oral, intravenous or subcutaneous administrations to animals. Similar to previous methods after blood sampling in various time intervals, the brain is taking out and after sectioning the frozen brain to suitable sections the radioactivity is measured. Intra vascular correction is needed here too. Obtaining the regional PS values is possible using this method and the resolution of obtained data is high because of the micrometer dimensioned studied sections (Bickel, 2005; Rooy et al., 2010).

4.2.5 Positron emission tomography
Positron emission tomography is a non-invasive method which is applicable in human. The suitable tracers are administered to the body and the emission is monitored using positron emission tomography scanners. The blood sampling is done in designed intervals and the brain and plasma distribution is measured using a curve fitting method. Similar to quantitative auto radiography the regional information about drug distribution is achievable using this method (Dash & Elmquist, 2003).

4.2.6 Intra cerebral microdialysis
Microdialysis is the only technique which is able to provide the concentration of CNS drug candidates in the interstitial fluid directly. A stereotaxic probe equipped with a semi permeable membrane implanted under anesthesia. The interior of the probe perfused with a physiological solution and samples are taken from freely moving animals and analyze using suitable separation techniques (commonly chromatographic systems) (Bickel, 2005; Alivajeh & Palmer, 2010). The studied compound can be administered orally, intravenously, subcutaneously or from other routes. This method is applicable for human and by implanting the probe in different regions of brain; specific data from different parts of brain (which have different properties) could be collected. The recovery of the probe is an important point in this method to get the absolute concentration data. Pharmacokinetic

parameters of CNS drug candidates including half-life, C_{max}, T_{max}, total exposure, volume of distribution, clearance, BBB influx and efflux rates for different brain regions and most importantly the $K_{p,uu}$ at steady state can be obtained and calculated using microdialysis driven data. These data can be used for pharmacodynamic studies and dosing regimens (Alivajeh & Palmer, 2010).

The methods reviewed in sections 4.2.1 to 4.2.6 give information about the overall exposure resulted from different passive or active influx and efflux systems.

4.2.7 Permeation mechanism study *in vivo*

During drug development the detailed information about the mechanism of permeation and possible efflux or metabolic instability are needed to design the structure of the desired drug and its delivery system. To get detailed information researchers have been used different methods such as: knockout or gene deficient animals for studying the effect of a specific transporter, special enzyme or transporter inhibitors (e.g. efflux inhibitors) or receptor antagonists to eliminate the desired transport effect from the study.

In order to study passive diffusion of drug candidates without interfering of other permeation mechanisms, a number of methods have been developed. For example, it is possible to use excess molar of unlabelled compound in order to saturate the transporters, enzymes or facilitated mechanisms. Also it is possible to use efflux transporters' inhibitors (e.g verapamil for P-gp). Beside these, by studying the Michaelis-Menten behaviour of drugs, it is possible to ensure that the permeation mechanism is passive diffusion (unsaturable) or not.

4.2.8 *Ex vivo*

Ex *vivo* experiments are developed to study drug candidates more reliably out of the body in the simulated physiologic condition (pH, temperature, buffer, nutrients, oxygen) which have the advantage of being applicable in post mortem human samples obtained by autopsy. The resulted data from these experiments have been shown acceptable correlation with *in vivo* experiments. Although in this method impossible experiments and studies in living organism can be conducted, but the differences between the living organism and the slices obtained by autopsy according to the degradation of some proteins should be take into account (Cardoso et al., 2010).

4.3 *In vitro*

In order to do more rigorous investigations on the complex mechanisms occurred in endothelial cell membranes and in intracellular compartments (e.g. active and passive efflux and influx) in the BBB of a living organism, *in vitro* methods can be used. *In vitro* models of BBB should be simple, reproducible and mimic the *in vivo* conditions (both normal and pathologic). Most of the *in vitro* models of BBB are based on endothelial cells as the foundation of BBB and different animals are used to prepare cell cultures. The results should be interpret carefully because of the differentiations (the lower tightness of the developed cell lines, the phenotype modification and the absence of intercellular contact and in vivo signallings occur during the cell isolation). But it is a reliable method for high throughput screening experiments, in order to compare the penetration ability of a set of compounds (Cardoso et al., 2010). The main categories of *in vitro* models include cell based and non cell based methods. Cell based models are simplification of *in vivo* system in which the brain and non brain derived cell cultures are used to study the permeation and transport of drug candidates. The brain derived cell cultures (primary endothelial cultures) show closest phenotype to the *in vivo* brain while their preparation and handling are more difficult than non-brain derived cell lines. Primary endothelial cultures prepared by isolating animal brain micro vessels and *seeding* in culture medium where the endothelial cells grow out and make suitable mono layers for experiments. In order to mimic the *in vivo* system more closely co-cultures included astrocytes have been developed which provide more physical and physiological features in comparison with primary cell cultures (Cardoso et al., 2010). Non brain derived models use the epithelial cell cultures (e.g. Caco 2) and modified epithelial cell cultures which are used for drug absorption studies in order to rank the permeability of CNS drug candidates. Non cell based *in vitro* models include the parallel artificial membrane permeability assay (PAMPA) and immobilized artificial membranes (IAMs) which used as HPLC columns and mimic the properties of biological membrane (Abbott, 2004). PAMPA models initially developed for study passive oral absorption and successfully applied in the pharmaceutical industry. Recently, it has been modified for using in BBB permeation studies and showed good correlation with *in vivo* findings (Mensch et al., 2010).

4.4 BBB permeation prediction methods (*in silico* methods)
In vivo, ex vivo and *in vitro* methods of assessing brain drug penetration leads to high quality data resemble most of the permeation mechanisms in BBB, but they are highly cost and time demanding and are not suitable for screening of large compound libraries. As soon as BBB studies have begun, attempts to predict the BBB permeation properties of drug candidates lead to primary structure activity relationships which later accepted as essential rules of CNS drug development. These structural features later used to develop quantitative relationships to predict the pharmacokinetic properties of CNS drugs. During years and improving the knowledge about the effect of different passive and active mechanisms of brain drug penetration, the prediction models improved and specific models to predict different aspects of BBB permeation have been developed. In order to develop a model first the prediction endpoint (dependent variable or experimental value) should be measured or obtained from the literature. The quality of these data is deterministic for developed model certainty. After selection of the data set, the inclusion of each point in data set should be evaluated and possible outliers should be determined. The next step is to split data set in training and test sets and measure or calculate the desired independent descriptors. The significant descriptors should be selected and the relationship between the dependent and independent variables should be developed using appropriate modelling method. While the model has been developed, its predictive ability along with other validation parameters should be calculated and the effect of selected descriptors on the experimental value should be defined. The details of each step are provided in following sections. Some commercial software have been developed to predict the brain drug penetration which can be used to get primary estimations about the CNS activity of a compound.

4.5 Prediction endpoints (Experimental data)
In order to get initial information about the BBB permeation of new drug entities, studying the existing information using different methods is more interesting than experimental

measurement. There are different (*in vivo* or *in vitro*) indicators which are able to evaluate the rate or extent of drug permeation to the BBB (see section 4.1.3). Among them logBB values have been used extensively for *in silico* methods in order to predict the extent of drug penetration to the brain and the related data sets can be found in the literature. Unbound drug fraction, logPS and BUI% have been used to develop the prediction methods, while some researchers used *in vitro* data (e.g. PAMPA derived P-gp binding affinity) for their studies (Dagenais et al., 2009). Beside these BBB+/- and CNS+/- data which have been extracted from logBB experiments and implications of brain disorders or targets about primary site of action of compounds respectively, were utilized for classification purposes (Klon, 2009). It seems that using the combined information derived from different indicators will be more useful than individual ones. The quality of selected data set should be considered according to the experimental method which used to obtain it (data set homogenesity). The homogenesity of logBB data sets have been questioned, but the studies showed that these combined data sets are applicable. Also the outliers should be determined using statistical methods or according to the experimental method. One of the most common statistical methods is to compute deviations of a single data point from mean dependent or independent variables or both of them and exclude highly deviated datum. In fact an applicability domain for each prediction method should be defined and the compounds out of this domain should be excluded from analyses. For experimental procedures it should be kept in mind that if special efflux inhibitors are used or not. In some methods, scientists are used unlabeled substrate to saturate the desired enzyme or transporter or receptor and the resulted data from these experiments should not be combined with others (Lavnevskij et al., 2010). The third point which should be kept in mind is that the number of the data points should be enough for developing statistical properties (e.g. regression coefficients) of the developed model and also for excluding a part of data as test set. If it is not possible the prediction capability of developed model cannot be evaluated and it will be applicable for the entire data set.

4.6 Descriptors

The structural features and physicochemical properties (Table 2) of the studied compounds should be extracted using the available experimental and computational methods (commercial software, fragment based methods, …). The most studied and evaluated descriptors to define the BBB permeation are those related with passive diffusion. Table 3 contains the details of most frequently used descriptors as well as their effects on BBB permeation. As can be seen from the table, the overall findings about the structural features (also known as the rule of five) of the CNS drug candidates are:

- High lipophilicity
- Low hydrogen binding
- Small molecular weight.

It should be noted that these rules should be used cautiously during drug design procedure. For example, although high lipophilicity increase the permeation rate but it causes the poor solubility, metabolic instability and higher membrane bounding which are not suitable properties for a drug candidate.

Descriptor	Topological descriptors Constitutional, Molecular properties, Quantum chemical, ACDLabs, free aqueous solubility energy
Software	Absolve, Dragon, Hyperchem, Volsurf, MOE, Cerius package

Table 2. Frequently used descriptors and software.

Property	The cutoff for BBB permeation
Molecular weight	< 400-500 Da
H bond donor	<3
H bond acceptor	<7
ClogP*	<7
logD7.4	1-3
Polar surface area	< 60-70 A$^{\circ 2}$
Rotatable bonds	<8
Flexibility	1.27
pKa	7.5-10.5
N+O	<6

* The studies showed that logPoct/water have poorer correlation with permeation data in comparision with ΔlogP or logD7.4. Recent studies showed that the ionization state of drug candidates in physiologic condition should be defined and the models should be developed accordingly (Lavenskij et al., 2009, 2010; Shayanfar et al., 2011).

Table 3. Descriptors used in rules of five methods and their cut off points (Di, 2008; Palmer, 2010)

4.7 Model development
After preparing a number of descriptors, the best descriptor or a combination of descriptors which are able to describe the desired dependent variable (prediction end point) should be selected. There are two approaches for descriptor selection:

4.7.1 Mechanistic approach
In this method, the studied property (e.g. BBB permeation) affecting parameters should be extracted from theoretical findings (several processes include in the overall result) and convert to mathematical representations. The provided descriptors depend on their effects (positive or negative, direct or inverse) on desired property should be correlated to the prediction end point and the resulted equation could be used for prediction purposes (Lavenskij et al., 2010).

4.7.2 Statistical approach
It is so important to exclude insignificant descriptors to prevent over fitting and biased results using a descriptor selection method. The number of descriptors depends on the modelling method. For simple multivariate regression methods, the number of descriptors depends on the number of data points, while for partial least square and principal component analyses methods it is not limited. In addition to the number of the descriptors

and their significances, the inter correlation between them should be checked and just one of the highly correlated descriptors should be kept in multiple linear regression methods, while this is not a problem for partial least square or principal component analyses. There are different methods for descriptor selection and more information can be found in the literature. It is better to keep the penetration mechanisms and approved relationships in mind in this step and avoids complete statistical methods.

4.8 Method development
As soon as the descriptors selected or provided in mechanistic approach, the model should be developed according to the purpose of the modelling. The *in silico* methods developed for following purposes in CNS drug studies:

4.8.1 Classification
It is important to know that if the desired compound is CNS active or not. To do this a border value should be defined for the scaled dependent variable. Different data sets have been used for these models:
- logBB data (BBB+/-),
- CNS active or inactive compounds (CNS+/-),
- P-gp substrate or non-substrate (Pgp+/-).

These models are applicable for screening studies (primary steps of CNS drug development) where the goal is to select the possible CNS active compounds from large compound libraries and in advanced steps of CNS drug studies where the possible reasons of efficacy failure are investigated. Different classification methods have been developed until now using different algorithms and descriptors. The review of these studies showed that the methods were more successful for CNS+ and BBB+ compounds than CNS- and BBB- ones. One reason for this approach is raised from efflux pumps which efflux some structurally suitable compounds from brain. Considering the efflux system substrates during method development will improve the prediction accuracy for these compounds. It should be noted that there is a difference between BBB+ and CNS+, since a drug could be penetrated into brain without measurable biological effect. However in some modelling studies these data were mixed up. It seems that in order to develop more accurate classifiers, some physiological properties of brain such as the extent of non-specific protein and tissue binding, the concentration of the target protein and specific receptors in the brain should be considered.

4.8.2 Permeability prediction (The rate and extent of penetration)
The logBB, $K_{p,uu}$ (for exposure extent studies) and logPS (for rate studies) have been frequently used to develop prediction models. The multiple linear regression and least square methods are among the most studied models providing simple and interpretable equations.

Detailed review of these equations could be found in the literature (Garg et al., 2008; Klon, 2009; Mehdipour & Hamidi, 2009; Shayanfar et al., 2011). The descriptors used for rules of five (Table 3) studies originally comprised from these equations and at least one of these descriptors or similar descriptors which provide relevant information can be found in these equations. In this regard, most of the time, medicinal chemists use the same descriptors to check the new data set or new methods. Lipophilicity descriptors, size and shape descriptors, ionization states of compounds, and polar surface area descriptors proved to have effect on BBB permeation. The complexity of BBB permeation encouraged scientists to check non linear methods applicability in this field and some exponential linear equations and neural networks have been successfully developed. Although neural networks provided more accurate predictions in comparison with linear ones, their interpretation and reproducibility are in question and their usefulness for developing universal models which can be applicable for chemists have not been approved yet. In fact the best model for a chemist is a model which is able to answer him/her what is the possible modification for desired property improvement and the un-interpretable models are not able to answer this question. Because of this, using less accurate but well defined models are preferred to complicate but accurate ones.

The studies of unbound fraction of the drug in brain ($K_{p,uu}$) showed that the previously accepted trend of permeation (higher permeation for more lipophilic compounds) which was raised from $\log BB$ and $\log PS$ studies are not the same for unbound fraction, and lipophilicity have inverse relation with it. These findings showed that the absolute values for the effective descriptors are not suitable and a balanced range of descriptors should be defined for them (Lavenskij et al., 2010).

4.9 Validation

In order to check the sensitivity, specificity, prediction capability, reproducibility, error margins and chance correlations for the developed models, some validation statistics should be provided and using these parameters researchers will be able to make decision on selecting or rejecting a model in comparison with others. The details of these parameters and their usefulness for evaluating the model have been reviewed. For classification methods the lower failure in localization of compounds (both positive and negative) is better and for predictive models the higher correlation coefficients (both for training and test sets and cross validation sets), lower prediction errors (less than about 1 log unit deviation and relative mean squared errors less than 0.3)and lower correlation coefficients (e.g. <0.2) for Y randomized data sets are acceptable. These parameters are not absolute and it would be possible to accept a low quality model in the absence of the better one.

4.10 Prediction using commercial software

Using the developed models, some software has been developed in order to calculate the BBB permeation or P-gp binding affinity which can be used for estimation of compound permeation. These predictions are included in the most of the ADME prediction software which could be found on internet.

5. Conclusion

The importance of BBB for reaching CNS drugs to their targets and also undesired penetration of non CNS drugs to avoid their CNS side effects are briefly discussed. Short review of measurement methods of drug's penetration to CNS is presented along with a summary of computational aspects used for modelling purposes.

The molecular and cellular properties of BBB have been reviewed and the role of its compartments in the regulating of drugs and xenobiotics penetration to the brain has been discussed. Working as a regulatory interface BBB is able to work as a physical and physiological barrier which prevents peripheral drugs to penetrate the brain and reduce their CNS side effects. This barrier activity causes some difficulties in CNS drug delivery and different measurement methods have been developed to study the rate and extent of drug delivery to the brain and the mechanism of delivery methods have studied using these methods. Beyond the experimental methods, prediction of these properties are studied in order to provide cheaper, simpler and more rapid methods for medicinal chemists who work in brain drug development field.

6. Acknowledgment

This work is dedicated to Professor Morteza Samini, Tehran University of Medical Sciences, Tehran, Iran, for his long life efforts in training pharmacy students in Iran.

7. References

Abbott, N. J. (2004). Prediction of blood-brain barrier permeation in drug discovery from in vivo, in vitro and in silico models. *Drug Discovery Today: Technologies*. Vol. 1, pp. 407-416.

Abbott, N. J. (2005). Physiology of the blood-brain barrier and its consequences for drug transport to the brain. *International Congress Series*. Vol. 1277, 3-18.

Abbott, N. J.; Rinnback, L. & Hansson, E. (2006). Astrocyte-endothelial interactions at the blood-brain barrier. *Nature Reviews Neuroscience*. Vol.7, pp. 41-53.

Alam, M. I.; Beg, S.; Samad, A.; Baboota, S.; Kohli, K.; Ali, J.; Ahuja, A. & Akbar, M. (2010). Strategy for effective brain drug delivery. *European Journal of Pharmaceutical Sciences*. Vol. 40, pp. 385-403.

Alavijeh, M. S. & Palmer, A. M. (2010). Measurement of the pharmacokinetics and pharmacodynamics of neuroactive compounds. *Neurobiology of Disease*. Vol. 37, pp. 38-47.

Ballabh, P.; Braun, A. & Nedergaard, M. (2004). The blood-brain barrier: An overview: Structure, regulation, and clinical implications. *Neurobiology of Disease*. Vol. 16. pp. 1-13.

Bickel, U. (2005). How to measure drug transport across the blood-brain barrier. *NeuroRx* Vol. 2, pp. 15-26.

Cardoso, F. L.; Brites, D. & Brito, M. A. (2010). Looking at the blood-brain barrier: Molecular anatomy and possible investigation approaches. *Brain Research Reviews*. Vol. 64, pp. 328-363.

Dagenais, C.; Avdeef, A.; Tsinman, O.; Dudley, A. & Beliveau, R. (2009). P-glycoprotein deficient mouse In situ blood-brain barrier permeability and its prediction using an incombo PAMPA model. *European Journal of Pharmaceutical Sciences*. Vol. 38, pp. 121-137.

Dash, A. K. & Elmquist, W. F. (2003). Separation methods that are capable of revealing blood-brain barrier permeability. *Journal of Chromatography B*. Vol. 797, pp. 241-254.

Eyal, S.; Hsiao, P. & Unadkat, J. D. (2009). Drug interactions at the blood-brain barrier: Fact or fantasy?. *Pharmacology & Therapeutics*. Vol. 123, pp. 80-104.

Fischer, H.; Gottschlich, R. & Seelig, A. (1998). Blood-brain barrier permeation: Molecular parameters governing passive diffusion. *Journal of Membrane Biology.* Vol. 165, pp. 201-211.

Hammarlund-Udenaes, M.; Friden, M.; Syvonen, S. & Gupta, A. (2008). On the rate and extent of drug delivery to the brain. *Pharmaceutical Research.* Vol. 25, 1737-1750.

Jeffrey, P. & Summerfield, S. (2010). Assessment of the blood-brain barrier in CNS drug discovery. *Neurobiology of Disease.* Vol. 37, pp. 33-37.

Kerns, E. H. & Di, L. (2008). Drug-like Properties: Concepts, Structure Design and Methods: from ADME to Toxicity Optimizati. *Academic Press,* 978-0-12-369520-8,

Klon, A. E. (2009). Computational models for central nervous system penetration. *Current Computer-Aided Drug Design.* Vol. 5, pp. 71-89.

Lajoie, P.; Nabi, I. R. & Kwang, W. J. (2010). Lipid Rafts, Caveolae, and Their Endocytosis. International Review of Cell and Molecular Biology, *Academic Press.* Vol. 282, pp. 135-163.

Lanevskij, K.; Japertas, P.; Didziapetris, R. & Petrauskas, A. (2009). Ionization-specific QSAR models of blood-brain penetration of drugs. *Chemistry and Biodiversity.* Vol. 6, pp. 2050-2054.

Lanevskij, K.; Japertas, P.; Didziapetris, R. & Petrauskas, A. (2010). Prediction of blood–brain barrier penetration by drugs. *Delivery to the Central Nervous System Drug.* Vol. 45, pp. 63-83.

Loscher, W. & Potschka, H. (2005). Role of drug efflux transporters in the brain for drug disposition and treatment of brain diseases. *Progress in Neurobiology.* Vol. 76, pp. 22-76.

Mehdipour, A. R. & Hamidi, M. (2009). Brain drug targeting: a computational approach for overcoming blood-brain barrier. *Drug Discovery Today.* Vol. 14, pp. 1030-1036.

Mensch, J.; Melis, A.; Mackie, C.; Verreck, G.; Brewster, M. E. & Augustijns, P. (2010). Evaluation of various PAMPA models to identify the most discriminating method for the prediction of BBB permeability. *European Journal of Pharmaceutics and Biopharmaceutics.* Vol. 74, pp. 495-502.

Mruk, D. D.; Su, L. & Cheng, C.Y. (2010). Emerging role for drug transporters at the blood testis barrier. *Trends in pharmacological sciences.* Vol. 32, pp. 99-106.

Palmer, A. M. (2010). The role of the blood-CNS barrier in CNS disorders and their treatment. *Neurobiology of Disease.* Vol. 37, pp. 3-12.

Pardridge, W. M. (1998). *Introduction to the blood-brain barrier: methodology, biology, and pathology.* Cambridge University PRESS. 0 521 58124 9 (hb).

Pardridge, W. M. (2007). Blood-brain barrier delivery. *Drug Discovery Today.* Vol. 12, pp. 54-61.

Prabha, G.; Jitender, V. & Nilanjan, R. (2008). *Drug Absorption Studies,* Springer. 978-0-387-74901-3

Prinz, M. & Mildner A. (2011). Microglia in the CNS: Immigrants from another world. *GLIA* Vol. 59, pp. 177-187.

Read, K. D. & Braggio, S. (2010). Assessing brain free fraction in early drug discovery. *Expert Opinion on Drug Metabolism and Toxicology.* Vol. 6, pp. 337-344.

Reichel, A. (2009). Addressing Central Nervous System (CNS) Penetration in Drug
    Discovery: Basics and Implications of the Evolving New Concept. *Chemistry &*
    Biodiversity. Vol. 6, pp. 2030-2049.
Rooy, I.; Cakir-Tascioglu, S.; Hennink, W. E.; Storm, G.; Schiffelers, R. M. & Mastrobattista,
    E. (2010). In vivo Methods to Study Uptake of Nanoparticles into the Brain.
    Pharmaceutical Research. DOI: 10.1007/s11095-010-0291-7.
Shayanfar, A.; Soltani, S.& Jouyban, A. (2011). Prediction of Blood–Brain Distribution: Effect
    ofIonization. *Biological and Pharmaceutical Bulletin*. Vol. 34, pp. 266-271.
Smith, Q. R. & Allen, D. D. (2003). In situ Brain Perfusion Technique. *Springer protocols*. Vol.
    89, pp. 209-218.
Ueno, M. (2009). Mechanisms of the penetration of blood-borne substances into the brain.
    Current Neuropharmacology. Vol. 7, pp. 142-149.

Diagnostic Accuracy and Interpretation of Urine Drug Testing for Pain Patients: An Evidence-Based Approach

Amadeo Pesce[1], Cameron West[1], Kathy Egan-City[1] and William Clarke[2]
[1]Millennium Research Institute,
[2]Johns Hopkins School of Medicine,
USA

1. Introduction

Pain is a complex disease. The complexities and co-morbidities of this disease include depression, anxiety, addiction, and other psychological diagnoses that lead to difficulties in management and aberrant behavior such as not taking medications as prescribed, taking additional medications, or illicit drugs. In the effort to provide the highest standard of care for their patients, pain physicians are required to continually assess patients for addiction and, if necessary, refer them to addictionologists for additional treatment (Chou et al., 2009).

1.1 Chronic opioid therapy

In this chapter we will refer to pain patients as those persons being treated with chronic opioid therapy for non-cancer-related pain. It is this patient population that has been associated with opiate abuse and diversion, and therefore monitoring these patients for drug use in a manner analogous to therapeutic drug monitoring is necessary. One of the most frequent complaints by patients seeing pain physicians is back pain, which is often associated with failed back surgery (Manchikanti et al., 2004; Michna et al., 2007). Currently opiate medications are one of the treatments of choice used by physicians to provide pain relief. These medications can induce euphoria as well as pain relief; because of this, opiates are frequently abused by this population, as well as the general population (National Survey on Drug Use and Health: Detailed Tables - Prevalence Estimates, Standard Errors, P Values, and Sample Sizes, 1995-2006; Webster & Dove, 2007). Additionally, these medications are associated with physical as well as psychological dependence and can pose addiction risks (Webster & Dove, 2007).

1.2 Pain treatment

One of the treatments of choice for chronic pain involves strong medications such as opioids, as well as additional or adjuvant medications (Chou et al., 2009; Trescot et al., 2006). Side effects of opioids include sedation, dizziness, nausea, vomiting, and constipation. Living day to day with any or all of these symptoms is challenging at the least and is compounded by the underlying pain these patients suffer from. Naturally, patients often attempt to minimize the side effects by taking less of the medication when side effects are particularly debilitating or unpleasant. "Chronic pain patients often adjust their dose of prescribed medication in response to changing levels of activity with no malicious or maladaptive intent. Although they may state that their pattern of use of medications is stable, this is often a statement made "on average" rather than a precise pattern of use. This is particularly evident with short-acting medications used in the treatment of breakthrough pain." (Gourlay & Heit, 2010b)

UDT is used to give confidence to both the physician and the patient that the patient is following the medication regimen and is therefore getting the most benefit from their treatment. In addition, the side effects of these medications often result in their misuse, underuse, and/or mixing of medications that are not prescribed (Manchikanti et al., 2004). This can also result in the social problems of abuse, misuse, or diversion of these medications. These factors require of pain physicians that they be particularly attentive to their prescribing practices. Adding to the complexity of managing pain patients is the fact that these medications are controlled substances and cannot be purchased over the counter, and so have high street value (Katz et al., 2003; National Prescription Drug Threat Assesment, 2009). This in turn requires of the physician that he or she determine whether patients under their care are compliant with their medication regime, binging on their medications, or diverting them for financial gain (Manchikanti et al., 2005, 2006a, 2006b).

1.3 Complications of pain treatment

Further compounding the situation, alcohol use is of major concern to the physician because alcohol-drug interactions can cause morbidity (Harmful Interactions: Mixing Alcohol with Medicines, 2007). Although physicians prohibit patient alcohol use during treatment with opiates or benzodiazepines, verbal contracts are commonly broken and therefore alcohol use must be monitored with (UDT) to manage the high risk of alcohol-drug reactions and mortality (Chou et al., 2009; Trescot et al., 2006). In addition, for reasons involving inadequate pain control, sleep deprivation, and psychological pathology, this patient population commonly takes other medications not prescribed by treating physicians as well as illicit drugs (Manchikanti et al., 2005, 2006a, 2006b). To respond to these potential problems, physicians traditionally relied upon behavioral assessment and pill counts to aid them in making treatment decisions. UDT has augmented these tools by providing physicians with objective, scientifically measurable outcomes to help them make decisions (Gourlay et al., 2010; Hammett-Stabler & Webster, 2008; Nafziger & Bertino, 2009; Reisfield et al., 2007). A detailed protocol of how to appropriately prescribe these controlled substances for this population is discussed in the book *Universal Precautions*, by Gourlay and Heit (Gourlay et al., 2005).

2. Urine drug testing

Traditionally, UDT has been associated with forensic testing, often referred to as workplace testing, to detect illicit drug use in employees. Workplace UDT has traditionally focused on identifying use of abused drugs including amphetamines (methamphetamine), cocaine, marijuana, phencyclidine (PCP), and heroin (opiates) (Federal Register - Mandatory Guidelines and Proposed Revisions to Mandatory Guidelines for Federal Workplace Drug Testing Programs [Federal Register], 2004). This type of testing is oriented toward determining positive results; that is, identifying the presence of an illicit substance. The reasoning behind this focus is obvious; a positive result for a prohibited substance is a cause for a consequence such as job dismissal (Federal Register, 2004). Testing for these drugs usually follows scheduled guidelines established by the Substance Abuse and Mental Health Services Administration (SAMHSA) (Federal Register, 2004). Analytically, the testing involves qualitative immunoassay screening followed by confirmation by mass spectrometry. Testing for patients on chronic opioid therapy is a different paradigm as both positive and negative results are important. It also requires assays that are more sensitive and can determine both the parent drug and one or more of its metabolites.

2.1 Immunoassays

Immunoassays are tests that are based on the ability of an antibody to bind with a drug (Feldkamp, 2010). Antibodies are made in such a way that they bind with a specific drug, such as morphine. In one approach, manufacturers of point of care (POC) devices embed test strips with antibodies and install them in devices designed to interact with urine specimens (Amedica Drug Screen Test Cup). A urine specimen with the drug in it (in this example, morphine) will displace the drug-indicator molecule on the test strip causing the morphine drug indicator line to disappear or change color. These test strips are then visually inspected by the person administering the test. The absence or presence of a line or the change in color, such as on a home pregnancy test, indicates whether the result is positive or negative. The immunoassay antibody binding reaction can be measured in other, more sophisticated ways than using test strips, such as reference laboratory analytical instruments (Olympus Au640 Product Information; Siemens V-Twin Analyzer Product Information; Thermo Fisher Mgc-240 Analyzer Product Information). However, the fundamental property of immunoassays is always the binding reaction of the antibody to the test drug (analyte).

2.2 Limitations of immunoassay

The qualitative immunoassay model of testing is only a partial UDT solution for the pain population (Gourlay et al., 2010; Hammett-Stabler & Webster, 2008; Nafziger & Bertino, 2009; Reisfield et al., 2007). There are a number of reasons for this. First, doctors treating patients for pain are concerned with negative as well as positive results. This is because a negative result can mean that a patient is not taking a prescribed medication. Second, workplace UDT assays do not fit the clinical medication regimen used in the treatment of pain patients and do not take into account the variable dosing often employed by pain patients as they try to balance their need for pain relief against the side effects of these medications (Gourlay & Heit, 2010a). In analytical terms this means that the cutoff for detection and quantitation (concentration of drug present) must be low enough to capture minimal use of the drug. Thirdly, the physicians need to have an exact indication of the medications the patients are taking. For example, a positive opiate test does not indicate whether the patient is on codeine, hydrocodone, morphine, or hydromorphone. That is, it measures the class not the particular drug. Each of these are specific medications the physician may choose to treat the patient with, so in order to establish compliance it is necessary to determine exactly which medication has been ingested and assure the patient is not taking additional opiates which could create an unsafe situation (Cone et al., 2008). Finally, if an immunoassay screening method is used, the antibody must detect all drugs of that particular class. Recent advances in designing opiate and benzodiazepine classes of drugs have resulted in agents which do not react well with the traditional antibodies. and are used in much lower concentrations than the earlier-designed drugs (Fraser, 2001). This complicates identification of these new agents by immunoassay.

3. Drugs observed in pain patients

Table 1 lists both licit and illicit drugs as well as alcohol and the frequency observed in the pain patient population tested by Millennium Laboratories. These observations are similar to those reported by Cone (Cone et al., 2008). The medications most commonly found in the urine of this population are clearly hydrocodone and oxycodone, followed by morphine and hydromorphone; codeine is not frequently prescribed for this population. Benzodiazepines are the next most prescribed group. Other opioid medications such as fentanyl, meperidine, tramadol, and propoxyphene are less frequently used. Use of the muscle relaxants carisoprodol is commonly seen. Marijuana is by far the most prevalent among the illicit drugs, followed by cocaine and methamphetamine. From the table it is clear that alcohol use is about 10% as measured by the presence of alcohol's metabolites ethyl glucuronide (EtG) and ethyl sulfate (EtS) (Crews et al., 2011a; Dahl et al., 2002; Helander & Beck, 2005; Helander et al., 1996; Schmitt et al., 1997; Stephanson et al., 2002; Wojcik & Hawthorne, 2007; Wurst et al., 2006; Wurst et al., 2004). These data show that in order to provide appropriate monitoring and decrease risk and mortality for this population, a broad test menu is needed. These same drugs are often abused and frequently found to be present though they had not been prescribed by the treating physician. Table 2 shows the frequency of these non-prescribed drugs in the pain patient population.

3.1 Need for urine drug testing
Many physicians prescribing opioids for non-cancer pain patients follow guidelines established by the American Pain Society (Chou et al., 2009). These guidelines specify the regular or periodic use of UDT as a component of treatment, including administering UDT upon assessing potential risk for substance abuse, misuse or addiction (Atluri & Sudarshan, 2003; Ives et al., 2006; Madras et al., 2009). Guidelines also suggest that doctors use UDT to monitor patient adherence to prescribed treatments and further state that periodic UDT is warranted because "the therapeutic benefits of these medications are not static and can be affected by changes in the underlying pain condition, coexisting disease, or in psychological or social circumstances" (Chou et al., 2009). In observation of these recommendations, many physicians use POC devices to obtain a real time, in-office assessment of patient compliance, illicit drug use and possible diversion (Manchikanti et al., 2006b, 2010).

3.2 Point of care testing
As mentioned previously, these POC devices are qualitative immunoassays that test for various drug classes as well as a few specific drugs. A typical POC device can measure 12 drugs or drug classes (Amedica Drug Screen Test Cup). The most commonly monitored agents are barbiturates, benzodiazepines, opiates, oxycodone, propoxyphene, methadone, tricyclic antidepressants and the illicit drugs methamphetamine, marijuana, cocaine, methylenedioxymethamphetamine (MDMA), and phencyclidine (PCP). The physicians use these screens to immediately detect adherence to regimen or non-adherence to the prescribed drug therapy. At that point they can elicit a more complete drug history, initiate a conversation assessing the need for additional medications not prescribed, or confront the

Drug Class	N Positive	% Positive	Mean (ng/mL)	Median (ng/mL)	Range (ng/mL)	Cutoff (ng/mL)
Alcohol	10,594	*10.0%*				
Ethyl Glucuronide	8,602	81.2%	59,827.9	7,220.1	500.47 - 5,942,830	500
Ethyl Sulfate	6,644	62.7%	18,660.7	3,546.1	500.17 - 1,565,150	500
Ethanol (Screen)	2,410	22.7%	735.1 mg/dL	68.6 mg/dL	20 - 151,316 mg/dL	20 mg/dL
Total Specimens Tested	**106,014**					
Amphetamines	7,005	*4.2%*				
Amphetamine	6,045	86.3%	8,471.2	2,790.2	100.31 - 409,816	100
Methamphetamine	1,178	16.8%	18,217.8	3,263.8	105.12 - 453,763	100
MDA	961	13.7%	1,771.1	844.5	101 - 416,68.9	100
MDMA	74	1.1%	5,328.2	1,260.6	120.14 - 40,395.3	100
Total Specimens Tested	**167,533**					
Barbiturates	4,797	*3.6%*				
Barbiturates (Screen)	4,797	100.0%	927.8	904.0	200 - 15,886	200
Total Specimens Tested	**133,032**					
Benzodiazepines	60,160	*35.6%*				
α-Hydroxyalprazolam	26,954	44.8%	479.9	177.3	20 - 55,249.1	20
Oxazepam	18,475	30.7%	2,036.0	617.4	40 - 203,128	40
7-Amino-Clonazepam	16,466	27.4%	674.6	287.0	20.01 - 47,501.7	20
Temazepam	15,647	26.0%	5,552.3	851.9	50 - 752,950	50
Nordiazepam	12,758	21.2%	693.9	281.5	40 - 25,864.3	40
Lorazepam	6,390	10.6%	1,583.1	681.2	40.09 - 63,170.8	40
Total Specimens Tested	**168,980**					
Buprenorphine	6,308	*6.0%*				
Buprenorphine	5,841	92.6%	313.0	75.1	10.01 - 58,691.5	10
Norbuprenorphine	4,237	67.2%	639.8	279.0	20 - 13,615.1	20
Total Specimens Tested	**104,972**					
Cannabinoids	11,752	*11.3%*				
cTHC	11,752	100.0%	579.6	153.1	15 - 25,960.3	15
Total Specimens Tested	**104,453**					
Carisoprodol	13,302	*16.4%*				
Meprobamate	13,188	99.1%	36,884.0	16,190.5	100.18 - 1,244,200	100
Carisoprodol	5,379	40.4%	2,931.9	455.0	100.1 - 648,442	100
Total Specimens Tested	**80,990**					
Cocaine	4,951	*3.0%*				
Cocaine metabolite	4,951	100.0%	12,372.5	627.1	50.05 - 342,160	50
Total Specimens Tested	**166,501**					

Table 1. Drug and Metabolite Prevalence, Positivity, and Concentrations. N = 184,049 patient specimens. Test dates: 10/01/09–4/29/10.

Drug Class	N Positive	% Positive	Mean (ng/mL)	Median (ng/mL)	Range (ng/mL)	Cutoff (ng/mL)
Fentanyl	13,141	*14.1%*				
Norfentanyl	11,589	88.2%	626.8	236.6	8 - 47,354.9	8
Fentanyl	9,283	70.6%	109.4	36.1	2 - 33,050.7	2
Total Specimens Tested	**93,526**					
Meperidine	6,310	*7.3%*				
Normeperidine	4,247	67.3%	1,456.3	339.5	50 - 276,993	50
Meperidine	2,522	40.0%	34,321.8	13,533.4	50.18 - 616,862	50
Total Specimens Tested	**86,344**					
Methadone	12,415	*11.0%*				
EDDP	12,109	97.5%	7,871.9	4,117.3	100.05 - 251,835	100
Methadone	11,792	95.0%	5,265.1	2,409.4	100.11 - 260,433	100
Total Specimens Tested	**113,073**					
Opiates	116,683	*64.6%*				
Hydrocodone	59,346	50.9%	2,564.4	859.9	50 - 477,876	50
Hydromorphone	51,205	43.9%	836.0	240.4	50 - 204,633	50
Oxymorphone	49,688	42.6%	5,760.2	1,298.6	50 - 1,512,220	50
Oxycodone	41,603	35.7%	11,207.3	2,124.5	50 - 5,947,380	50
Morphine	21,400	18.3%	29,611.8	9,600.3	50.06 - 1,995,940	50
Codeine	3,686	3.2%	4,752.0	828.4	50.01 - 233,036	50
6-Acetylmorphine	465	0.4%	1,108.8	275.7	10.01 - 24,069.1	10
Total Specimens Tested	**180,487**					
Phencyclidine	23	*0.02%*				
Phencyclidine	23	100.0%	539.4	87.5	10.89 - 3,718.53	10
Total Specimens Tested	**104,137**					
Propoxyphene	6,397	*4.8%*				
Norpropoxyphene	6,395	100.0%	5,524.3	2,026.9	100 - 167,037	100
Propoxyphene	2,780	43.5%	1,919.5	583.6	100 - 178,006	100
Total Specimens Tested	**133,992**					
Tapentadol	277	*0.4%*				
Tapentadol	277	100.0%	11,557.1	6,870.3	52.05 - 492,895	50
Total Specimens Tested	**66,797**					
Tramadol	6,521	*12.1%*				
Tramadol	6,521	100.0%	19,288.0	8,191.4	100 - 601,928	100
Total Specimens Tested	**54,111**					

Table 1. (continued). Drug and Metabolite Prevalence, Positivity, and Concentrations. N = 184,049 patient specimens. Test dates: 10/01/09–4/29/10.

DRUG CATEGORY	OCCURRENCES	% of TOTAL
Benzodiazepine	14,559	28.32%
Illicit Drugs	6,769	13.17%
Natural and Semi-Synthetic Opioids	13,241	25.75%
Other	11,514	22.39%
Stimulants	954	1.86%
Synthetic Opioids	4,379	8.52%
TOTALS	**51,416**	**100.00%**
Total Creatinine Tests	69,888	
Total RADAR C Positives	51,416	
% POSITIVE	**73.57%**	
Benzodiazepine	*14,559*	
7-Amino-Clonazepam	3,864	
Alpha-Hydroxyalprazolam	5,543	
Lorazepam	1,079	
Nordiazepam	1,907	
Oxazepam	1,803	
Temazepam	363	
Illicit Drugs	*6,769*	
6-MAM (Heroin metabolite)	165	
Cocaine metabolite	1,710	
Methamphetamine	320	
MDMA	17	
cTHC (Marijuana metabolite)	4,546	
Phencyclidine	11	
Natural and Semi-Synthetic Opioids	*13,241*	
Buprenorphine	809	
Codeine	692	
Hydrocodone	5,138	
Hydromorphone	1,789	
Morphine	1,317	
Norbuprenorphine	73	
Oxycodone	2,618	
Oxymorphone	805	
Other	*11,514*	
Carisoprodol	735	
Ethyl Glucuronide	5,320	
Ethyl Sulfate	4,820	
Meprobamate	639	
Stimulants	*954*	
Amphetamine	954	
Synthetic Opioids	*4,379*	
EDDP (Methadone metabolite)	1,381	
Fentanyl	729	
Meperidine	29	
Methadone	271	
Norfentanyl	204	
Normeperidine	55	
Norpropoxyphene	898	
Propoxyphene	25	
Tapentadol	17	
Tramadol	770	

Table 2. Incidence of Non-prescribed Use of Prescription Medications and Illicit Drugs.

patient about illicit drug use. Point of care devices are extremely useful because they provide physicians with immediate information, particularly on initial patient intake. Of course, like many CLIA-waived (or simple) test devices, they do have limitations, inasmuch as they require that a person visually inspect them in order to interpret the results. For this reason as well as the fact that these units are not 100% accurate, manufacturers of POC devices recommend that doctors not confront patients without first confirming the POC results (Table 3) (Amedica Drug Screen Test Cup). Table 3 lists a number of known drugs or agents that cause false positive results in POC immunoassays. In contrast with POC immunoassay tests, which only show a positive or negative result, laboratory-based immunoassays are often semi-quantitative (Feldkamp, 2010). This means that a positive result for morphine will also indicate approximately how much morphine is in the specimen. These immunoassays have quality control and proficiency testing surveys that make the results more objective and reliable than those obtained using POC devices (American Proficiency Institute 2011 Catalog of Programs, 2011; College of American Pathologists 2011 Surveys and Anatomic Pathology Education Programs, 2011).

POCT Kit Abbreviation	Drug or Drug Class	Target Drugs[1]	Compounds That May Cause A False Positive[1]
THC	Marijuana	Marijuana and Marinol (contains THC),	Prilosec, Protonix , efavirenz, NSAIDs
COC	Cocaine	Cocaine	Unknown/Infrequent
OPI300[2]	Opiates	Codeine, morphine, hydrocodone, hydromorphone. Also, poppy seeds that contain morphine.	Oxycodone
AMP	Amphetamines	Amphetamine, Adderall. Occasionally: benzphetamine, selegiline, Vicks Nasal Inhaler[4]	Phenylpropanolamine, ephedrine, pseudoephedrine, ranitidine, phentermine
MET	Methamphetamine	Methamphetamine. Occasionally: benzphetamine, selegilene, Vicks Nasal Inhaler[4]	Adderal, phenylpropanolamine, ephedrine, pseudoephedrine, ranitidine, phentermine
PCP	Phencyclidine	Phencyclidine	Venlafaxine, dextromethorphan, diphenhydramine
MDMA	Methylenedioxymethamphetamine	Methylenedioxymethamphetamine	Phenylpropanolamine, ephedrine, pseudoephedrine, ranitidine, phentermine
BAR	Barbiturates	Butalbital, phenobarbital, secobarbital, amobarbital and other barbiturates	Unknown/Infrequent

BZO	Benzodiaze-pines	Oxazepam, nordiazepam, temazepam, alprazolam and other benzodiazepines to varying degrees	Oxaprozin, sertaline
MTD	Methadone	Methadone	Verapamil, quetiapine
TCA	Tricyclic Antidepres-sants	Amitriptyline, nortriptyline, imipramine, desipramine, doxepin and other tricyclics to varying degrees.	Cyclobenzaprine, carbamazepine, diphenhydramine
OXY[3]	Oxycodone	Oxycodone and oxymorphone	Codeine, morphine, hydrocodone and hydromorphone

Table 3. False Positive Results: Immunoassay Cross Reactants.
[1] While most immunoassays are highly selective for their target compounds, cross reactive compounds and adulterants, particularly when present at high concentrations may result in a false positive. Additional cross reactants have been reported and cross reactivity may vary between immunoassay manufacturers and lot to lot. The manufacturers of point of care test devices recommend that positive results should be confirmed by mass spectrometry.
[2] OPI300 is an assay to detect codeine, morphine, hydrocodone and hydromorphone. Oxycodone may give a positive at higher concentrations.
[3] OXY is an assay to detect Oxycodone. Other opiates, esp. codeine, morphine, hydrocodone and hydromorphone may give a positive result at higher concentrations.
[4] Adderall contains amphetamine. Benzphetamine (Didrex) is metabolized to d-amphetamine and d-methamphetamine. Selegiline (Eldepryl) is metabolized to l-amphetamine and l-methamphetamine. Vick's Inhaler contains l-methamphetamine.

3.3 Determining appropriate UDT cutoffs
Sensitivity of detection currently used in many immunoassays may not be appropriate for the pain patient. This is because manufacturers set cutoffs for assays to identify overdose in emergency unit settings (Fraser & Zamecnik, 2003; Fraser, 2001; Hattab et al., 2000; Wingert, 1997). There is a need to establish appropriate cutoffs for patients on clinical doses of their medications rather than the high concentrations encountered in overdose situations. Specifically, studies have been conducted that better identify the appropriate cutoff for the pain patient population (Pesce et al., 2011).
One definition of appropriate cutoff levels is one that captures 97.5% or more of the population on a specific drug (Pesce et al., 2011). An example of the importance of setting appropriate cutoffs is for the drug clonazepam (West et al., 2010b). When measured by immunoassay using a nominal cutoff of 200 ng/mL, only 28% of the patients on the drug were determined to be compliant. When the same samples were measured by LC-MS/MS technique using a cutoff of 200 ng/mL, the group was found to be 70% compliant. Finally, when the LC-MS/MS cutoff was lowered to 40 ng/mL the group was 87% compliant. This study showed that first the immunoassay was insensitive in that the nominal 200 ng/mL cutoff did not apply to clonazepam, and second, a lower cutoff was needed to appropriately categorize compliance. Other studies have shown the need for lower cutoffs for pain medications (Mikel et al., 2009; Pesce et al., 2010a). As the consequences to the patient of dismissal from a practice can be very large and even life-changing (e.g., loss of insurance, loss of job or income), it is essential that physicians do not unjustifiably dismiss even a

single patient who is compliant with their medication regimens. This can be avoided by using appropriate cutoffs.

In an attempt to better define appropriate cutoffs for the pain patient population, the quantitative urine drug test results were examined for the prescription medications listed in Table 4. Using the criterion that the cutoffs should capture 97.5% of the examined population and employing the LC-MS/MS cutoffs listed in Table 4 showed it was possible to meet this standard (Pesce et al., 2011). One limitation of this approach is that the time after last dose and the dose itself were not known for these subjects. Regardless of the limitations of the study, the lower cutoffs provide results that can clearly identify compliance more accurately than other methods.

Drug	Analytical Cutoff (ng/mL)	Lower 2.5%	
		Estimated New Cutoff (Raw, ng/mL)	CR Normalized Cutoff (µg/g creatinine)
7-Amino-Clonazepam	10	19	15
Alpha-Hydroxyalprazolam	10	15	11
Amphetamine	50	76	59
Buprenorphine	5	7	5
Carisoprodol	50	56	35
Codeine	25	29	15
Fentanyl	1	2	2
Hydrocodone	25	41	31
Hydromorphone	25	34	26
Lorazepam	20	30	25
Meperidine	25	88	28
Meprobamate	50	92	113
Methadone	50	89	74
Morphine	25	59	52
Oxycodone	25	45	46
Oxymorphone	25	44	38
Propoxyphene	50	60	42
Tapentadol	25	42	58
Tramadol	50	147	70

Table 4. Medication Cutoff Values. Modified with permission from Pesce et al., 2011.

As stated earlier, illicit drug use is common in this population (Madras et al., 2009; Schuckman et al., 2008). It stands to reason that identifying the appropriate illicit drug cutoffs for UDT is equally important. Using the same criterion as stated above, cutoffs for marijuana, cocaine, and methamphetamine have also been determined (Table 5) (West et al., 2011a). The lowering of these illicit drug cutoffs consistent with the latest SAMHSA guidelines in which the cocaine and amphetamine cutoffs were lowered to capture more illicit drug users (Federal Register, 2004).

Drug	Lower 2.5%	
	Raw (ng/mL)	CR Normalized (ng/mg CR)
Cocaine	29.6	17
Marijuana	9.5	6.2
Methamphetamine	56.1	33.5

Table 5. Illicit Drug Cutoff Values. Modified with permission from West et al., 2011a.

3.4 Confirmatory testing: mass spectrometry

Physicians dealing with pain patients not following the treatment plan or using illicit or non-prescribed medications, have difficulty with these situations (Jung & Reidenberg, 2007). The doctor must be absolutely confident that the test data from both the POC and laboratory conducting further testing is correct. By having positive results obtained in their offices as well as confirmatory laboratory data, physicians can confidently discuss expectations and behavioral changes with patients. Questions about laboratory mix-up of specimens or laboratory error can be dismissed.

Many laboratories performing UDT on the pain patient population typically test specimens by immunoassay and then follow this with confirmation by mass spectrometry (Cone et al., 2008). Mass spectrometry is an analytical technique that separates molecules based on their weight (mass) and fragmentation pattern. Identification is based on the fact that each drug has a specific mass and breakdown in the same way that each person has a specific fingerprint. A mass spectrometry instrument is usually coupled to a chromatographic column, in which the test drug, for example morphine, is separated from other components in the urine before submitting the sample into the mass spectrometer. The mass spectrometer identifies the test drug by its position in the chromatogram, the specific weight of the molecule, and by its fragmentation pattern. This technology is virtually foolproof. Mass spectrometry techniques are divided into two methods: gas chromatography-mass spectrometry (GC-MS) and liquid chromatography-tandem mass spectrometry (LC-MS/MS). Of the two, the newer LC-MS/MS is considered the gold standard, for reasons we will describe later (Siuzdak, 2006).

In cases where the physician wants the results immediately (within hours), confirmatory mass-spectrometry methods used at the most modern diagnostic laboratories provide results within 24-30 hours. As stated above, the major limitations of immunoassays are inappropriate cutoffs (sensitivity), varying specificity for individual drugs, and cross-reactivity with other agents producing both false-negative and false-positive results (Manchikanti et al., 2008). The term cross reactivity is used to describe the reaction of an antibody with a chemical that is not the original immunizing drug. The reaction is poor because the affinity is much worse than the original drug. By poor we mean that at the same concentration of the original drug the test compound does not bind as well. However, as the concentration of the test compound is increased it eventually saturates the antibody binding site giving a positive test result.

3.5 Test menu requirement

As mentioned earlier a broader clinical laboratory UDT menu is necessary to accurately monitor the pain patient population. Smaller hospitals as well as physician offices cannot meet this requirement. One reason for this is that immunoassays require separate analytical channels for each assay and this limits the number of tests a smaller laboratory may have in its menu (Olympus Au640 Product Information; Siemens V-Twin Analyzer Product Information; Thermo Fisher Mgc-240 Analyzer Product Information). Another reason is that certain drug tests may not exist for the laboratory's specific instruments, and the addition of another instrument is financially prohibitive, particularly if that instrument is a mass spectrometer (Agilent Technologies, Inc.). Many physicians treating the pain patient population send specimens to reference laboratories specifically designed to provide the required test menu to meet these needs. Tests for new drugs (i.e., tapentadol) (Nucynta - Tapentadol, 2010) or new illicit substances (i.e., K2, spice) (Sobolevsky et al., 2010; Vardakou et al., 2010) encountered in the pain patient population can be rapidly set up and validated on LC-MS/MS instrumentation. Therefore, this analytical technique is supplementing screening by immunoassay. Because of the limitations of immunoassays, confirmatory testing is essential for accurate clinical assessment of medication usage. With confirmatory testing, physicians have specific evidence of what medications a patient is or isn't taking. This assures the doctor that he or she is not discharging a patient inappropriately, and that care is appropriate and not limited.. The laboratories with the most advanced technology can eliminate the immunoassay step saving both the patient and the insurer money.

3.6 Mass spectrometry as the gold standard for testing

At this point in time, mass spectrometry is considered the method of choice for UDT analysis in pain management. This is because mass spectrometry offers the chromatographic separation and mass fragmentation patterns that are specific for the test medications such as opiates and benzodiazepines (Mohsin et al., 2007). In addition, this analytic approach uses isotope dilution to quantify the amount of drug in the urine specimen; isotope dilution is considered the gold standard for determining how much of a drug is in a specimen (quantitation) (Federal Register, 2004). This ability to quantify the amount of drug in urine has been proposed as a method of detecting drug abuse (Pesce et al., 2010c). However, it is important to note that it is not possible to relate the quantitative excretion of a drug to the drug dosage (Nafziger & Bertino, 2009). Quantitation of drugs using immunoassay technology is problematic, particularly if the antibody reagent cross reacts with multiple structurally related drugs; if the urine drug sample contains more than one drug in a class (i.e., hydrocodone and hydromorphone), the antibody reaction will vary with each drug present in the solution. This means that the assay cannot distinguish between the two drugs and give a reliable calculation of the amount of either drug present (Feldkamp, 2010).

Of the two commonly used mass spectrometry methods, LC-MS/MS offers several advantages over GC-MS (Mikel et al., 2010). These include the ability to discriminate a larger number of drugs in each test run, the very small amount of urine specimen required (as little as 25 microliters, or one drop), and the ability to use a sample that is neither derivatized nor extracted. This in turn has made possible the analysis of hundreds of urine specimens per day for a single mass spectrometer. Advances in the automated handling of specimens and bar coding allow for the accurate processing of thousands of samples per day. This method of analysis can provide physicians with results more rapidly than by GC-MS (Mikel et al., 2010).

4. Interpretation of UDT results

The accurate interpretation of test results requires an understanding of the usefulness and limitations of immunoassays (Gourlay et al., 2010; Hammett-Stabler & Webster, 2008; Manchikanti et al., 2010; Nafziger & Bertino, 2009; Reisfield et al., 2007), a knowledge of opiate metabolism, and awareness of the expected ratios of the parent drug and its metabolites in urine (Reisfield et al., 2007). In addition, small amount of impurities in medications detectable by mass spectrometry can complicate the interpretation of UDT results. For example, codeine is present in morphine preparations and hydrocodone is present in oxycodone preparations (Evans et al., 2009; West et al., 2009, 2011b). Physicians who aren't aware of the presence of these impurities may wrongly dismiss a patient because he or she tested positive for codeine or hydrocodone when it was not prescribed. The presence of both parent drug and its metabolite in a urine sample readily measured by mass spectrometry can reassure the physician that the patient is taking the medication and that it is being metabolized appropriately. Also, for some drugs such as carisoprodol, fentanyl, or buprenorphine, only the metabolite may be observed. It is imperative that physicians prescribing these medications use a reference laboratory that is able to measure both the parent drug and its corresponding metabolite and be able to present interpretive results for the physician (Heltsley et al., 2010).

Creatinine is a metabolic breakdown product that is present in urine. The amount of creatinine excreted into urine is nearly constant for any individual. Reference laboratories calculate the amount of drug excreted per gram of creatinine, which allows the monitoring of excreted medication or illicit drug over time. This information is useful to physicians in certain circumstances because some drugs, such as nordiazepam remain in the system long after a person stops taking them. A UDT result that is not corrected for creatinine may show that the patient is more positive for the drug than on a previous test, even though the patient has in fact stopped taking it. Except for changes in the patient's renal status, or loss from adipose tissue due to dieting, this conflicting result may be due to the second urine being more concentrated than the first. A creatinine-corrected value will correct for a patient's hydration on the day of the test and show a decrease in the amount of nordiazepam in the urine, thus supporting the patient's claim that he or she has stopped taking the drug. It is important that reference laboratories not only provide creatinine-corrected results but that they give doctors or staff help in interpreting the data (Cone et al., 2009). It is also important for the physician to know if a patient has attempted to obscure UDT results by diluting a urine specimen. To accomplish this, he or she must have a grasp of creatinine and specific gravity UDT validity tests (Wu, 2001). Laboratory staff who interface with clients should provide this information when questions arise.

5. Monitoring ethanol use in pain patients

As stated earlier, alcohol (ethanol) use among pain patients is a significant problem because of the risk for drug-drug interaction with opioid medication. For doctors to understand UDT ethanol results, it is essential that they understand ethanol metabolism and the formation of the ethanol byproducts ethyl glucuronide and ethyl sulfate (Crews et al., 2011a; Crews et al., 2011b; Dahl et al., 2002; Helander & Beck, 2005; Helander et al., 1996; Rosano & Lin, 2008; Schmitt et al., 1997; Stephanson et al., 2002; Wojcik & Hawthorne, 2007; Wurst et al., 2006; Wurst et al., 2004). This is because false positive ethanol results can result from fermentation of glucose from diabetic patient samples (Crews et al., 2011b). Crews et al. reported that about 1/3 of the ethanol positive samples were due to fermentation. Misinterpretation of these results can have grave consequences as doctors may establish a contract with a patient that he or she abstain from any alcohol use while being treated with opioid medication; therefore, a positive finding for alcohol use can result in dismissal from the practice (Federal Register, 2004).

6. When to use UDT

Urine drug testing must be tailored to fit the pain patient's clinical history. For the intake visit, the patient is advised as to the necessity for UDT and is typically requested to provide a urine specimen. If the patient fails to do this, he or she may be immediately dismissed from the practice. In some practices, the urine specimen is tested by a POC device at the time of the appointment and the results are compared to the patient reported history.   If necessary, discrepancies are discussed. As a matter of course, a portion of the POC urine sample is sent to the reference laboratory to confirm the POC test results, test for additional medications, and, at the discretion of the physician, to test for the prescribed medications, non-prescribed medications and illicit drugs at lower cutoff levels than those provided by the POC test.

For many established pain patients, quarterly or semi-annual UDT is considered appropriate. It is best if this is done on a random basis. The strongest recommendation for doing UDT is adding additional medications to the regimen or changing medications. Urine drug testing may also be administered if a patient changes their behavior or exhibits addiction tendencies such as complaining of running out of medications early (Chou et al., 2009; Trescot et al., 2006). Testing may be conducted as frequently as every office visit for some patients who exhibit unusual behavior, have a history of abuse, or if illicit or non-prescription drugs were found to be present on a previous test. Gourlay, D. & Heit, H. (2010a).

7. Purposes and costs of UDT

As stated earlier, the purpose of UDT (as well as the relative costs) may be broken down into three components: testing prescribed medications for compliance; testing for non-prescribed medications; and testing for illicit drugs. At the time when the forensic model of drug testing was instituted the vast majority of people who died from drugs died from the use of illicit drugs. At this point in time more people die from prescription medications than by illicit drugs (Hall et al., 2008; Krausz et al., 1996; Okie, 2010). There are now 13 or more classes of drugs that are used to treat pain. Pain patients are on an average using three of these drugs (Kuehn, 2007; Okie, 2010). Therefore, for every 100 patients, 300 confirmations by mass spectroscopy are required. This is more than a 100-fold increase in the number of tests needed to serve this patient population compared to workplace testing. This represents a radical change in UDT model from the forensic model used at the time when the purpose of drug testing was to root out the one or two percent of drug-using professional drivers. It is important that legislators and payors for UDT services understand the shift from the forensic UDT model to the clinical model. Currently the insurance reimbursement codes and categories do not accurately reflect the costs associated with these new clinical drug testing requirements (*Cpt Current Procedural Technology*, 2010).

7.1 Cost effectiveness of UDT
It is also important to discuss the cost-effectiveness of UDT. The National Institute on Drug Abuse (NIDA) states that the cost of not treating an addict is $56,000/year. An example of

effective treatment for heroin addiction is the methadone maintenance program, which has an average cost of $4,700/per patient/per year (Principles of Drug Addiction Treatment: A Research-Based Guide, 2009). Based on these figures, every dollar invested in drug treatment programs yields a return of about 12 times this amount. The goal then should be detecting untreated drug abuse. Urine drug testing helps accomplish this goal.

There are two aspects of drug abuse in the pain patient population; one is the use of illicit drugs, and the other more prevalent aspect is abuse of the prescribed and non-prescribed medications. Combined, these two facets of abuse may approach 20-30% of the patients on chronic opioid therapy. Using this percentage of patients and factoring the $56,000/patient cost, this means that on average each of these patients may actually be costing society and insurers $16,800 more annually than what is estimated by only calculating costs of office visits and medications. If clinical UDT is performed 2-4 times per year for each patient reimbursed at $500 per UDT, this represents a cost of $1000-$2000 per patient per year. This is in contrast to the $16,800 referenced above. It seems clear that using UDT to detect these patients should significantly reduce the cost of care as well as the costs to society (Wall et al., 2000).

7.2 Social costs of drug abuse

In light of the fact that providing the highest standard of care is one of the basic tenets of the medical profession, it is important to note that several studies have shown that untreated opioid-abusing patients have significantly higher societal cost (Wall et al., 2000) and mortality rate (between 2 and 10 times) than the comparative general population (Hall et al., 2008; Oyefeso et al., 1999). Based on this data alone, the use of UDT should be justified for pain patients.

8. Conclusions

8.1 When and how to test

Pain is a complex disease and chronic opioid therapy is one of the treatments of choice. Urine drug testing is one of the ways to measure patient adherence to the treatment regimen. At the intake office visit it is important for the physician to be able to make immediate assessment of the patient to validate their reported history and to determine the overt presence of illicit drugs or non-prescribed medications. Either a POC device or in-office immunoassay analyzer should be used for this purpose. A portion of the patient's urine specimen should be sent to a reference laboratory for analysis using lower cutoffs and a much extended test menu such as those listed in Tables 1 and 2. As stated earlier, this will give the physician further confidence that the patient's history is valid and provide measurable evidence for informed clinical decision making. In addition, alcohol use, which cannot easily be detected by the POC devices, can be identified as a risk factor.

8.2 Ongoing testing

At subsequent visits UDT will provide the physician with evidence of patient compliance with prescribed medications (West et al., 2010a) and eliminate the potential for abuse of non-prescribed medications or illicit drugs (Pesce et al., 2010b). For this purpose, depending upon clinical judgment, the test menu does not have to be quite as extensive. Tests for rarely-observed illicit drugs such as MDMA and PCP may not be included. Similarly, tests for rarely-prescribed or removed medications such as propoxyphene may not be included. If intake visit UDT showed that the patient was observed to be taking a non-prescribed medication or illicit drug then subsequent visit UDT's should include tests for those agents. Because of the potential for morbidity from alcohol-medication interactions, it may be necessary to continue to monitor certain patients for ethanol and its metabolites.

8.3 Minimum analytical requirements

When monitoring for opioid medication compliance, the testing method should be able to differentiate between codeine, morphine, hydrocodone, norhydrocodone, and hydromorphone. The test should also be able to differentiate between oxycodone, noroxycodone, and oxymorphone. This will allow the physician to determine that the opiate the patient is taking is in fact the one being prescribed and that the patient is metabolizing the medication properly (Pesce et al., 2010a). A similar case can be made for the testing of benzodiazepines. The method should be able to detect at low concentrations and differentiate between alpha-hydroxyalprazolam, 7-aminoclonazepam, lorazepam, nordiazepam, temazepam, and oxazepam. This will allow the doctor to see that the patient is taking the prescribed benzodiazepine and allay any concerns about doctor shopping. Frequency of UDT should be based on the physician's observations of the patient's behavior as well as suggested guidelines. For those patients whose behavior is not of concern, some guidelines suggest UDT between two and four times per year on a random basis (Chou et al., 2009; Trescot et al., 2006). For those patients with non-compliant behavior or a history of addiction, testing should be done as often as every office visit (Chou et al., 2009; Trescot et al., 2006).

9. References

Agilent Technologies, Inc. 5301 Stevens Creek Blvd, Santa Clara, CA 95051, USA. Thermo Fisher Scientific. 81 Wyman St, Waltham, MA 02454, USA.

Amedica Drug Screen Test Cup. Hayward, CA: Amedica Biotech, Inc.

American Proficiency Institute 2011 Catalog of Programs. Traverse City, MI: American Proficiency Institute, 2011.

Atluri, S. & Sudarshan, G. (2003). Evaluation of Abnormal Urine Drug Screens among Patients with Chronic Non-Malignant Pain Treated with Opioids. *Pain Physician*, Vol.6, No.4, pp.407-409,

Chou, R., Fanciullo, G., Fine, P., Adler, J., Ballantyne, J., Davies, P., Donovan, M., Fishbain, D., Foley, K., Fudin, J., Gilson, A., Kelter, A., Mauskop, A., O'Connor, P., Passik, S., Pasternak, G., Portenoy, R., Rich, B., Roberts, R., Todd, K. & Miaskowski, C. (2009). Clinical Guidelines for the Use of Chronic Opioid Therapy in Chronic Noncancer Pain. *The Journal of Pain*, Vol.10, No.2, (February 2009), pp.113-130, 1526-5900

College of American Pathologists 2011 Surveys and Anatomic Pathology Education Programs. Northfield, IL: College of American Pathologists, 2011.

Cone, E., Caplan, Y., Black, D., Robert, T. & Moser, F. (2008). Urine Drug Testing of Chronic Pain Patients: Licit and Illicit Drug Patterns. *Journal of Analytical Toxicology*, Vol.32, No.8, (October 2008), pp.530-543, ISSN 1945-2403

Cone, E., Caplan, Y., Moser, F., Robert, T., Shelby, M. & Black, D. (2009). Normalization of Urinary Drug Concentrations with Specific Gravity and Creatinine. *Journal of Analytical Toxicology*, Vol.33, No.1, (January-February 2009), pp.1-7, ISSN 1945-2403

Cpt Current Procedural Technology. (2010). (Professional ed.), American Medical Association, Chicago, IL

Crews, B., Latyshev, S., Mikel, C., Almazan, P., West, R., Pesce, A. & West, C. (2011a). Improved Detection of Ethyl Glucuronide and Ethyl Sulfate in a Pain Management Population Using High-Throughput Lc-Ms/Ms. *Journal of Opioid Management,* Vol.6, No.6, (Novenber-December 2010), pp.415-421, ISSN 1551-7489

Crews, B., West, R., Gutierrez, R., Latyshev, S., Mikel, C., Almazan, P., Pesce, A., West, C. & Rosenthal, M. (2011b). An Improved Method of Determining Ethanol Use in a Chronic Pain Population. *Journal of Opioid Management,* Vol.In Press, (n.d.), ISSN 1551-7489

Dahl, H., Stephanson, N., Beck, O. & Helander, A. (2002). Comparison of Urinary Excretion Characteristics of Ethanol and Ethyl Glucuronide. *Journal of Analytical Toxicology,* Vol.26, No.4, (May-June 2002), pp.201-204, ISSN 1945-2403

Evans, M., Kriger, S., Gunn, J. & Schwilke, E. (2009). Anomalous Opiate Detection in Compliance Monitoring. *Practical Pain Management,* Vol.9, No.7, (September 2009), pp.54-55,

Federal Register - Mandatory Guidelines and Proposed Revisions to Mandatory Guidelines for Federal Workplace Drug Testing Programs. Substance Abuse and Mental Health Services Administration. Rockville, MD: Department of Health and Human Services, 2004;69(71).

Feldkamp, C.S. (2010). Immunological Reactions, In: *Clinical Chemistry: Theory, Analysis, and Correlation,* L. A. Kaplan and A. J. Pesce, pp. 151-179, Mosby, St. Louis

Fraser, A. & Zamecnik, J. (2003). Impact of Lowering the Screening and Confirmation Cutoff Values for Urine Drug Testing Based on Dilution Indicators. *Therapeutic Drug Monitoring,* Vol.25, No.6, (December 2003), pp.723-727, ISSN 1536-3694

Fraser, A.D. (2001). Psychotropic Agents: The Benzodiazepines, In: *The Clinical Toxicology Laboratory: Contemporary Practice of Poisoning Evaluation,* L. C. Shaw, T. C. Kwong, T. G. Rosano, P. J. Orsolak, B. A. Wolf and B. Magnani, pp. 211-221, American Association for Clinical Chemistry, Inc., Washington, DC

Gourlay, D. & Heit, H. (2010a). The Art and Science of Urine Drug Testing. *The Clinical Journal of Pain,* Vol.26, No.4, (May 2010), pp.358, ISSN 0749-8047

Gourlay, D., Heit, H. & Almahrezi, A. (2005). Universal Precautions in Pain Medicine: A Rational Approach to the Treatment of Chronic Pain. *Pain Medicine,* Vol.6, No.2, (March-April 2010), pp.107-112, ISSN 1526-4637

Gourlay, D., Heit, H. & Caplan, Y. Urine Drug Testing in Clinical Practice: The Art and Science of Patient Care. California Academy of Family Physicians. Stamford, CT: PharmaCom Group, Inc., 2010.

Gourlay, D. & Heit, H.A. (2010b). The Art and Science of Urine Drug Testing. *Clin J Pain,* Vol.26, No.4, pp.358,

Hall, A., Logan, J., Toblin, R., Kaplan, J., Kraner, J., Bixler, D., Crosby, A. & Paulozzi, L. (2008). Patterns of Abuse among Unintentional Pharmaceutical Overdose Fatalities. *JAMA,* Vol.300, No.22, (December 2008), pp.2613-2620, ISSN 1538-3598

Hammett-Stabler, C. & Webster, L. A Clinical Guide to Urine Drug Testing: Augmenting Pain Management and Enhancing Patient Care. University of Medicine and

Dentistry of New Jersay - Center for Continuing and Outreach Education. Stamford, CT: PharmaCom Group, Inc, 2008.

Harmful Interactions: Mixing Alcohol with Medicines. National Institute on Alcohol Abuse and Alcoholism. Bethesda, MD: National Institutes of Health, 2007.

Hattab, E., Goldberger, B., Johannsen, L., Kindland, P., Ticino, F., Chronister, C. & Bertholf, R. (2000). Modification of Screening Immunoassays to Detect Sub-Threshold Concentrations of Cocaine, Cannabinoids, and Opiates in Urine: Use for Detecting Maternal and Neonatal Drug Exposures. *Annals of Clinical and Laboratory Science*, Vol.31, No.1, (January 2000), pp.85-91, ISSN 1550-8080

Helander, A. & Beck, O. (2005). Ethyl Sulfate: A Metabolite of Ethanol in Humans and a Potential Biomarker of Acute Alcohol Intake. *Journal of Analytical Toxicology*, Vol.29, No.5, (July-August 2005), pp.270-274, ISSN 1945-2403

Helander, A., Beck, O. & Jones, A. (1996). Laboratory Testing for Recent Alcohol Consumption: Comparison of Ethanol, Methanol, and 5-Hydroxytryptophol. *Clinical Chemistry*, Vol.42, No.4, (April 1996), pp.618-624, ISSN 1530-8561

Heltsley, R., Zichterman, A., Black, D., Cawthon, B., Robert, T., Moser, F., Caplan, Y. & Cone, E. (2010). Urine Drug Testing of Chronic Pain Patients. Ii. Prevalence Patterns of Prescription Opiates and Metabolites. *Journal of Analytical Toxicology*, Vol.34, No.1, (January-February 2010), pp.32-38, ISSN 1945-2403

Ives, T., Chelminski, P., Hammett-Stabler, C., Malone, R., Perhac, J., Potisek, N., Shilliday, B., DeWalt, D. & Pignone, M. (2006). Predictors of Opioid Misuse in Patients with Chronic Pain: A Prospective Cohort Study. *BMC Health Services Research*, Vol.6, No.1, (April 2006), pp.46, ISSN 1472-6963

Jung, B. & Reidenberg, M. (2007). Physicians Being Deceived. *Pain Medicine*, Vol.8, No.5, (July-August 2007), pp.433-437, ISSN 1526-4637

Katz, N., Sherburne, S., Beach, M., Rose, R., Vielguth, J., Bradley, J. & Fanciullo, G. (2003). Behavioral Monitoring and Urine Toxicology Testing in Patients Receiving Long-Term Opioid Therapy. *Anesthesia and Analgesia*, Vol.97, No.4, (October 2003), pp.1097-1102, ISSN 1526-7598

Krausz, M., Degkwit, P., Haasen, C. & Verthein, U. (1996). Opioid Addiction and Suicidality. *Crisis*, Vol.17, No.4, pp.175-181,

Kuehn, B.M. (2007). Opioid Prescriptions Soar: Increase in Legitimate Use as Well as Abuse. *JAMA*, Vol.297, No.3, pp.249-251, 0098-7484 1538-3598

Madras, B., Compton, W., Avula, D., Stegbauer, T., Stein, J. & Clark, H. (2009). Screening, Brief Interventions, Referral to Treatment (Sbirt) for Illicit Drug and Alcohol Use at Multiple Healthcare Sites: Comparison at Intake and 6 Months Later. *Drug and Alcohol Dependence*, Vol.99, No.1-3, (January 2009), pp.280-295, ISSN 1879-0046

Manchikanti, L., Atluri, S., Trescot, A. & Giordano, J. (2008). Monitoring Opioid Adherence in Chronic Pain Patients: Tools, Techniques, and Utility. *Pain Physician*, Vol.11, No.2, (March 2008), pp.S155-S180, ISSN 1533-3159

Manchikanti, L., Cash, K., Damron, K., Manchukonda, R., Pampati, V. & McManus, C. (2006a). Controlled Substance Abuse and Illicit Drug Use in Chronic Pain Patients: An Evaluation of Multiple Variables. *Pain Physician*, Vol.9, No.3, (July 2006), pp.215-226, ISSN 1533-3159

Manchikanti, L., Damron, K., McManus, C. & Barnhill, R. (2004). Patterns of Illicit Drug Use and Opioid Abuse in Patients with Chronic Pain at Initial Evaluation: A Prospective, Observational Study. *Pain Physician*, Vol.7, No.4, (October 2004), pp.431-437, ISSN 1533-3159

Manchikanti, L., Malla, Y., Wargo, B., Cash, K., Pampati, V., Damron, K., McManus, C. & Brandon, D. (2010). Protocol for Accuracy of Point of Care (Poc) or in-Office Urine Drug Testing (Immunoassay) in Chronic Pain Patients: A Prospective Analysis of Immunoassay and Liquid Chromatography Tandem Mass Spectometry (Lc/Ms/Ms). *Pain Physician*, Vol.13, No.1, (January 2010), pp.E1-E22, ISSN 1533-3159

Manchikanti, L., Manchukonda, R., Pampati, V., Damron, K., Brandon, D., Cash, K. & McManus, C. (2006b). Does Random Urine Drug Testing Reduce Illicit Drug Use in Chronic Pain Patients Receiving Opioids? *Pain Physician*, Vol.9, No.2, (April 2006), pp.123-129, ISSN 1533-3159

Manchikanti, L., Manchukonda, R., Pampati, V. & Damron, K.S. (2005). Evaluation of Abuse of Prescription and Illicit Drugs in Chronic Pain Patients Receiving Short-Acting (Hydrocodone) or Long-Acting (Methadone) Opioids. *Pain Physician*, Vol.8, No.3, pp.257-261,

Michna, E., Jamison, R., Pham, L., Ross, E., Janfaza, D., Nedeljkovic, S., Narang, S., Palombi, D. & Wasan, A. (2007). Urine Toxicology Screening among Chronic Pain Patients on Opioid Therapy: Frequency and Predictability of Abnormal Findings. *The Clinical Journal of Pain*, Vol.23, No.2, (February 2007), pp.173-179, ISSN 1536-5409

Mikel, C., Almazan, P., West, R., Crews, B., Latyshev, S., Pesce, A. & West, C. (2009). Lc-Ms/Ms Extends the Range of Drug Analysis in Pain Patients. *Therapeutic Drug Monitoring*, Vol.31, No.6, (December 2009), pp.746-748, ISSN 1536-3694

Mikel, C., Pesce, A. & West, C. (2010). A Tale of Two Drug Testing Technologies: Gc-Ms and Lc-Ms/Ms. *Pain Physician*, Vol.13, No.1, pp.91-92,

Mohsin, S., Yang, Y. & Zumwalt, M. Quantitative Analysis of Opiates in Urine Using Rrht Lc/Ms/Ms. Santa Clara, CA: Agilent Technologies, Inc., 2007.

Nafziger, A. & Bertino, J., Jr. (2009). Utility and Application of Urine Drug Testing in Chronic Pain Management with Opioids. *The Clinical Journal of Pain*, Vol.25, No.1, (January 2009), pp.73-79, ISSN 1536-5409

National Prescription Drug Threat Assesment. U.S. Department of Justice. Johnstown, PA: National Drug Intelligence Center, 2009.

National Survey on Drug Use and Health: Detailed Tables - Prevalence Estimates, Standard Errors, P Values, and Sample Sizes. Substance Abuse and Mental Health Services Administration. Rockville, MD: Department of Health and Human Services, 1995-2006.

Nucynta - Tapentadol. (2010). December 3, 2010, Available from: <www.nucynta.com>

Okie, S. (2010). A Flood of Opioids, a Rising Tide of Deaths. *The New England Journal of Medicine*, Vol.363, No.21, (November 2010), pp.1981-1985, ISSN 1533-4406

Olympus Au640 Product Information. Brea, CA: Beckman Coulter, Inc. Lab Systems and Routine Testing.

Oyefeso, A., Ghodse, H., Clancy, C., Corkery, J. & Goldfinch, R. (1999). Drug Abuse-Related Mortality: A Study of Teenage Addicts over a 20-Year Period. *Social Psychiatry and Psychiatric Epidemiology*, Vol.34, No.8, (August 1999), pp.437-441, ISSN 1433-9285

Pesce, A., Rosenthal, M., West, R., West, C., Crews, B., Mikel, C., Almazan, P. & Latyshev, S. (2010a). An Evaluation of the Diagnostic Accuracy of Liquid Chromatography-Tandem Mass Spectrometry Versus Immunoassay Drug Testing in Pain Patients. *Pain Physician*, Vol.13, No.3, pp.273-281,

Pesce, A., West, C., Rosenthal, M., West, R., Crews, B., Mikel, C., Almazan, P., Latyshev, S. & Horn, P. (2010b). Marijuana Correlates with Use of Other Illicit Drugs in a Pain Patient Population. *Pain Physician*, Vol.13, No.3, pp.283-287,

Pesce, A., West, C., West, R., Crews, B., Mikel, C., Almazan, P., Latyshev, S., Rosenthal, M. & Horn, P. (2010c). Reference Intervals: A Novel Approach to Detect Drug Abuse in a Pain Patient Population. *Journal of Opioid Management*, Vol.6, No.5, (September-October 2010), pp.341-350, ISSN 1551-7489

Pesce, A., West, C., West, R., Crews, B., Mikel, C., Rosenthal, M., Almazan, P. & Latyshev, S. (2011). Determination of Medication Cutoff Values in a Pain Patient Population. *Journal of Opioid Management*, Vol.In Press, (n.d.), ISSN 1551-7489

Principles of Drug Addiction Treatment: A Research-Based Guide. National Institue on Drug Abuse. Bethesda, MD: Department of Health and Human Services, 2009.

Reisfield, G., Salazar, E. & Bertholf, R. (2007). Rational Use and Interpretation of Urine Drug Testing in Chronic Opioid Therapy. *Annals of Clinical and Laboratory Science*, Vol.37, No.4, (Autumn 2007), pp.301-314, ISSN 1550-8080

Rosano, T. & Lin, J. (2008). Ethyl Glucuronide Excretion in Humans Following Oral Administration of and Dermal Exposure to Ethanol. *Journal of Analytical Toxicology*, Vol.32, No.8, (October 2008), pp.594-600, ISSN 1945-2403

Schmitt, G., Droenner, P., Skopp, G. & Aderjan, R. (1997). Ethyl Glucuronide Concentration in Serum of Human Volunteers, Teetotalers, and Suspected Drinking Drivers. *Journal of Forensic Sciences*, Vol.42, No.6, (November 1997), pp.1099-1102, ISSN 1556-4029

Schuckman, H., Hazelett, S., Powell, C. & Steer, S. (2008). A Validation of Self-Reported Substance Use with Biochemical Testing among Patients Presenting to the Emergency Department Seeking Treatment for Backache, Headache, and Toothache. *Substance Use and Misuse*, Vol.43, No.5, (n.d.), pp.589-595, ISSN 1433-9285

Siemens V-Twin Analyzer Product Information. Hermosa Beach, CA: Siemens Healthcare Diagnostic, Inc.

Siuzdak, G. (2006). *The Expanding Role of Mass Spectrometry in Biotechnology* (2nd ed.), MCC Press, San Diego, CA

Sobolevsky, T., Prasolov, I. & Rodchenkov, G. (2010). Detection of Jwh-018 Metabolites in Smoking Mixture Post-Administration Urine. *Forensic Science International*, Vol.200, No.1-3, (July 2010), pp.141-147, ISSN 1872-6283

Stephanson, N., Dahl, H., A., H. & Beck, O. (2002). Direct Quantification of Ethyl Glucuronide in Clinical Urine Samples by Liquid Chromatography-Mass

Spectrometry. *Therapeutic Drug Monitoring,* Vol.24, No.5, (October 2002), pp.645-651, ISSN 1536-3694

Thermo Fisher Mgc-240 Analyzer Product Information. Franklin, MA: Thermo Fisher Scientific.

Trescot, A., Boswell, M., Atluri, S., Hansen, H., Deer, T., Abdi, S., Jasper, J., Singh, V., Jordan, A., Johnson, B., Cicala, R., Dunbar, E., Helm, S., II, Varley, K., Suchdev, P., Swicegood, J., Calodney, A., Ogoke, B., Minore, W. & Manchikanti, L. (2006). Opioid Guidelines in the Management of Chronic Non-Cancer Pain. *Pain Physician,* Vol.9, No.1, (January 2006), pp.1-40, ISSN 1533-3159

Vardakou, I., Pistos, C. & Spiliopoulou, C. (2010). Spice Drugs as a New Trend: Mode of Action, Identification and Legislation. *Toxicology Letters,* Vol.197, No.3, (September 2010), pp.157-162, ISSN 1879-3169

Wall, R., Rehm, J., Fischer, B., Brands, B., Gliksman, L., Stewart, J., Medved, W. & Blake, J. (2000). Social Costs of Untreated Opioid Dependence. *Journal of Urban Health,* Vol.77, No.4, (December 2000), pp.688-722, ISSN 1468-2869

Webster, L. & Dove, B. (2007). *Avoiding Opioid Abuse While Managing Pain: A Guide for Practitioners,* Sunrise River Press, North Branch, MN

West, R., Crews, B., Mikel, C., Almazan, P., Latyshev, S., Pesce, A. & West, C. (2009). Anomalous Observations of Codeine in Patients on Morphine. *Therapeutic Drug Monitoring,* Vol.31, No.6, (December 2009), pp.776-778, ISSN 1536-3694

West, R., Pesce, A., Crews, B., Mikel, C., Rosenthal, M., Almazan, P., Latyshev, S. & West, C. (2011a). Determination of Illicit Drug Cutoff Values in a Pain Patient Population. *Clinica Chimica Acta,* Vol.In Press, (n.d.), ISSN 1873-3492

West, R., Pesce, A., Mikel, C., Rosenthal, M., Latyshev, S., Crews, B. & Almazan, P. (2010a). Observations of Medication Compliance by Measurement of Urinary Drug Concentrations in a Pain Management Population. *Journal of Opioid Management,* Vol.6, No.4, (July-August 2010), pp.253-257, ISSN 1551-7489

West, R., Pesce, A., West, C., Crews, B., Mikel, C., Almazan, P., Rosenthal, M. & Latyshev, S. (2010b). Comparison of Clonazepam Compliance by Measurement of Urinary Concentration by Immunoassay and Lc-Ms/Ms in Pain Management Population. *Pain Physician,* Vol.13, No.1, pp.71-78,

West, R., West, C., Crews, B., Almazan, P., Latyshev, S., Rosenthal, M., Pesce, A. & Mikel, C. (2011b). Anomalous Observations of Hydrocodone in Patients on Oxycodone. *Clinica Chimica Acta,* Vol.412, No.1-2, (January 2011), pp.29-32, ISSN 1873-3492

Wingert, W. (1997). Lowering Cutoffs for Initial and Confirmation Testing for Cocaine and Marijuana: Large-Scale Study of Effects on the Rates of Drug-Positive Results. *Clinical Chemistry,* Vol.43, No.1, (January 1997), pp.100-103, ISSN 1530-8561

Wojcik, M. & Hawthorne, J. (2007). Sensitivity of Commercial Ethyl Glucuronide (Etg) Testing in Screening for Alcohol Abstinence. *Alcohol and Alcoholism,* Vol.42, No.4, (July-August 2007), pp.317-320, ISSN 1464-3502

Wu, A.H.B. (2001). Urine Adulteration before Testing for Drugs of Abuse, In: *The Clinical Toxicology Laboratory: Contemporary Practice of Poisoning Evaluation,* L. C. Shaw, T. C. Kwong, T. G. Rosano, P. J. Orsolak, B. A. Wolf and B. Magnani, pp. 157-171, American Association for Clinical Chemistry, Inc., Washington, DC

Wurst, F., Dresen, S., Allen, J., Wiesbeck, G., Graf, M. & Weinmann, W. (2006). Ethyl Sulphate: A Direct Ethanol Metabolite Reflecting Recent Alcohol Consumption. *Addiction*, Vol.101, No.2, (February 2006), pp.204-211, ISSN 1360-0443

Wurst, F., Wiesbeck, G., Metzger, J., Weinmann, W. & Graf, M. (2004). On Sensitivity, Specificity, and the Influence of Various Parameters on Ethyl Glucuronide Levels in Urine - Results from the Who/Isbra Study. *Alcoholism, Clinical and Experimental Research*, Vol.28, No.8, (August 2004), pp.1220-1228, ISSN 1530-0277

3

Multi-Well Engineered Heart Tissue for Drug Screening and Predictive Toxicology

Alexandra Eder, Arne Hansen and Thomas Eschenhagen
Department of Experimental Pharmacology and Toxicology,
University Medical Centre Hamburg-Eppendorf,
Germany

1. Introduction

Drug development is time- and cost-intensive and, overall, inefficient. Only one out of an estimated 10.000 new chemical entities (NCEs) finally enters the market. The later the failure occurs, the higher are the costs. It is for this reason that preclinical development aims at identifying the potential for failure as early as possible and with high sensitivity. On the other hand, high sensitivity generally also means low specificity, suggesting that many potentially successful NCEs are currently excluded from further development. Common reasons for exclusion are adverse drug reactions (ADR). Among the various ADRs, cardiac toxicities and arrhythmias play an important role, because they represent about 21% of all ADRs (Lasser et al., 2002) and are frequently lethal. The single most important mechanism in this context is the prolongation of cardiac repolarization bearing a proarrhythmic potential. These interferences can be visualized by standard ECGs as a prolongation of the QT-interval. Such a prolongation is called "long QT-syndrome" (LQT-syndrome) and is associated with *Torsade-de-Pointes* (TdP) arrhythmias and sudden cardiac death. In the past, several prominent drugs had to be withdrawn from the market due to TdP in humans, e.g. astemizole, terfenadine, cisapride, sparfloxacin, grepafloxacin and recently clobutinol (Silomat). Moreover, numerous drugs are still on the market that are associated with the potential to cause LQT and TdP, including widely prescribed drugs such as the antibiotic erythromycin.

Given the fatal consequences of LQT and TdP in healthy patients without any cardiac disposition, the regulatory bodies (FDA, EMEA and others) have decided some years ago to require testing for LQT to be an obligatory part of preclinical development of any NCE. Several tests have been developed and some of them are routinely used. The three major (but by far not exclusive) tests in the field are the HERG test, rabbit Purkinje fibers and telemetry in dogs. These tests have different advantages and disadvantages and are generally employed subsequently. The HERG test can be considered an obligatory test for all NCEs and it is unlikely that any company further develops a compound that showed major inhibitory activity in this test (of a single ion channel activity). However, examples exist of successful drugs on the market that are potent inhibitors of the HERG current without ever giving rise to TdP arrhythmia (e.g. verapamil, azithromycin). Thus, the predictive value of the HERG test is limited. Reasons lie, among others, in its inability to give an integrated readout of effects of drugs on the electrophysiology of the intact cardiac myocyte or the intact heart as a multicellular organ consisting of a functional syncytium of cardiac myocytes and all other cardiac cell types that make up normal heart tissue (e.g. fibroblasts, endothelial cells and smooth muscle cells).

1.1 Cardiac tissue engineering

Over the past decade, techniques have been developed to generate cardiac tissue-like 3-dimensional constructs in vitro (Eschenhagen & Zimmermann, 2005). The field of cardiac tissue engineering opened the possibility for many applications. Artificial hart constructs may serve as means for cell-based cardiac repair and as improved in vitro models for predictive toxicology and target validation, taking advantage of a more physiological cellular environment. Previous studies used different approaches to construct engineered tissues: Cell seeding onto solid, preformed scaffolds (Carrier et al., 1999; Engelmayr et al., 2008; Leor et al., 2000; Li et al., 2000; Ott et al., 2008; Radisic et al., 2004), matrix-free generation of tissues from stackable cell sheets (Shimizu et al., 2002) or the generation of constructs in preformed casting moulds using hydrogels such as collagen I, matrigel, fibronectin or fibrin (Bian et al., 2009; Eschenhagen et al., 1997; Huang et al., 2007; Naito et al., 2006; Zimmermann et al., 2002). The hydrogel technique has been shown to be suitable for both, cardiac repair in vivo (Zimmermann et al., 2006) and target validation in vitro (El-Armouche et al., 2007). Circular engineered heart tissues (EHTs) were made by casting neonatal rat heart cells, collagen I and matrigel into circular casting moulds and develop a high degree of cellular differentiation, longitudinal orientation, intercellular coupling and force generation (Zimmerman et al., 2002). It turned out that several factors improve tissue quality and force generation of EHT such as phasic (Fink et al., 2000) or auxotonic stretch, increased ambient oxygen concentration during culture and supplementation with insulin (Zimmermann et al., 2006). Others demonstrated beneficial effects of electrical stimulation (Radisic et al., 2004). The possibility to generate cardiac myocytes from human embryonic stem cells (Kehat et al., 2001) or induced pluripotent stem cells (Zhang et al., 2009) have opened the realistic and exciting perspective to use these techniques for the validation of hypotheses and testing drugs in healthy and diseased human heart muscles (Zimmermann & Eschenhagen 2007).

The current techniques to generate engineered cardiac tissues are either not suitable for this purpose (stacked cell sheet technique) or exhibit drawbacks that limit their usefulness. Extensive handling steps preclude routine execution of large series in an at least medium through put scale and are always a source of variability. Furthermore, the EHT technique in the ring format requires relatively high numbers of cells and turned out to be difficult to miniaturize.

In this chapter we describe a new EHT technique that was driven by the intention to miniaturize the EHT-format for multi-well-testing and automated evaluation and to determine the suitability of EHTs for drug screening and predictive toxicology. The main results have been published in a recent original paper (Hansen et al. 2010). An essentiel change was to use fibrin(ogen) instead of collagen I as a matrix. Fibrinogen is part of the blood clotting cascade. It is a glycoprotein with a size of 340 kDa. Physiologically it achieves plasma concentrations of 1.5 to 4 g/l and can be relative easily purified from different species. An important mechanical property is its nonlinear elasticity. Due to this, fibrin polymers have a high elastic modulus under shear stress combined with a beneficial softness in comparison to other filamentous biopolymers (Janmey et al., 2009). The final properties of fibrin are mainly governed by the concentrations of fibrinogen and thrombin. Additionally fibrin properties can be affected by the introduction of bonds by plasma transglutaminase (factor XIII; Janmey et al., 2009). In contrast to other extracellular matrices, the *in vitro* polymerisation of fibrin is very close to the *in vivo* fibrin polymer. Fibrin gels are fully degradable by fibrinolytic enzymes like plasmin. All together, the mechanical and biological properties, its availability from autologous sources in addition to the possibility to covalently bind growth or other factors (Hubbell 2003) make fibrin an interesting compound for tissue engineering approaches.

2. Methods

2.1 Cell isolation
Total heart cells (excluding the atria) were isolated from neonatal Wistar rats (postnatal day 0 to 3) by a fractionated DNase/Trypsin digestion protocol as previously described (Eschenhagen & Zimmermann, 2005). The resulting cell populations were immediately subjected to FBME generation. Experimental procedures were reviewed and approved by Ethics Committee, Hamburg University.

2.2 Manufacturing teflon spacers and sylgard posts racks
For the generation of fibrin-based mini-EHTs (FBMEs), Teflon spacer and silicone post racks were used. The Teflon spacers were important for the casting molds. They had the following geometry (Figure: 1B): length 12 mm, width 3 mm, height 13.5 mm. Sylgard 184 silicone elastomer (Dow Corning) was used for the production of silicone post racks, which were needed for culturing the FBMEs. The silicone post racks were made in custom-made Teflon casting molds. According to the manufacture's instructions, the 2-component Sylgard 184 was degassed under vacuum conditions before casting. The final silicone post racks consisted of 4 pairs of posts, having a little plate at their end. The racks had the following geometry (Figure 1A): length/width of rack: 79x18.5 mm, length of posts 12 mm, diameter 1 mm, plate diameter 2 mm, distance (center-center) 8.5 mm. They were initially self-made and currently industrial-made. Silicone post racks can be autoclaved and reused for several times.

2.3 Generation of fibrin-based mini-EHTs
The reconstitution mixture for the generation of fibrin-based mini-EHTs was prepared on ice as follows (final concentration): 4.1×10^6 cells/ml, 5 mg/ml bovine fibrinogen (Sigma F4753, stock solution: 200 mg/ml in 0.9% NaCl supplemented with 0.5 µg/mg aprotinin), 3 U/ml bovine thrombin (Sigma T7513, stock solution: 100 U/ml). To ensure isotonic conditions, one additional fibrinogen and thrombin volume of 2x DMEM was added. Ordinary 24-well cell culture plates were used as casting molds. After 1.6 ml of sterile 2% agarose (Invitrogen 15510-027) in PBS was pipetted into each well, the Teflon spacers could be placed. After the agarose was solidified, the Teflon spacers were removed. The silicone posts racks were placed onto the cell culture dish with each pair of silicone posts reaching into one of the preformed casting molds (geometry: 12x3x4 mm). The reconstitution mix was carefully resuspended. For each FBME 100 µl of the mixture was mixed briefly with an appropriate volume of thrombin and pipetted into an agarose slot. To ensure complete polymerization of the fibrinogen, the constructs were placed into a humidified cell culture incubator (37 °C, 7% CO_2, 40% O_2) for 2 hours. Before transferring the silicone posts racks to

a new medium-filled culture plate, every construct was covered with DMEM (300 µl) to ease the removal. FBMEs were maintained in 37 °C, 7% CO_2, 40% O_2 in a humidified cell culture incubator. Media was changed on Mondays, Wednesdays and Fridays. FBME medium consisted of DMEM (Biochrom F0415) supplemented with 10% horse serum (Gibco 26050), 2% chick embryo extract (self-made), 1% penicillin/streptomycin (Gibco 15140), insulin (Sigma I9278, 10 µg/ml) and aprotinin (Sigma A1153, 33 µg/ml).

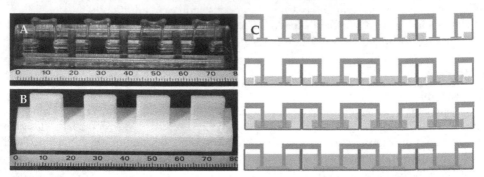

Fig. 1. Illustration of the experimental setup for casting and cultivation and photography of a silicone post rack with four FBMEs. Silicone post rack with four FBMEs (turned upside down, scale in millimetres; A). Teflon spacer for the generation of agarose casting molds (turned upside down, scale in millimetres; B). Illustration of FBME generation (C). First lane: Casting molds are made using Teflon spacers and agarose in a 24-well cell culture dish. Silicone posts racks are placed onto the culture dish, with each pair of posts reaching into a mold. Second lane: Mastermix is pipetted into each mold. Third lane: After 2 h the fibrin is polymerized and the silicone posts are embedded in the hydrogel. FBMEs can be transferred into a new medium-filled 24-well culture plate. Fourth lane: FBMEs are maintained in culture for 15 to 30 days (Hansen et al. 2010).

2.4 Video-optical analyses

The setup for video-optical analyses consisted of a cell culture incubator-like unit, in which gas conditions, humidity and temperature could be controlled. This device was equipped with a glass roof for monitoring purposes. A Basler CCD-camera (Type A 602f-2) was attached to an XYZ-device (IAI Corporation) and positioned above the glassroof in a PC-controlled manner. Light-emitting diodes (LEDs) were placed underneath the cell culture dish. Illumination of a single LED was synchronized with the video-optical recording procedure in order to minimize heating of the cell culture medium by LED waste heat. Figure 2A shows a schematic picture of the whole setup and 2B shows a 24 well cell culture plate with six silicone posts racks and with one FBME in every well (view from above). For the video-optical analyses a customized software package developed by Consulting Team Machine Vision (ctmv.de; Pforzheim, Germany) was used. This software is based on figure recognition and is able to identify the FBME's shape in a fully automated manner. In brief, the system automatically places measuring points at the top and bottom end of the contracting muscle strip. Due to the contraction, the distance in between the moving silicone posts changes. These changes are determined and recorded by the software over time. Based on post geometry, elastic modulus of the Sylgard 184 (2.6 kPa) and the delta value of post distance (post deflection), the developed force was calculated based on a recently published equation (Vandenburgh et al. 2008). The recorded contractions are filtered and identified as such by certain peak criteria (e.g. threshold value, minimal force and minimum relaxation). Besides average force, the software calculates values for frequency, fractional shortening, contraction- and relaxation time (bpm, T1 and T2, respectively) based on the recognized contraction peaks. T1 and T2 were determined at 20% of peak maximum. Reports with an overview of the environmental information (temperature, gas, humidity) in the cell culture like unit plus all calculated parameters are automatically generated after each run. These underlie two levels of quality control: pictures are taken at the beginning and the end of each recording. Blue squares indicate top and bottom end of each respective FBME where the software placed the points for the measurement (Figure 2D). Contractions are recorded as force development over time. Identified peaks, which are included in the calculation, are marked with green squares (Figure 2C). The effort to analyse a 24-well plate with contracting muscle strips is limited to defining the XYZ-coordinates for each well once before starting a series of measurements.

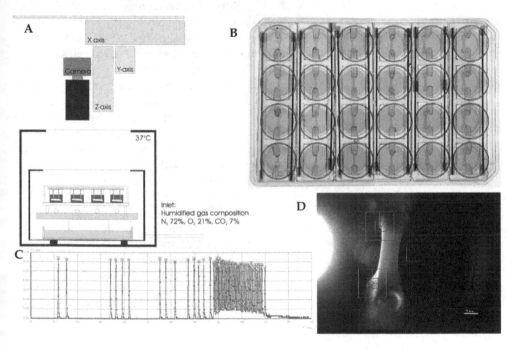

Fig. 2. Illustration of the experimental setup for video-optical recordings of FBME, a 24 well cell culture dish with FBMEs, a magnified view of a single FBME as recorded by the video camera and an example of a contraction pattern (one FBME for 60 s). A shows a schematic picture of the experimental setup for video-optical recordings. In B a 24 well cell culture dish with FBMEs is shown (view from above). The original contraction pattern of one FBME over time (60 s, C). Image of a contractile muscle strip from an automatically generated report (D). Blue squares indicate positions automatically recognized by the software at top and bottom end of the FBME. Green squares mark the recognized contraction peaks which are included for the calculation of several parameters (Hansen et al. 2010).

3. Results

3.1 General aspects of the new technique

We developed a new technique for the generation and evaluation of contractile cardiac tissue from neonatal rat heart cells *in vitro* (Hansen et al. 2010). In this method, isolated heart cells are mixed with fibrinogen, thrombin and medium and pipetted into rectangular casting moulds made from 2%-agarose in ordinary 24-well cell culture plates. Due to the polymerisation of the fibrin, the gel is fixed to both silicone posts. After 2 h at 37 °C the constructs can be transferred to new culture dishes and maintained under cell culture conditions for several days. Figure 1C demonstrates this procedure in a schematic way. During cultivation, the cells inside the gel spread along the force lines and form extensive cell-cell contacts, the hydrogel is remodelled and degraded. These processes are accompanied by marked condensation of the constructs and deflection of the silicone posts towards each other. The initial length of a FBME directly after casting is 8.5 mm and the mean final length 6.5 mm. The post deflection differs between individual FBMEs, likely reflecting their degree of cardiac tissue development. In consequence, each FBME is exposed to an "individually optimized preload". With this simplified method, 48-72 FBMEs can be routinely generated out of one cell preparation (30 rat hearts). Figure 2B illustrates a typical 24 well plate with silicone posts racks and FBMEs. Fibrin is affected by proteases in the culture medium. To decrease degradation, the protease inhibitor aprotinin at a concentration of 33 µg/ml is added to the medium. This inhibitor markedly reduces fibrinolysis but cannot entirely stop it. To further protect the hydrogel from proteolysis tranexamic acid, another protease inhibitor, can be added to the medium. The combination of both inhibitors results in improved stability and allows longer cultivation periods. Tranexamic acid-treated FBMEs have a markedly increased diameter (final width 1.3 to 1.4 mm [Figure 2C and 8D] instead of 0.2 to 1.0 mm in its absence [Figure 4A]).

3.2 Morphology and beating activity

Directly after casting, FBMEs appeared as a soft fibrin-block fixed at the end of the silicone posts and exhibiting the dimensions of the casting moulds (12x3xx mm). Within this clot, the heart cells were round and amorphous but homogeneously distributed throughout the gel (Figure 3A). During the first days after casting, cells spread, elongated along force lines, started to beat as single cells and finally in the form of synchronously beating areas on day 4 to 5. The further development was characterized by matrix remodelling and degradation. This lead to a marked reduction of the size (from 3 mm to 1-2 mm width in the presence and 0.2-1 mm in the absence of tranexamic acid) and increased cell-density. Between day 5 and day 7 the cardiomyocytes formed small groups (Figure 3B through E). Coherent beating of the muscle construct started around day 7 to 9. By day 10 the generated force was sufficient to rhythmically deflect the silicone posts. Measurements were routinely performed between day 14 to 16. At this point the cardiomyocytes finally appeared as spindle-shaped cells with an approximately length of 100 to 200 µm and a diameter of 10 to 20 µm (Figure 3F).

Hematoxylin/eosin-stained paraffin sections of mature FBMEs (day 15) showed a dense network of longitudinally aligned cells throughout the gel (Figure 4A). No clear evidence for cell density gradient from peripheral to central areas of the gel could be found, arguing against a significant inhomogeneity of oxygen and nutrient supply.

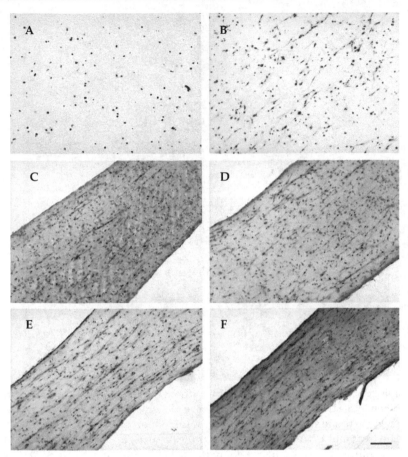

Fig. 3. Histological analysis of FBMEs. FBMEs were cultured with aprotinin plus tranexamic acid. For histological analysis they were fixed with formaldehyde at indicated time points, embedded with paraffin and the sections were HE-stained (10x magnification). A Day 0: cells are present as single, round and amorphous cell suspension in fibrin matrix; B day 3: cells spread out along force lines. C day 6, D day 9: degradation of extracellular matrix, cells spread and align with neighbouring cells. E day 12, F day 15: extended degradation of extracellular matrix, the cellular density is increased; cells align and show orientation along force lines. Scale bar 100 μm (Hansen et al. 2010).

Whole-mount FBMEs were also analysed by immunofluorescent staining. The pictures showed a dense network of regularly cross striated, α-actinin-positive, longitudinally aligned cardiomyocytes. The elongated cells had well developed sarcomeric structures reaching into the periphery of the cytoplasm. Cardiomyocytes were also characterized by connexion-43 positive structures, the gap junctions. In contrast to the *in vivo* situation connexion-positivity was mostly localized on lateral parts of the cell membrane, but not clustered at the border to connecting cells. Moreover, the immunfluorescence showed lectin-positive endothelial cells intermingled with cardiomycytes and forming primitive tube-like structures (Figure 4).

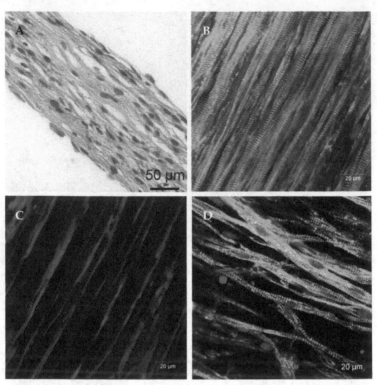

Fig. 4. Histological analysis of FBMEs (day 15, without tranexamic acid). A, HE-stained paraffin section. Note the almost complete absence of extracellular matrix and well-developed cardiac tissue structure. B, Merged immunofluorescence staining for α-actinin (green), lectin (red) and DRAQ5 (blue; 63x magnification). C, Lectin-positive structures alone (63x magnification). D, Connexin-43 (red), phalloidin (green) and DRAQ5 (blue; 63x magnification). Scale bar 50 μm (A) and 20 μM (B-D; Hansen et al. 2010).

3.3 DNA/RNA content, histone H3 phosphorylation and caspase-3 activity

To further investigate cell survival in FBMEs during culture, the histological data were supported by measurements on a molecular biological level. The DNA/RNA content, histone H3 phosphorylation as well as the caspase-3-activity were analysed. The DNA content dropped by 20% between day 0 and day 3. Thereafter it remained stable for at least two weeks (Figure 5A). Investigations of histone H3 phosphorylation as a marker of proliferative activity and caspase-3 activity as a marker for apoptosis in FBMEs were well in line with these observations. Histone H3 phosphorylation level was initially very low and further decreased over time (Figure 5C). Caspase-3 activity was high directly after cell preparation and dropped during culture even below detectable levels (Figure 5D). After an initial drop of the RNA-content during the first three days of 50% it remained, like the DNA content, more or less stable for at least two weeks (Figure 5B). In summary, these data suggest that some of the cells died within the first three days after casting, likely as a consequence of cell damage during the isolation procedure. Thereafter the cell population remained essentially stable in FBMEs.

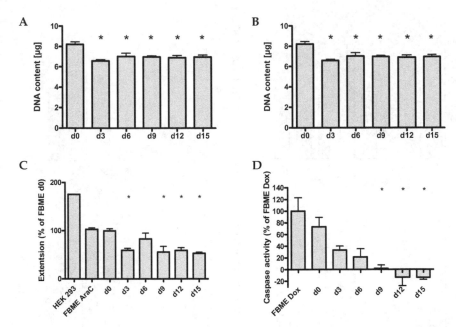

Fig. 5. DNA and total RNA content of FBMEs. A DNA content of FBMEs over time (n=4). B Total RNA content over time (n=4). * p<0.05 vs. d0 (Student's t test). Bars show means +/- SD. C, D Concentration of phosphorylated histone H3 (C) and caspase-3 activity (D) in FBMEs over time of cultivation. Day 0 represents freshly solidified FBMEs 2 h after casting. Proliferating HEK293 cells and AraC-treated FBMEs served as positive and negative controls for proliferation, respectively. Doxorubicin-treated FBMEs served as positive controls for caspase-3 activity. Bars show mean +/-SEM, n=4. * p<0.05 vs. d0 (Student's t test; Hansen et al. 2010).

3.4 Cardiac marker gene expression over time

To get an idea about cardiomyocyte maturation in FBMEs, transcript levels of known cardiac marker genes (α-actinin, SR Ca^{2+}-ATPase [SERCA], α- and β-myosin heavy chain [α-/β-MHC], Na^+/Ca^{2+}-exchanger [NCX], titin) were analysed over time. To avoid bias due to the effect of the drop of overall cell count after preparation, all values were normalized to the mRNA concentration of the cardiac myocyte-specific protein calsequestrin 2. Values were additionally compared to intact adult (ARH) and neonatal rat hearts (NRHT; Figure 6). In the first phase (day 0 to day 6), which represents the time when the single cells spread, formed clusters and started to beat, the transcript levels seemed to be relatively stable. In the second phase (day 9 to day 12) the expression levels reached their maximum concomitantly with the start of rhythmical deflection of the silicone posts by the FBMEs. In the third phase (day 12 to day 15) transcript levels generally decreased. Some cardiac markers (α-actinin, SERCA, α-MHC) reached a comparable level to native myocardium on day 15. Other (β-MHC, titin and NCX) remained several fold higher, indicating higher remodelling activity.

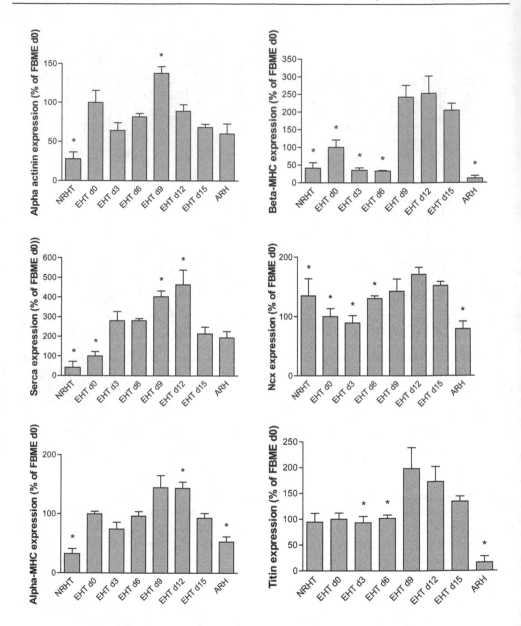

Fig. 6. RT-qPCR of FBMEs in comparison to neonatal (NRHT) and adult rat heart (ART). ΔΔCT values were generated by normalisation to the mRNA of cardiac specific protein calsequestrin 2 (average CT values for normalisation were as follows: d0: 20.8, d3: 20.4, d6: 20.6, d9: 21.3, d12: 21.6, d15: 20.5). Figures show relative expression compared to day 0. Each bar represents results from 4 biological replicates (each measured 3 times). * p<0.05 vs. day 15 (Student's t test). Bars show means +/- SEM (Hansen et al. 2010).

3.5 Non quantitative ion channel expression profile

Ion channels play an important role as targets of proarrhythmic drugs. To determine whether the principal ion channel subunits known from human hearts are expressed in rat FBMEs transcripts of 23 ion channel α-subunits (7 calcium channels, 6 sodium channels, 10 potassium channels) were amplified from total RNA of FBMEs and a nonfailing human heart sample by RT-PCR (35 cycles). 22/23 transcripts were amplified from both sources, one channel (CacnA1I) was neither amplified in FBMEs nor in the nonfailing human heart (Figure 7).

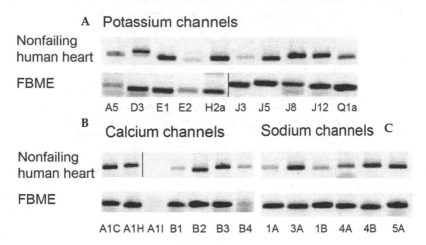

Fig. 7. Agarose gel of the PCR-products of 23 ion channel subunits. The ion channel profile of FBMEs was compared to the expression profile of a nonfailing human heart. Potassium channels (A), calcium channel (B) and sodium channels (C) showed qualitatively similar results (descriptions indicate the related gene for each channel subunit; for further information see table 1; Hansen et al. 2010).

3.6 Robustness and reproducibility of the new method

To determine robustness and reproducibility or the assay, we generated 6 independent series of FBMEs (1-2 24-well plates each, total number 192 FBMEs) and analysed them under standard conditions (culture medium with insulin, aprotinin and tranexamic acid; measurements done by video-optical recordings). Two FBMEs could not be transferred from the casting moulds, 4 FBMEs were not recognized by the software and 17 did not beat during the recording time (60 s) at day 15. Thus, the total success rate was 89% (169/192; Figure 8). Contraction parameters were examined and compared among different series. These results showed that the average force per series (day 15) was between 0.11 and 0.22 mN (series SD 7.6%), the contraction time (T1=time to peak) ranged between 66 and 81 ms (series SD 41%), relaxation time (T2=time to 80% relaxation) between 67 and 88 ms (series SD 25%), frequency between 162 and 20 beats per minute (series SD 109%), construct diameter between 1.3 and 1.4 mm (series SD 9.9%) and length between 5.6 and 6.7 mm (series SD 16.7%). The relatively large size in FBME diameter in these examinations could be attributed to the use of tranexamic acid.

Family	Abbre-viation	Description
KCN	A5	Voltage-gated channel subunit Kv1.5
	D3	Voltage-gated channel subunit Kv4.3
	E1	Potential voltage-gated channel subunit beta (KvLQT1; ERG; function: I_{Ks} or $_{Kr}$)
	E2	Potential voltage-gated channel subunit beta (minK-related peptide 1; KvLQT1; ERG; function: I_{Ks} or I_{Kr})
	H2a	I_{Kr} producing rapid voltage-gated channel subunit beta (ether-a-go-go-related gene (ERG) channel 1)
	J3	G protein-activated inward rectifier channel 1 (Kir3.1)
	J5	G protein-activated inward rectifier channel 4 (Kir3.4)
	J8	ATP-sensitive inward rectifier channel 8 (Kir6.1)
	J12	ATP-sensitive inward rectifier channel 12 (Kir2.2)
	Q1a	I_{Ks} producing slow voltage-gated channel subunit alpha (KvLQT1)
CACN	A1C	Voltage-dependent subunit alpha-1C (L-type)
	A1H	Voltage-dependent subunit alpha-1H (T-type)
	A1I	Voltage-dependent subunit alpha-1I (T-type)
	B1	Voltage-dependent subunit beta-1 (L-type)
	B2	Voltage-dependent subunit beta-2 (L-type)
	B3	Voltage-dependent subunit beta-3 (L-type)
	B4	Voltage-dependent subunit beta-4 (L-type)
SCN	1A	Voltage-gated channel protein type-1 subunit alpha
	3A	Voltage-gated channel protein type-3 subunit alpha
	1B	Voltage-gated channel subunit beta-1
	4A	Voltage-gated channel protein type 4 subunit alpha
	4B	Voltage-gated channel subunit beta-4
	5A	Voltage-gated channel protein type-5 subunit alpha

Table 1. Overview of the analysed ion channels shown in figure 7.

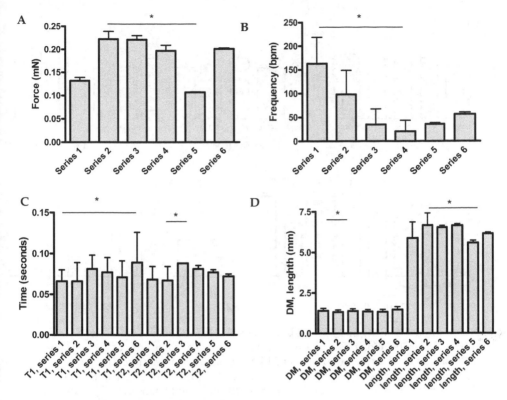

Fig. 8. Reproducibility of the assay. FBMEs were generated at 6 different time points (series 1-6) and spontaneous activity was recorded on day 15. Parameters of contractility (A: force, B: frequency, C: contraction time T1, relaxation time T2) and construct dimensions (D) were averaged and compared. Minimal and maximal values were used to test for significant differences and are indicated with * p<0.05 (Student's t test). Bars show means +/- SD. Analysed FBMEs for each series were: Series 1: n=21, series 2: n=24, series 3: n=20, series 4: n=18, series 5: n=39, series 6: n=47 (Hansen et al. 2010).

3.7 Cardiotoxic and proarrhythmic effects of drugs

To determine whether the new method could be used for the detection of cardiotoxic and proarrhythmic drug effects, well characterized compounds with known cardiotoxic and repolarization-inhibitory effects were tested. The cardiotoxic drug doxorubicin was applied in different concentrations (0.1-1.000 nmol/L) for up to 96 h. Doxorubicin-treated FBMEs showed time- and concentration-dependent changes in contractile force. Very low concentrations of doxorubicin (1-10 nmol/L) led to a trend towards an increase in contractile force, 100 nmol/L induced a transient increase in contractile force after 24 h which was followed by a decrease at 72 and 96 h (Figure 9). In the presence of 1 μmol/L doxorubicin all FBMEs stopped to beat after 3 days.

To examine a repolarization-inhibitory effect on FBMEs, the experimental I_{Ks}-blocker chromanol 293B as well as the clinically used drugs quinidine and erythromycin were

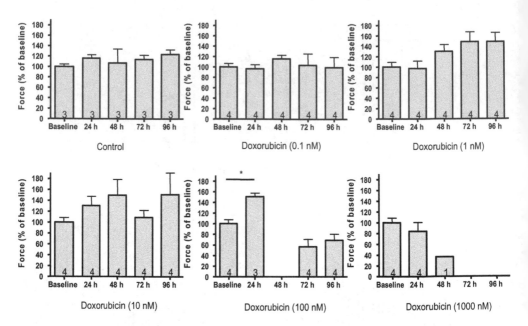

Fig. 9. Doxorubicin toxicity on FBMEs. FBMEs were incubated in the presence of doxorubicin (0.1-1000 nM, starting at day 13 of culture), average forces were determined daily. While doxorubicin at 0.1 μM increased force after 24 hours, higher concentrations (1 μM) lead to a time-dependent reduction in force development. * p<0.05 (Student's t test). Bars show means ⁻ +/- SEM, number of evaluated (beating) constructs as indicated (Hansen et al. 2010).

tested. All three compounds induced a concentration-dependent delay in relaxation time (T2; Figure 10). In the presence of chromanol 293B, FBMEs already showed a prolongation of T2 at a concentration of 1 μmol/L. At 100 μmol/L chromanol, T2 was 7-fold longer than control, resulting in a "church-like" configuration of the twith (Figure 10). Quinidine and erythromycin, both associated with arrhythmias in clinical applications, also extended the relaxation time at high concentrations (100 μmol/L). Time of contraction was not affected by any of the compounds.

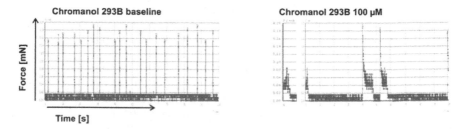

Fig. 10. Chromanol 293B-induced "church-like" contraction pattern. Cutout of the original contraction recordings in the presence and absence of Chromanol 293B (100 μM; modified from: Hansen et al. 2010).

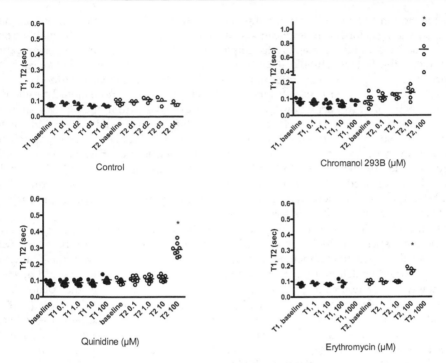

Fig. 11. Effect of repolarisation inhibitors on FBME contraction (T1) and relaxation time (T2). FBMEs were incubated with increasing concentrations of the indicated compounds (1-2 h) and evaluated before application of drug (baseline) and after each concentration. Note the absence of effect of all compounds on T1 and the concentration-dependent increase in T2 with chromanol, quinidine and erythromycin (at 1000 µM of erythromycin FBMEs discontinued contractile activity). A typical alteration of contraction peak morphology with increasing concentrations of quinidine, chromanol and erythromycin is shown in supplementary figure 5. * p<0.05 (Student's t test). Bars show means +/- SEM, each spot represents one analysed FBME (Hansen et al. 2010).

4. Conclusion

In this book chapter we describe a recently developed method (Hansen et al. 2010) to generate miniaturized, fibrin-based EHTs (FBMEs) in a 24-well format and determine their contractile activity in an automated manner. This technique turned out to be robust and highly reproducible. Its main advantages are its simplicity in terms of handling, the standard 24-well format, its robustness and the high content automated readout of contractile activity. Compared to previously EHT-protocols (Eschenhagen et al. 1997, Zimmermann et al. 2002), three major changes were introduced. (i) Collagen I was replaced by fibrinogen and thrombin. Due to the fast fibrin-polymerisation, the heart cells were homogenously distributed throughout the entire hydrogel. Polymerisation occurs in minutes and allows transfer of the constructs from the casting moulds to a new medium-filled culture dish after two hours. Moreover, fast solidification allowed 50% higher cell concentration (0.6x10[6]/150 µl versus 2.5x10[6]/900 µl), because it prevents accumulation of cells at the bottom of the casting moulds with detrimental consequences. Fibrin has additional advantages for future applications, such as transplantations. It is available from autologoues sources and has the ability to couple covalently growth-promoting, angiogenic or other interesting factors (Hubble 2003). (ii) The original ring-format was changed to a stripe-format. This step was very important because it allowed miniaturization (volume reduced from 900 to 150 µl), the use of standard 24-well plates and automation. The silicone racks with 4 pairs of posts each allow simple transfer of FBMEs from one plate to another and thus reduce the number of nonstandardized handling steps to a minimum. Moreover, the silicone posts subject the growing muscle construct to an individually optimized preload and allow them to perform contractile work against the elastic properties of the post. (iii) Video-optical measurements of contractile parameters further improved the whole technique. They superseded the manual transfer for measurements as it was required in former EHT-protocols. Additionally, video-optical recordings allowed simple, reproducible, standardized measurements of large series in a short spell.

The new stripe-format was inspired by a previously described method for generating skeletal muscle tissues (Vandenburgh et al. 2008). Turning the silicone posts up side down was the major difference to this method and simplified handling. In this way the quality of the constructs could be determine with an ordinary microscope or even by eye and opened the possibility for automated video-optical recordings from above the plate. This experimental setup, in combination with fibrin, has several important features. (i) It is simple and not longer addicted to some kind of special dish because standard 24-well cell culture plates can be used. In the beginning silicone posts racks were self-made, which turned out to relevantly limit reproducibility. We therefore have the racks industrial made now, which makes the method robust and highly reproducible (Figure 8). (ii) FBMEs exhibit an excellent cardiac tissue development (Figure 4). Several factors are likely to contribute to these beneficial effects. As outlined above, the fast polymerisation of fibrin allowed higher cell concentrations and lead to homogenous cell distribution throughout the hydrogel. Another reason was that cell survival appeared very high in the current fibrin-based format. Moreover, proliferative activity (of non-myocytes) was very low (Figure 5), making the system stable over prolonged periods. The stable mRNA expression pattern of cardiac markers (α-actinin, α-MHC, titin, calsequestrin 2 and SERCA) may be an additional hint for a relatively stable system. Interestingly, the fetal gene marker β-MHC showed a several fold decrease within in the first six days. This phase was associated with cell spreading and contractions on a cellular level. Later, between day 6 and day 9 there was a ~5-fold increase of the β-MHC mRNA expression, coinciding with the beginning of macroscopic contractions. A third positive effect of the described new technique is the optimized mechanical load on the cardiomyocytes. The mechanical load is produced by the resistance of the silicon posts and adapted individually for each FBME. If the tonic (diastolic force) of the construct is high, post deflection by the FBMEs is stronger and *vice versa*. Furthermore, the FBMEs can perform contractile work against an elastic resistance. These circumstances mimic in some ways the *in vivo* situation in which the beating heart needs to work against the afterload induced by the total peripheric resistance. This kind of optimized "auxotonic" load in contrast to motorized phasic stretch improves tissue development as shown earlier in other EHT-studies (Zimmermann et al. 2006).

Regarding the development of a drug screening, miniaturization, reduction of nonstandardized steps during the procedure and an automated, objective readout were very important. The miniaturization to a 24-well format reduced the cell number by a factor of

~4. Additionally, pilot experiments could show that a further miniaturization to a 96-well format would be possible. At this point the 24-well format turned out to be a good compromise between miniaturization and ease of handling. FBMEs do not longer need to be manually transferred as single tissues because the entire silicon racks were handled. In contrast to that, circular EHTs needed to be manually transferred from the casting mould to a motorized stretcher and finally from the stretcher to the organ bath for the measurements. Compared to this method, the video-optical recordings were simple and robust. To confirm the calculated forces, isometric measurements were exemplarily done in the organ bath in parallel and showed that the calculated forces were roughly in the range of the measured ones (0.3 vs. 0.9 mN). The threefold difference could indicate a systematic error, but more likely reflects optimized conditions in the organ bath (preload optimization, electrical pacing and isometric versus auxotonic contraction). A force of 0.9 mN (organ bath) and a diameter of 0.2 mm (Figure 4A; without tranexamic acid) results in a relative force development of 28.7 mN/mm^2. This is still lower than values in an intact muscle (50 mN/mm^2), but point in the right direction. The development of a software which works by automated figure recognition was important in two aspects. On the one hand, it is time-saving since it calculates all important contractile parameters automatically. On the other hand, it provides an objective readout.

Initial experiments to determine the suitability of FBMEs to detect either cardiotoxic or proarrhythmic effects looked promising. The known cardiotoxic drug doxorubicin suppressed contractile activity at the highest concentration (1.000 nmol/L) and increased force at lower concentrations (100 nmol/L) and earlier time points (24 h). This may be due to the reactive oxygen species-generating effect of this compound, which at later time points and/or higher concentrations turned into toxicity.

Three known proarrhythmic drugs caused a concentration-dependent prolongation of relaxation time in FBMEs. Chromanol 293B is an experimental I_{Ks}-blocker with an IC_{50}-value of 8 µmol/L in H9c2 cells (Lo et al. 2005). A concentration of 100 µmol/L was needed to fully block I_{Ks} in these cells. This correspond well to the relaxation-prolonging effect in FBMEs, which was visible at 10 µmol/L and marked at 100 µmol/L (Figure 10) matching quite well the published data (Lo et al. 2005). Quinidine, known as a class IA antiarrhythmic drug according to Vaughan-Williams classification (Vaughan-Williams 1975), also blocks I_{Ks} and I_{Kr} with EC_{50} values of 10 µmol/L and 300 nmol/L, respectively (Lo et al. 2005; Redfern et al. 2003). In FBMEs, quinidine prolonged relaxation time at 100 µmol/L. This is not an entirely different range in comparison with the determined IC_{50} for quinidine on I_{Ks} but far away from I_{Kr}-IC_{50}. This argues again for the role of I_{Ks} in FBME-repolarisation. Erythromycin, a clinically used antibiotic, which is associated with *Torsades-de-Pointes* arrhythmias and increased lethality in men (Ray et al. 2004), inhibits I_{Kr} but not I_{Ks} in dogs (Antzelevitch et al. 1996) and increases action potential duration in rat ventricular cardiomyocytes (IC_{50} 60 µmol/L; Hanada et al. 2003). In FBMEs erythromycin caused an increase in relaxation time at concentrations of 100 µmol/L and above. Even though the channel subunits for both I_{Kr} and I_{Ks} are expressed on mRNA-level in FBMEs (Figure 7), their role in repolarisation of rat cardiomyocytes is still controversial (Regan et al. 2005). In any case, the observation that the prototype proarrhythmic drugs specifically affected relaxation time in FBMEs indicates that this parameter may be useful as a surrogate of repolarisation. However, the detailed mechanisms behind the cardiotoxic and proarrhythmic effects are still unclear and need to be further investigated in follow up studies.

The presented technique still has a number of important limitations with regard to drug screening. (i) The cell preparation cannot be fully standardized. In particular, the age of newborn rats varies from 0-3 days and has significant impact of the quality of FBMEs, most likely explaining part of the variability between series (Figure 6). (ii) The system is not well suited to determine acute positive or negative inotropic effects because measurements are done under spontaneous beating, leading to confounding effects of concomitant negative or positive chronotropic effects. We are working on a system which allows measurements to be done under continuous pacing. (iii) Histological observations showed spindle-shaped cardiomyocytes and a predominantly lateral orientation of connexion-43-postive gap junctions. This suggests that cardiomyocytes, despite functional, molecular and morphological indices of advanced maturation, do not reach an adult phenotype. (iv) Our assay system exclusively monitors alterations in contractile activity and does not directly determine calcium transients or action potential duration. We believe that relaxation time is a good surrogate parameter of action potential, but the direct proof is still lacking. (v) Finally, rodents are known to be poor models for detecting proarrhythmic drug effects because mechanisms governing their action potential differ considerably from that in humans. For example, I_{Kr} plays a relatively minor role in rodents, but a major one in humans (Regan et al. 2005). Our present results suggest that proarrhythmic drug effects can still be monitored in this system, but much more work is necessary to determine which ion channel or combination of ion channels have to be blocked to see changes in relaxation time and/or arrhythmias in FBMEs.

Thus, validation of the new system will require testing of a large number of drugs that are known to cause cardiac arrhythmias in humans and those that are known to be free of arrhythmic side effects, including those that have effects on HERG but are not associated with *Torsades-de-Pointes* arrhythmias. Moreover, a number of randomly chosen new chemical entities should be analysed to obtain an estimate how many non selected compounds give a signal. These studies are currently under way.

5. References

Antzelevitch, C.; Sun, Z. Q.; Zhang, Z. Q. & Yan, G. X (1996). Cellular and ionic mechanisms underlying erythromycin-induced long QT intervals and torsade de pointes. *Journal of the American College of Cardiology*; 28:1836-48

Bian, W.; Liau, B.; Badie, N. & Bursac, N. (2009). Mesoscopic hydrogel molding to control the 3D geometry of bioartificial muscle tissues. *Nature Protocols*; 4:1522-34

Carrier, R. L.; Papadaki, M.; Rupnick, M.; Schoen, F.J.; Bursac, N.; Langer, R.; Freed, L. E. & Vunjak-Novakovic, G. (1999). Cardiac tissue engineering: cell seeding, cultivation parameters, and tissue construct characterization. *Biotechnology Bioengineerening*; 64:580–589

El-Armouche A, Singh J, Naito H, Wittköpper K, Didié M, Laatsch A, Zimmermann WH, Eschenhagen T. (2007). Adenovirus-delivered short hairpin RNA targeting PKCalpha improves contractile function in reconstituted heart tissue. *Journal of Molecular Cell Cardiology*; 43:371-6

Engelmayr, G. C. Jr; Cheng, M.; Bettinger C. J.; Borenstein J.T.; Langer, R. & Freed L. E. (2008). Accordion-like honeycombs for tissue engineering of cardiac anisotropy. *Nature Materials.*; 7:1003–1010

Eschenhagen, T.; Fink, C.; Remmers, U.; Scholz, H.; Wattchow, J.; Weil J.; Zimmermann, W.; Dohmen, H. H.; Schafer, H.; Bishopric, N.; Wakatsuki, T. & Elson, E. L. (1997). Three-dimensional reconstitution of embryonic cardiac myocytes in a collagen matrix: a new heart muscle model system. *The FASEB Journal*; 11:683–694

Eschenhagen, T. & Zimmermann, W.H. (2005). Engineering myocardial tissue. *Circulation Research.*; 97:1220-31

Fink, C.; Ergün, S.; Kralisch, D.; Remmers, U.; Weil, J. & Eschenhagen, T. (2000). Chronic stretch of engineered heart tissue induces hypertrophy and functional improvement. *The FASEB Journal*; 14:669-79

Hanada, E.; Ohtani, H.; Hirota, M.; Uemura, N.; Nakaya, H.; Kotaki, H.; Sato, H.; Yamada, Y. & Iga, T. (2003). Inhibitory effect of erythromycin on potassium currents in rat ventricular myocytes in comparison with disopyramide. *The Journal of Pharmacy and Pharmacology*; 55:995-1002

Hansen, A.; Eder, A.; Bönstrup, B.; Flato, M.; Mewe, M.; Schaaf, S.; Aksehirlioglu, B.; Schwörer, A.; Uebeler, J. & Eschenhagen T. (2010). Development of a drug screening platform based on engineered heart tissue. *Circulation Research*; 107(1):35-44.

Huang, Y.C.; Khait, L. & Birla, R. K. (2007). Contractile three-dimensional bioengineered heart muscle for myocardial regeneration. *Journal of Biomedical Material Research Part A*; 80:719–731

Hubbell, J. A. (2003). Materials as morphogenetic guides in tissue engineering. *Current Opinion in Biotechnology*; 14:551-8

Janmey, P. A.; Winer, J. P. & Weisel, J.W. (2009). Fibrin gels and their clinical and bioengineering applications. *Journal of the Royal Society Interface*; 6:1-10

Kehat, I.; Kenyagin-Karsenti, D.; Snir, M.; Segev, H.; Amit, M.; Gepstein, A.; Livne, E.; Binah, O.; Itskovitz-Eldor, J. & Gepstein, L. (2001). Human embryonic stem cells can differentiate into myocytes with structural and functional properties of cardiomyocytes. *Journal of Clinical Investigation*; 108:407-14

Lasser, K. E.; Allen, P. D.; Woolhandler, S. J.; Himmelstein, D. U.; Wolfe, S. M. & Bohr D. H. (2002). Timing of new black box warnings and withdrawals for prescription medications. *JAMA*; 287(17):2215-20

Leor, J.; Aboulafia-Etzion, S.; Dar, A.; Shapiro, L.; Barbash, I. M.; Battler, A.; Granot, Y. & Cohen, S. (2000). Bioengineered cardiac grafts a new approach to repair the infarcted myocardium? *Circulation*; 102:III56–IIII61

Li, R. K.; Yau, T. M.; Weisel, R. D.; Mickle, D. A.; Sakai, T.; Choi, A. & Jia, Z. Q. (2000). Construction of a bioengineered cardiac graft. *Journal of Thoracic and Cardiovascular Surg*ery;119:368–375

Lo, Y. C.; Yang, S. R.; Huang, M.H.; Liu, Y. C. & Wu, S. N. (2005). Characterization of chromanol 293B-induced block of the delayed-rectifier K+ current in heart-derived H9c2 cells. *Life Sciences*;76:2275-2286

Naito, H.; Melnychenko, I.; Didie, M.; Schneiderbanger, K.; Schubert, P.; Rosenkranz, S.; Eschenhagen, T. & Zimmermann, W. H. (2006). Optimizing engineered heart tissue for therapeutic applications as surrogate heart muscle. *Circulation*; 114:I72–I78

Ott, H.C.; Matthiesen, T. S.; Goh, S. K.; Black, L. D.; Kren, S. M.; Netoff, T. I. & Taylor, D. A. (2008). Perfusion-decellularized matrix: using nature's platform to engineer a bioartificial heart. *Nature Medicine*; 14:213–221

Radisic, M.; Park, H.; Shing, H.; Consi, T.; Schoen, F. J.; Langer, R.; Freed, L. E. & Vunjak-Novakovic, G. (2004). Functional assembly of engineered myocardium by electrical stimulation of cardiac myocytes cultured on scaffolds. *PNAS*; 101:18129–18134

Ray, W. A.; Murray, K. T.; Meredith, S.; Narasimhulu, S. S.; Hall K. & Stein C. M. (2004). Oral erythromycin and the risk of sudden death from cardiac causes. *The New England Journal of Medicine*; 351(11):1089-96

Redfern, W. S.; Carlsson, L.; Davis, A. S.; Lynch, W. G.; MacKenzie I.;Palethorpe, S.; Siegl, P. K.; Strang, I.; Sullivan, A. T.; Wallis, R.; Camm, A. J. & Hammond, T. G. (2003). Relationship between preclinical cardiac electrophysiology, clinical QT interval prolongation and torsade de pointes for a broad range of drugs: evidence for a provisional safety margin in drug development. *Cardiovascular Research*; 58(1):32-45.

Regan, C. P.; Cresswell, H. K.; Zhang, R. & Lynch J. J. (2005). Novel method to assess cardiac electrophysiology in the rat. *Journal of Cardiovascular Pharmacology*; 46(1):68-75.

Shimizu, T.; Yamato, M.; Isoi, Y.; Akutsu, T.; Setomaru, T.; Abe, K.; Kikuchi, A.; Umezu, M. & Okano, T. (2002). Fabrication of pulsatile cardiac tissue grafts using a novel 3-dimensional cell sheet manipulation technique and temperature-responsive cell culture surfaces. *Circulation Research*; 90:e40

Vandenburgh, H.; Shansky, J.; Benesch-Lee, F.; Barbata, V.; Reid, J.; Thorrez, L.; Valentini, R. & Crawford, G. (2008). Drug-screening platform based on the contractility of tissue-engineered muscle. *Muscle Nerve*; 37:438-447

Vaughan-Williams E., M. (1975). Classificationof antidysrhythmic drugs. Pharmacology & therapeutics; 1(1):115-38.

Zhang, J.; Wilson, G. F.; Soerens, A. G.; Koonce, C. H.; Yu, J.; Palecek S. P.; Thomson J. A. & Kamp, T. J. (2009). Functional cardiomyocytes derived from human induced pluripotent stem cells. *Circulation Research*; 104:e30-41

Zimmermann, W. H.; Schneiderbanger, K.; Schubert, P.; Didie, M.; Munzel, F.; Heubach, J. F.; Kostin, S.; Neuhuber, W. L. & Eschenhagen, T. (2002). Tissue engineering of a differentiated cardiac muscle construct. *Circulation Research*; 90:223–230

Zimmermann, W. H.; Melnychenko, I.; Wasmeier, G.; Didié, M.; Naito, H.; Nixdorff, U.; Hess, A.; Budinsky, L.; Brune, K.; Michaelis, B.; Dhein, S.; Schwoerer, A.; Ehmke, H. & Eschenhagen, T. (2006). Engineered heart tissue grafts improve systolic and diastolic function in infarcted rat hearts. *Nature Medicine*; 12:452-8

Zimmermann, W. H. & Eschenhagen, T. (2007). Embryonic stem cells for cardiac muscle engineering. *Trends in Cardiovascular Medicine*; 17:134-40

4

Experimental and Computational Methods Pertaining to Surface Tension of Pharmaceuticals

Abolghasem Jouyban[1] and Anahita Fathi-Azarbayjani[2]
*[1]Drug Applied Research Center and Faculty of Pharmacy,
Tabriz University of Medical Sciences, Tabriz,
[2]Faculty of Medicine, Urmia University of Medical Sciences, Urmia,
Iran*

1. Introduction

The molecules of a fluid experiences attractive forces exerted on it by all its neighboring molecules. In the bulk of the liquid, molecules are attracted equally in all directions resulting in a net force of zero. Molecules at or near the surface experience attractive force which tends to pull them to the interior. Surface chemistry deals with thermodynamic and kinetic parameters that take place between two different coexisting phases at equilibrium. Surface tension, γ is free energy of the surface at any air/fluid interface defined as force per unit length or energy per unit area. The latter term, also called surface energy, is more useful in thermodynamics and it applies to solids as well as liquid surfaces. The surface free energy of a liquid is measured by its surface tension and the surface free energy of a solid can be revealed by contact angle measurements. The surface tension measurement depends very markedly upon the presence of impurities in the liquid, temperature and pressure changes (Buckton, 1988).

Surface tension is a phenomenon that we see in our everyday life. Human biological fluids, e.g. serum, urine, gastric juice, amniotic liquid, cerebrospinal and alveolar lining liquid contain numerous low-and high-molecular weight surfactants, proteins and lipids that adsorb at liquid interface. The physicochemical processes that take place in these interfaces are extremely important for the vital function of body organs and have a great impact on pharmacodynamic parameters of drug molecules (Kazakov et al., 2000; Trukhin et al., 2001). Drug substances are usually administered as part of a formulation in combination with excipients that have varied and specialized pharmaceutical functions. The design of drug formulation is based on the principles of pharmacokinetic, biopharmaceutic and pharmaceutical technology. The pharmaceutical industry has directed its attention mainly to the quality and processability of active pharmaceutical products which is reflected in various physicochemical parameters. The drug and pharmaceutical materials require extensive characterization and testing of their stability, physico-chemical properties, effectiveness, palatability and ease of administration to ensure drug efficacy. Among the important characteristics are the drug dissolution and solubility in gastrointestinal tract, intestinal absorption, drug distribution and drug-plasma protein binding. By applying special surface treatments such as contact angle and surface tension measurements to pharmaceutical compounds, drug distribution, dissolution behavior and release pattern in various body fluids can be improved (Hancock et al., 1997; Ho et al., 2010).

Surface tension can influence the development, prediction and performance of pharmaceutical products and help to solve industrial problems and improve products quality. Due to the importance of this phenomenon in drug formulations, there is a growing need for specific interfacial consideration that can be used routinely to solve pharmaceutical problems and improve product quality and stability. In order to meet challenges and develop new and better performing pharmaceutical products, knowledge of surface tension and its measurements techniques is of utmost importance. Amongst many techniques used for characterizing the surface energies of pharmaceuticals are the surface tension measurements, contact angle and wettability tests (Buckton, 1988; Chamarthy et al., 2009; Puri et al., 2010). The objective of this chapter is to introduce experimental and computational methods of surface tension measurment in the pharmaceutical industry.

2. Standard methods and instrumentations of surface tension measurement

Surface tension is a very complicated property of a liquid and it depends upon many variables such as temperature, composition of the solution, measurement time, materials of the apparatus and viscosity of the liquid. When a new surface is being formed, surface active chemicals diffuse to the surface and align. During this process, the surface tension is changing rapidly and continuously. Dynamic surface tension measurements allows track of these changes. When the process reaches equilibrium, static surface tension is obtained by measuring the maximum force at a liquid/gas interface on a sample where the net forces on the line is zero during the test time. Pure fluids and solvents have a single surface tension value and are measured with these devices (Drelich et al. 2002, Thiessen and Man, 1999).

There are a number of commonly available methods for measuring surface tension of liquids. Each has its advantages and limitations. The choice of a method depends on the nature of system to be studied and its stability, the degree of accuracy required, the condition under which its tension is to be measured and possibly on the ability of the instrument to automate the measurements. Realistically the surface tension values of a liquid will vary depending upon the method used (Thiessen and Man, 1999). The following section describes the most used methods for measuring static and dynamic surface and interfacial tension of liquid mixtures as well as semi solids and solids (a summary of the methods is shown in Table 1).

2.1 Wilhelmy plate method

The Wilhelmy plate consists of a thin glass, platinum plate or pre-wetted paper, usually on the order of a few centimeters square, attached to an electrobalance via thin metal wire and is used to measure equilibrium interfacial tension at an air-liquid or liquid-liquid interface (Figure 1). The metal plate must be cleaned from organic contaminants or test solutions, therefore the plate is flamed before the experiment to avoid contamination and to help maintain good wetting of the plate by the test liquid. The plate is then immersed and retracted into and out of the test solution contained in a beaker on a mechanical stage. During these cycles the force acting on the plate vs. depth of immersion are recorded. The meniscus formed at the solid–liquid interface is characterized by the contact angle. Two contact angles are measured, an advancing contact angle and a receding contact angle and the surface tension is calculated from the resulting force. The wetting force is monitored with time and this method is specially suited to check static surface tension value which in some cases is more than 4 h, hence the measurements are assumed to represent equilibrium. The main drawback of this method is that the surface age (time taken from surface formation till measurement) is not taken into account. When working with viscous liquids it takes time for a viscous material to flow from the dipped portion of the plate. Thus the surface tension will decrease initially till it reaches a pleatue once the excess liquid has flowed from the plate, therefore this method is not suited for highly viscous solutions (Avranas and Taspoulos, 2000; Krishnan et al., 2005; Santos and Castanho, 2004). The static wetting force on the plate is used to calculate the static surface tension (γ) using the Wilhelmy equation:

$$\gamma = \frac{F}{l.\cos\theta} \tag{1}$$

where F is the difference in wetting force upon immersion and withdrawal in mN/m, l is the wetted perimeter of the Wilhelmy plate and θ is the advancing or receding contact angle between the liquid phase and the plate. The contact angle θ of most liquids against platinum plate or clean glass is often assumed to be zero. This method does not require other correction factors such as fluid density. This method can be used to measure the contact angle and wetting properties of solid surfaces, where the platinum ring plate is replaced by the test surface (Avranas and Tasopoulos, 2000; Krishnan et al., 2005; Santos and Castanho, 2004; Sipahi, 2001; Tan et al., 2005).

The static contact angle, θ, is an important parameter in many industries including pharmaceutics. Contact angle measurements span every pharmaceutical field, from fluid dynamic to powder and tablet (Muster and Prestidge, 2002), adhesion and spray-drying of various drug delivery systems (Millqvist-Fureby et al., 1999) to the detection of impurities in the solutions of surface active compounds (Al-Maaieh and Aburub, 2007). It is of particular interest in powders, because the formulations are dependent on the contact angle. Contact angle measurements can be performed using various methods including Wilhelmy plate method, capillary rise method, goniometer and sessile drop method (Dingles and Harris, 2005). Among the interfacial tensiometry methods, the Wilhelmy plate method has been extensively developed and used by scientists in the pharmaceutical industry. The equipment used in this method is commercially available at several companies. With this technique it is possible to measure and control interfacial properties in granulation and tabletting, (Dreu et al., 2005) polymeric surfactants, emulsions and foams, protein-phospholipid interaction (Oritz et al., 2003), interfacial tension of topical skin formulations (Vejnovic et al., 2010), bioadhesive forces between mucosal tissue and microsphere drug delivery system (Vasir et al., 2003).

2.2 Du Noüy ring method

Du Noüy ring method is a traditional method used to measure static surface or interfacial tension. The measurement simply requires the ring to be wetted by the liquid and then pulled through the interface while measuring the force exerted on the ring (see Figure 1). Wetting properties of the surface or interface have little influence on this measuring technique. As in the case of Wilhelmy plate, the ring, with a diameter of 2-3 cm, is usually made up of platinum or iridium is submerged into liquid and then pulled through the liquid-air interface. Maximum pull exerted on the ring by the surface is measured which is directly proportional to the surface tension value at equilibrium (Bodour and Miller-Maier, 1998). The ring is submerged into the solution and then slowly pulled through the liquid-air interface to detach from the interface with a force that is correlated to the surface tension. With this method, it is possible to measure the interfacial tension at both liquid-air and liquid-liquid interfaces. Surface tension can be calculated using the equation below:

$$\gamma = \frac{F}{p \cos \theta} f \qquad (2)$$

where p is the perimeter of the three-phase contact line, f is the correction factor (because additional volume of liquid is lifted during the detachment of the ring from the interface) between each measurement. The platinum wire ring was rinsed three times with water, later with acetone as was blow dried (Drelich et al., 2002).

One major difference between the Du Noüy ring method and Wilhelmy's plate is the way in which the surface tension measurement is carried out. The ring moves through the interface whereas the plate is static at the interface, therefore there is no disturbance at the interface and this method is the recommended geometry for studying time dependent characteristics. Both ring and plate geometries can be used with the force balance type of tensiometer. A single instrument is normally capable of performing either Wilherlmy plate or du Noüy ring measurements (Thiessen and Man, 1999).

The surface tension measured by du Noüy method has been utilized in pharmaceutical research, for example, in the measurement of emulsion stability (Ishii et al., 1988; Takamura et al., 1984) and development of a dissolution media to simulate the physiological environment of the gastric region (Luner et al., 2001). This method can be used for characterization of pharmaceutical formulations such as plasticizer and polymer coating and surface tension calculation of various surfactant solutions and their CMC values (Palma et al., 2002) at the point of intersection of the interfacial tension value versus surfactant concentration plot (de la Maza, 1998; Korhonen et al., 2004; Zelkó et al., 2002).

2.3 Maximum bubble pressure method

The maximum bubble pressure method involves flow of a gas bubble (typically air or nitrogen) at a constant rate and blows them through a capillary with a known diameter which is submerged in the sample liquid. The pressure inside of the gas bubble increases until the bubble becomes hemispherical and its radius corresponds to the radius of the capillary. Beyond this the bubble is unstable and grows explosively until it detaches itself from the capillary and a new bubble is formed. The method is based on the continuous measurement of the applied pressure versus bubble rate formed at the end of the capillary. Figure 1 shows each step of bubble formation and corresponding change of bubble radius. The dynamic surface tension can be directly calculated by Young-LaPlace equation:

$$\gamma = \frac{\Delta P_{max} R}{2} \qquad (3)$$

where ΔP_{max} is the maximum pressure difference and R is the capillary radius (Drelich et al., 2002; Hallowell and Hirt, 1994; Fainerman et al., 2006). This method is one of the most popular techniques to measure the dynamic surface tension of various surfactants around and above their CMC value where adsorption is rapid (Christov et al., 2006). In the maximum bubble pressure method, a single interfacial tension value is drawn from each bubble formed. This device is the only available method capable of measuring surface tension in milliseconds time range. This method is particularly useful in measuring surface tension of highly concentrated surfactant solutions (Mischuk et al., 2000) and molten metals (Drelich et al., 2002).

2.4 Drop volume/weight method

Among the conventional methods of surface tension measurement, drop shape techniques have proven to be reliable and easy to handle. This method weighs the mass of the liquid drop or the volume of the drop that falls off a capillary tip of known diameter when pumped very slowly. The weight of the drop falling off the capillary correlates with the interfacial tension and is measured by balancing it against a known gravitational force through the following equation:

$$W = V\Delta\rho g = 2\pi r f \tag{4}$$

where $\Delta\rho$ is the difference in the density of the heavy phase and the light phase, g is the gravitational constant (g=9.81652 m/s^2), r is the radius of the capillary tip and f denotes the empirical drop correction factor introduced by Harkins and Brown. The correction factor is required because only a portion of the drop falls from the capillary tip during detachment and this corrects the deviation of the drop volume from its ideal value (Drelich et al., 2002; Gunde et al., 2001). Impurity of active pharmaceutical solutions (Al-Maaieh and Aburub 2007), emulsion stability (Rangsansarid and Fukada, 2007), potency of local anesthetics (Matsuki et al., 1998), stability of biphasic aqueous systems (Mishima et al., 1998) and surface active properties of drugs (Deo et al., 2004) have been evaluated using this technique.

2.5 Pendant drop method

Most of surface tension measurement techniques have limitations and only a few are suitable for protein solutions and high viscous solutions such as polymers blends. As discussed earlier, the Wilhelmy plate technique requires the establishment of a zero contact angle of the liquid at the plate which is difficult to guarantee with systems involving protein solutions and polymeric solutions with high viscosity. Du Noüy ring method, the drop volume technique or the maximum bubble method also lack dynamic control (Chen et al., 1999). In general, the equilibrium static methods such as sessile drop, spinning drop or a pendant drop method are most commonly used for measuring surface tension of molten metals and viscous solutions (Arashiro and Demarquette, 1999).

The pendent drop technique is capable of producing highly accurate static as well as dynamic interfacial tensions and contact angle measurements. This method is mostly used for the surface tension measurements of metals, alloys and polymers. In this method geometry of the drop is analyzed optically. The increased accuracy and simplicity of this ground based method allow ultra low surface tension, temperature and time dependence of interfacial tension as well as surface tension measurements at elevated pressures (Chen et al., 1999).

A typical pendant drop apparatus (see Figure 1) consists of three parts:

1. An experimental compartment, which includes a microsyringe to produce a pendent drop of a solution at the tip of a capillary, to measure the maximum volume of the drop at reservoir conditions (pressure and temperature).
2. A viewing system to visualize the drop; this part consist of an accurate video system and magnification factor for the image in both the x and y direction.
3. A data acquisition system to compute the surface tension from the digital image of the pendant drop (via Laplace's equation).

The accuracy of the surface tension measurements is highly dependent on the imaging system. Images of the drop can be captured automatically at certain frequencies over a period of several hours depending on the time duration of the test. These digitized pendant drop images can be stored on the computer to calculate the surface tension values as a function of the length of time (Arashiro and Demarquette, 1999; Gunde et al., 2001; Semmler and Kohler, 1999).

This method involves the determination of the profile of a drop of one liquid suspended in another liquid at mechanical equilibrium. This is done by the balance between gravity and surface forces. The equation of Bashforth and Adams which is based on Laplace's equation relates the drop profile to the interfacial tension. This is the most widely used method to date which is given below:

$$\gamma = \frac{\Delta\rho g D_e^2}{H} \tag{5}$$

where g is gravitational constant, $\Delta\rho$ is the difference in densities between tile drop and its surroundings and D is the equatorial diameter of the drop at the apex and H is the shape factor that contains the properties of the fluid (Arashiro and Demarquette, 1999; Dingle et al., 2005; Hernández-Baltazar and Gracia-Fadrique, 2005).

Dynamic surface tension of biological fluids (Trukhin et al., 2001), surfactants and protein complexes (Krägel et al., 2003) and surface tension of viscous solutions are some of the examples which employ this method to measure surface tension.

2.6 Sessile drop method

The sessile drop method is based on the analysis of the profile of the drop placed on a solid substrate (see Figure 1). The solid may be a flat horizontal plate, a tilted plate, a vertical plate, or the walls of a thin tube (capillary). This method for contact angle determination is, in principle, simple, but great care must be taken to make accurate measurements. When the contact angle is small, a sessile drop is difficult to observe, therefore it is recommended that substrates used in sessile drop measurements be poorly wetted by the drop and should have a contact angle greater than 90 degrees. The liquid is contained in a syringe from which a droplet is deposited onto the substrate, and a high resolution camera captures the image. The drop can then be analyzed either by eye (using a protractor) or using image analysis software to calculate contact angle, surface and interfacial tension, wettability and absorption (Allen, 2003; Dingle and Harris, 2005).

The sessile drop technique can be used to measure contact angle between solid, liquid and vapor phases and characterize the solid surface properties by solving Young's equation:

$$\cos\theta_c = \frac{\gamma_{SL} - \gamma_{SV}}{\gamma_{LV}} \tag{6}$$

where equilibrium contact angle, cos θ_c is related to the interfacial energy of the three involved surfaces; solid-liquid, γ_{SL}, solid-vapor, γ_{SV} and liquid-vapor γ_{LV}. If θ is less than 90°, the liquid is said to wet the solid. A zero contact angle represents complete wetting. If θ is greater than 90° then it is said to be non-wetting (Bachmann et al., 2000; Dingle and Harris, 2005; Muster and Prestidge, 2002).

The most widely employed method for contact angle studies is to measure the angle of a sessile drop resting on a flat solid surface using a goniometer-microscope equipped with an angle-measuring eyepiece or a video camera equipped with a suitable magnifying lens, interfaces with a computer and an image-analysis software to determine the tangent value precisely on the captured image. Contact angles are obtained at intervals over a period of time. The sessile drop method for contact angle determination is, in principle, simple, but great care must be taken to make accurate measurements. The error associated with this instrument varies based on user expertise. This method employs a single point on the contact line to measure the surface tension, therefore it is not a suitable technique in studying rough and heterogenous surfaces. To obtain reproducible and accurate measurements with rough surfaces it is advantageous to use the Wilhelmy plate method. An advantage of of the sessile drop method is that, the large solid surface allows multiple droplet evaluation. Reproducibility of the surface measured contact angle values will reflect the heterogeneity of the surface's energy properties (Allen, 2003; Dingle and Harris, 2005; Drelich et al., 2002; Ho et al., 2010).

Contact angle is one of the most widely used techniques in the surface characterization and wettability of pharmaceuticals formulations. The sessile drop technique is commonly used for estimating contact angle of pharmaceutical powders (Buckton, 1993), drug-carrier adhesion (Podczeck et al., 1996), compaction and granulation (Puri et al., 2010), emulsion stability (Hansen and Fagerheim, 1998), human biological fluids (Noordman et al., 1999) and dynamic wettability properties of contact lens hydrogels (Ketelson et al., 2005).

2.7 Spinning drop method

Spinning drop method is based on the profile analysis of rotating liquid drop or thread where a drop of the less dense phase is put into another heavy phase contained in a horizontal tube. The tube is then spun about its longitudinal axis causing the lower density fluid to centrifuge to the center and form an elongated drop (see Figure 1). The diameter of a drop within a heavy phase is measured while the tube is spun at a constant speed. For each speed of rotation the drop attains equilibrium where the shape of the drop is a balance between interfacial tension and the pressure difference between the phases. With this method the interfacial tension can easily be calculated from Vonnegut's Equation:

$$\gamma = \frac{1}{4}r^3 \Delta\rho\omega^2 \tag{7}$$

where r denotes the radius of the cylindrical drop, $\Delta\rho$ is the density difference between the drop and the surrounding fluid and ω is the rotational velocity (Drelich et al., 2002; Hu and Joseph, 1994; Seifert and Wendorff, 1992).

This technique has many advantages when compared to the other methods. The centrifugal force used for determining the shape of the interface can be changed at will, however pendant drop and the sessile drop use gravity as the deforming force. This technique is ideal for measuring ultralow interfacial tensions down to 10^{-6} mN/m. Time and temperature-dependent surface tension can be studied using this technique (Seifert and Wendorff, 1992).

Design and manufacturing of a spinning drop device are simple in principle and this method is widely used to study the interfacial tensions of many systems, e.g., polymer melts, organic solvents (Jon et al., 1986; Schoolenberg et al., 1998) and surfactants and emulsions (El-Aaseer et al., 1984; Martin and Velankar, 2008).

2.8 Capillary rise method

The origin of this method dates to one century ago, however it is still a subject of interest due to the widespread application in the pharmacy and it is considered the standard method for determining the surface tension and wettability of a liquid. This method is capable of very good accuracy in measurement when suitable precautions are taken. But in practice it suffers from the fact that the calibration of the capillary diameter is tedious. This method is based on measuring the penetration time needed for a liquid to rise to a certain height when the end of a capillary is immersed into the solution (see Figure 1). According to the rising speed, the contact angle may be calculated (Ramírez-Flores et al., 2010; Xue et al., 2006).

The Lucas– Washburn elucidated the dynamics of capillary rise by using the Poiseuille equation for capillary penetration of liquids using the pressure difference across the invading liquid meniscus. When the meniscus is ideally 'hemi-cylindrical' concave in shape, the height at which the solution reaches inside the capillary is related to the surface tension. The wicking of a solvent vertically through a powder is described by Washburn equation:

$$x^2 = \frac{r\gamma \cos\theta}{2\eta} t \tag{8}$$

where t is the time required for solvent to rise x millimeters above the solvent through the MPs, γ and η are the surface tension and viscosity of the solvent, cos θ is the cosine of the contact angle and r is the internal radius of the capillary (Norris et al., 1999; Ramírez-Flores et al., 2010; Xue et al., 2006).

The wetting of small particles and porous materials is a very important phenomenon in pharmaceutical technologies for wettability studies of drug powder and drug manufacturing with related processes. There are a number of available methods, however capillary rise method is a routine measurement for contact angle study of powder and porous materials (Ramírez-Flores et al., 2010; Galet et al., 2010; Xue et al., 2006). Contact angle method for powders can be classified into those which require compaction, and those which utilize penetration of liquid through an uncompacted bed. Powder penetration technique can be measured with the capillary rise method. However it has been found that this method tends to overestimate the contact angle value. An alternative method is to measure the contact angle on a compacted powder surface with the use of sessile drop technique. Disadvantage of the sessile drop method is that compaction may change the characteristics of the powder surface; also it requires the compact powder to be fully wetted by the test liquid. These problems may cause this method to underestimate the angle value. In such circumstances, Wilhelmy plate method allows calculation of contact angle without the need to pre-saturate the powder (Buckton et al., 1995).

2.9 Atomic force microscopy

Many engineered surfaces and pharmaceutical products cannot be melted, dissolved, or fractured; therefore their surface/interfacial tension cannot be determined through any of the conventional techniques. These conventional techniques are applicable to macroscopic solids with flat and homogenous surface and inert substrate, whereas for microscale surfaces with increased surface-to-volume ratio, or sensitive substrates another method needs to be employed. Atomic force microscopy (AFM) is a well-known tool capable of surface characterization at the atomic scale. This technique can be used to produce high resolution images and can offers contact angle studies for macroscopic surfaces and adhesion force measurements for microscopic and submicroscopic surfaces (Cuenot et al., 2004; Drelich et al., 2004). AFM can also provide information on other surface properties such as stiffness, friction, or elasticity (Alonso and Goldmann, 2003). Atomic force microscope works by scanning the samples surface using a fine tip attached to a cantilever in the equipment. The AFM can be operated in the contact (tip touching the sample) and tapping modes (tip oscillating rapidly above the sample). Thus, a topological or force map of the surface can be constructed which allows us to determine the structural information and surface properties such as surface tension (Edwardson and Henderson 2004; Handojo et al., 2009). The force required to pull the tip off the substrate surface is called pull-off or adhesion force (F) which is directly related to the surface tension of the sample (Drelich et al., 2004):

$$\gamma = \frac{F}{2c\pi R} \tag{9}$$

where R is the radius of the particle (probing tip) and c is a constant which depends on the model of the AFM (Drelich et al., 2004).

Atomic force microscopy allows imaging and measurement of biological and biomaterial samples, ligand-receptor interaction, protein adsorption and folding (Alonso and Goldmann, 2003; Edwardson and Henderson, 2004). This device is fast becoming a valuable tool in the pharmaceutical industry and is used in formulation and surface characterization of liposome vesicles (Maeda et al., 2002), microparticle preparation and biomaterials (Méndez-Vilas et al., 2006), surface characterization of parenteral nutrition bags (Realdon et al., 2003), wetting properties of human hair (Dupres et al., 2004) and other applications are discussed elsewhere (Santos and Castanho, 2004).

2.10 Oscilating jet method

The oscillating jet method consists of forcing a stream of liquid under constant pressure through an orifice. By adjusting the osciallation frequency, the liquid vibrates to forms a jet having a series of stationary waves which depends chiefly on the characteristics of the orifice, its position, wave number, rate of flow and the surface tension of the liquid (Chang and Franses, 1995; Defay and Pétré, 1962; Stückrad et al., 1993; Thomas and Potter, 1975). Surface tension can be calculated using Bohr equation:

$$\gamma = \frac{2 \times 10^3 \rho f^2 (1 + 1.542 b^2 / r^2) \psi}{3r\lambda^2 + 5\pi^2 r^3} \tag{10}$$

where γ is the surface tension on the wave surface (mN/m), f is the flow rate (m³/sec), ρ is the density of solution (kg/m3), λ is the wavelength of oscillation (m), r is the stream radius (m) , b/r is the wave amplitude, and Ψ differs from unity by about 1 part in 1000 (Thomas and Potter, 1975; Zhang and Zao, 1989).

This method can be employed to measure surface tension versus surface age (dynamic surface tension) for surface age varying between 0.1 and 0.001 second of surfactant solutions and surface elastisity (Defay and Hommelen, 1958; Warszynski et al., 1998). Oscillating bubble method is a similar method in which surface is periodically changed and the resulting surface tension variation is measured. Results have shown that surface tension measurements obtained using these methods are similar in value (Lunkenheimer et al., 1990).

2.11 Other methods of surface tension measurement

Laser light-scattering method is a non-invasive technique which is able to measure low values of surface tension without perturbing the interfacial thermal equilibrium (Jon et al., 1986; Huang, 1997). This method takes advantage of microscopic interfacial roughness caused by thermal fluctuations of a liquid surface and can be used to measure soft matter systems including microemulsions and bilayer lipid membranes (Cicuta and Hopkinson, 2004).

Langmuir trough methods can be used to study monolayers of surfactants and lipid solutions. In this method lipid solution is applied dropwise at the water surface with a micro liter syringe. This technique allows accurate measurement of surface and interfacial pressure and measurement of dilatational rheology of interfacial film and like Wilhelmy method this technique is independent of contact angle. Langmuir method can be used to measure equilibrium and dynamic surface tension of alveolar surfactant and lipid monolayers (Aveyard et al., 2000; Hills, 1985).

Pulsating bubble surfactometer can be used for studying the dynamic surface tension behavior of surfactants under constant or pulsating area. This method employs a sensitive transducer to determine the pressure difference across the bubble surface. A known area is pulsated sinosoidally resulting in a range of radius from which the surface tension is calculated. This method has been used for the interfacial measurement of soaps, surfactants and protein solutions and lung surfactant drugs (Chang et al., 1996; Coltharp and Franses, 1996).

The inclined plate method involves flowing a thin layer of surfactant solution over an inclined plate method. Surfactant molecules in the bulk adsorb at the interface and surface tension can be obtained from the flow rate of surfactant solution. However, since a Wilhelmy plate is used to measure the surface tension of the flowing surfactant solution, the lag time may introduce some errors during measurement, therefore, proper care is needed to orient the plate parallel to the flowing solution (Chang and Franses, 1995).

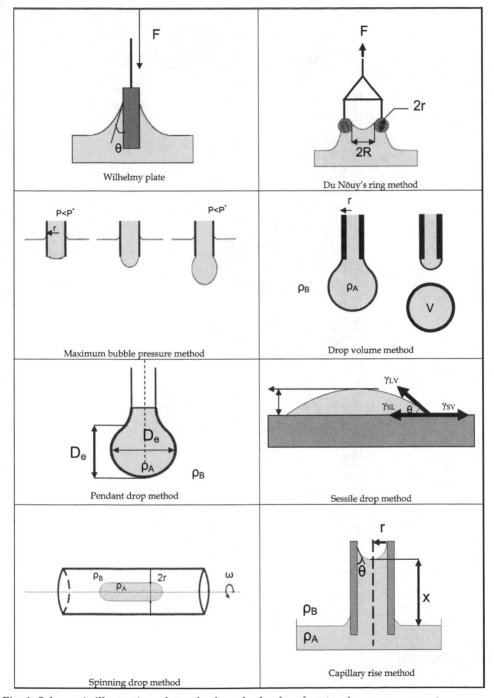

Fig. 1. Schematic illustration of standard methods of surface tension measurement.

Method involves measure of γ with:	Method	Accuracy mN/m	Suitability for surfactant solutions	Suitability for two-liquid systems	Suitability for viscous liquids	Suitability for contact angle measurement	Commercial availability	Instrument type
Microbalance	Wilhelmy plate	~0.1	Limited	Good	Good	Good	Yes	Manual
	Du Noüy ring	~0.1	Limited	Reduced accuracy	Not recommended	Not applicable	Yes	Manual
Capillary pressure	Maximum bubble pressure	0.1-0.3	Very good	Very good	Not recommended	Not applicable	Yes	Automatic
Equilibrium between capillary and gravity	Capillary rise	<<0.1	Very good	Very good, But experimentally difficult	Not recommended	Good	Not	Manual
	Drop volume/weight	0.1-0.2	Limited	Good	Not recommended	Not applicable	Yes	Automatic
Gravity-distorted drop	Pendant drop	~0.1	Very good	Very Good	Not recommended	Not applicable	Yes	Manual/Automatic
	Sessile drop	~0.1	Good	Very Good	Good	Good	Not	Manual/Automatic
Centrifugal forces	Spinning drop	0.1	Good	Very Good	Good	Not applicable	Yes	Manual
Resonance frequency	Atomic Force Microscopy	0.1	Good	Very Good	Good	Good	Yes	Automatic

*Drelich et al., 2002
*Thiessen and Man, 1999
*Fainerman et al., 2006
* Xue et al., 2006

Table 1. Accuracy and suitability of classic techniques used in surface tension measurement.

3. Computational methods of surface tension measurements

Modeling of physicochemical properties such as surface tension is needed in the pharmaceutical research. Experimental data on surface tension of liquid mixtures are very scarce in the literature, therefore theoretical methods of their prediction are found to be very useful. Reliable methods of surface tension prediction are useful in design of new materials and will undoubtfuly save laborious experimental measurement time. Surface tension of a liquid mixture is not a simple function of the surface tension of pure components, and is based on the assumption that the composition of the bulk phase is different from the composition of the adjacent vapor-liquid interface. There are various computational techniques in which the surface tension is evaluated through its thermodynamic definition or with the use of empirical equations. Most models require surface tension of the pure components. Models differ in the way in which the molar surface area and the activitycoefficients of the components are calculated (Bezerra et al., 2010; Pandey and Srivastava,2010). Evaluation of the performance of the models is calculated through average absolute deviation, AAD (%) for M data points using equation 11:

$$AAD(\%) = 100 \left[\sum_{i=1}^{M} \frac{\left| \left(\gamma_{exp} - \gamma_{calc} \right) / \gamma_{exp} \right|}{M} \right] \qquad (11)$$

With this, the reported experimental values of surface tension obtained using experimental methods are compared with predicted surface tension values from the proposed model.
The following topics present some literature models proposed for correlation and prediction of surface tension of liquid mixtures and solid surfaces.

3.1 Surface thermodynamic theory

The thermodynamic methods are based on the fact that surface layer between the bulk liquid and vapor phases has its own composition which affect the surface tension of the mixture. The number of the surface active molecules that reside on the surface can be calculated by the Gibbs adsorption equation:

$$\Gamma = -\frac{1}{RT} \frac{D\gamma}{d\ln c} \qquad (12)$$

where Γ is the surface excess or surface concentration in moles per unit area of surface, c is the concentration of the substance in the bulk solution, γ is the surface tension, differential $d\gamma/dc$ show the change in surface tension with change in concentration, R is the gas constant and T is the temperature (Ramírez-Verduzco et al., 2006). Butler developed an application of Gibbs energy based on the assumption that the surface layer can be treated thermodynamically as a separate phase from the bulk phase. Some important thermodynamic-based equations were developed from the Butler equation and have been studied for their ability to correlate the surface tension of non-ideal mixtures. Sprow and Prausnitz developed an equation to correlate the surface tension of binary and multicomponent liquid mixtures by employing UNIFAC to calculate the activity coefficients of the individual components at the interface and in the bulk of the liquid. The predictive method of Sprow and Prausnitz was applied to 4 systems including binary and ternary systems of water, ethyl butyrate/propionate and methanol at a constant temperature with an AAD value of less than 3.0 % (Kijevcanin et al., 2004; Rafati and Ghasemian, 2008).

Shereshefsky (1967) presented a model for the surface tension of binary solutions which is able to compute the excess properties and free energy changes in the surface region. This model was applied to 100 aqueous and 200 non-aqueous binary solutions at constant temperature. The agreement between the calculated and the experimental data is found to be very good with AAD of ~ 1.8% for aqueous and ~ 0.6% for non-aqueous systems (Tahery et al., 2005).

Guggenheim (1945) derived an equation for the surface tension as a function of heat for ideal solutions. Hildebrand and Scott extended this model for mixtures with dissimilar molecules. Eberhart (1966) employed a statistical thermodynamic approach and developed a one-parameter equation for binary liquid mixtures with good accuracy (Tahery et al., 2005).

A two-parameter equation was developed based on Wilson theory (Fu et al., 1986). This model was trained for a large number of systems and was able to correlate the data of 251 binary systems with an ADD of 0.5%. Li and co-workers extended that model and used the UNIFAC group contribution method to propose another two-parameter model to calculate the surface tension of binary mixtures (Kijevcanin et al., 2004; Li et al., 1990; Tahery et al., 2005).

Li and Lu have developed a predictive model for the surface tension of real mixtures on the basis of Davis theory and tested it against molecular dynamics simulation of the surface tension of the Lennard–Jones fluid. The proposed method was found to be suitable for obtaining surface tension values (Davis, 1975; Li and Lu, 2001).

The gradient theory of fluid interfaces is applied to compute the surface tension of various binary and ternary mixtures made up of gas (carbon dioxide, nitrogen or methane) and hydrocarbons. This model employs the Helmholtz energy density of the bulk homogeneous fluid and the influence parameters of the interfacial inhomogeneous fluid to correlate the surface tension of various pure fluids, binary mixtures and binary and ternary mixtures of gas and liquid hydrocarbons with good results. This method is predictive and is able to estimate surface tension values of gas mixtures with satisfactory results (Lin et al., 2007; Miqueu, 2004).

3.2 Empirical and correlative theories

MacLeod proposed an empirical method based on the temperature-independent constant K, between density ρ, and surface tension γ:

$$\gamma^{1/4} = K.\rho \tag{13}$$

Sugden slightly modified MacLeod's original expression to give a constant which he called the parachor (Sugden, 1924). Escobeo and Mansoori generated a model based on statistical mechanics for the prediction of surface tension of pure solvent using the equation of state. This model is shown to represent the experimental surface tension data of 94 pure solvent within 1.1 AAD% across all temperature ranges (Escobedo and Mansoori, 1996). Later they extended the same conformal solution theory to the case of mixtures of organic liquids. This equation was applied to 55 binary mixtures and the AAD was 0.5 % (Escobedo and Mansoori, 1998). However these equations are complicated and require critical temperature, critical pressure as well as critical compressibility and acentric factor. Therefore this model requires complex computational procedures which may not be suitable in pharmaceutical research.

There are a few models where the surface tension of the pure liquid is not required. Panday and co workers have extended Brick-Bird corresponding-state model, Goldsack-Sarvas volume fraction statistics and Sanchez method to multicomponent systems. These approaches require the values of thermal expansivity, isothermal compressibility and critical constants of pure components (Pandey et al., 2008).

Redlich-Kister equation expresses the excess energy thermodynamic properties which consist of a function of the mole fraction of each component and an interaction parameter (Redlich and Kister, 1948). An extension of this model was proposed which is able to correlate surface tension with the composition of the conjugate liquid (Fleming and Vinatieri, 1979).

Studies concerning temperature effect on the surface tension of aqueous and non-aqueous solutions are limited. Some of the models require many experimental parameters leading to low precision and accuracy in surface tension prediction. The Jouyban-Acree model was proposed based on the extension of the Redlich-Kister model as:

$$\ln \gamma_{m,T} = f_1 \ln \gamma_{1,T} + f_2 \ln \gamma_{2,T} + \frac{f_1 f_2}{T} \sum_{i=0}^{2} K_i \left(f_1 - f_2 \right)^i \tag{14}$$

where $\gamma_{m,T}$, $\gamma_{1,T}$, $\gamma_{2,T}$ are the surface tension of the mixture and solvents 1 and 2, respectively and f_1 and f_2 are the volume fractions of the solvents and K_i are the model constant calculated using a no intercept least square method. This model is able to correlate surface tension of binary and ternary mixtures at various temperatures with AAD of 4.1 and 1.4 % respectively (Jouyban et al., 2004a; 2004b). This equation can be extended to correlate different physicochemical properties of solvent mixtures; including acid dissociation constant, dielectric constant, and drug solubility in water-cosolvent mixtures (Jouyban et al., 1999; 2002; 2004a).

Neural network (NN) modeling in quantitative structure-property relationship (QSPR) studies allows prediction of various physicochemical properties from the molecular structure. Reliable methods for prediction of basic physicochemical properties would save time consuming experimental studies. Kauffman and Jurs reported a predictive NN model for surface tension of 213 common organic solvents using 8 descriptors. The root mean square error of the test sets were 2.89 mN/m (Taskinen and Yliruusi, 2003; Kauffman and Jurs, 2001).

3.3 Surface tension of immiscible fluids and solids

Surface tension calculation of immiscible fluids is possible by introducing repulsion between the neighboring particles of different fluids which has been employed in the macro-scale particle method. However equation of state is also possible for this type of measurement (Zhou et al., 2008).

Determination of the surface tension of solids is crucial in pharmaceutical powders and tableting. Amongst the various approaches to estimate the contact angle of solids is the Young equation (see equation 6). This method requires an ideal, flat and homogenous surface, whereas real measurements are carried out on rough and heterogeneous surfaces, on which the typical contact angle measured is an advancing contact angle which is larger than Young's equilibrium contact angle. The surface tension of a solid cannot be easily estimated from the Young's equation because of the two unknown parameters γ_{SV}, γ_{SL}. In order to calculate these quantities, equation of state (EQS) was proposed (Li and Neumann,

1990). However many researchers have criticized this equation for its thermodynamic analysis (Johnson and Dettre, 1989; Lee, 1993). Another approach is the geometrical methods for measuring surface tension of solids including Owen Wendt and van Oss theory. These methods decompose the surface tension into different components (Owens and Wendt, 1969; van Oss et al., 1986). Ahadian and colleagues compared the surface tension of 41 artificial solid surfaces as predicted by the equation of state and compared it to the values obtained by van Oss theory and Owen Wendt equation. Results indicate that equation of state was capable of good predictability, whereas the geometric methods are limited to higher range surface tension value of solid surfaces (Ahadian et al.,2007).

4. Conclusion

Measurements of surface rheological characteristics are of great importance for the pharmaceutical industry. Many of pharmaceutical processes depend on the cohesive and adhesive interactions between the materials used during the preparation of the product. Understanding and determination of surface free energies of both liquid and solid surfaces plays a key role in characterization of materials during their development, formulation and manufacturing of pharmaceutical applications. The chemical activity, adsorption, dissolution, and bioavailability of a drug may depend on the surface of the molecule.

There are several experimental approaches that one can employ to evaluate interfacial tension and large differences can exist among measurement methods. While one method may be proven useful for a number of applications, there are several restrictions that detract from its applicability in a specific system. The choice of the method depends on the nature of the interface, the rheology of the liquid(s), the range of temperature and pressure, ease of analysis, accuracy, precision, surface age, cost and convenience of the probing instrument. Most equilibrium methods may be used to measure dynamic tension, and there are certain methods by which one can measure solely dynamic tension. Most methods involve measurement of forces, interface shapes, pressure differences, or flow rates. Commonly used methods for measuring interfacial tension of various solutions as well as solid systems are mentioned in this chapter.

To facilitate an in-depth process understanding, a combination of experimental and computational design may be integrated in interfacial tension of compounds. Providing a simple method of correlating and predicting the interfacial properties of materials would be of great interest for pharmaceutical technology. There are various computational techniques in which the surface tension is evaluated through its thermodynamic definition or empirical equations. These methods require input data and several adjustable parameters obtained from multicomponent system and the pure component. Some of these equations on a thermodynamic basis are the two-parameter model for liquid mixtures. With these methods calculation of the free-energy between the two systems is a challenge to be accurately determined and these methods are difficult to implement at relatively high temperature due to stability problems. Empirical equations may be used to correlate and predict surface tension using one or two parameters. Some of these models may have limited range of applicability and may require a lot of experimental data. For practical use it is very important that the surface tension of multicomponent system can be predicted from the composition of the conjugate phases and some predictable physical parameters without any adjustable parameters.

In essence, an attempt has been made in this chapter to review and examine the performance of computational and experimental techniques in which surface tension are evaluated.

5. Acknowledgment

This work is dedicated to the spirit of Professor Fathollah Fathi-Azarbayjani, for believing that great things are born from tiny sparks of inspiration.

6. References

Ahadian, S.; Moradian, S.; Sharif, F.; Amani Tehran, M. & Mohseni, M. (2007). Application of artificial neural network (ANN) in order to predict the surface free energy of powders using the capillary rise method. *Colloids and Surfaces A: Physicochemical and Engineering Aspects*, Vol. 302, pp. 280-285.

Al-Maaieh, A. & Aburub, A. (2007). Surface activity of a non-micelle forming compound containing a surface-active impurity. *International Journal of Pharmaceutics*, Vol. 334, pp. 125-128.

Allen, J.S. (2003). An analytical solution for determination of small contact angles from sessile drops of arbitrary size. *Journal of Colloid and Interface Science*, Vol. 261, pp. 481-489.

Alonso, J.L. & Goldmann, W.H. (2003). Feeling the forces: atomic force microscopy in cell biology. *Life Sciences*, Vol. 72, pp. 2553-2560.

Arashiro, E.Y. & Demarquette, N.R. (1999). Use of the pendant drop method to measure interfacial tension between molten polymers. *Materials Research*, Vol. 2, pp. 23-32.

Aveyard, R.; Clint, J.H.; Nees, D. & Quirke, N. (2000). Structure and collapse of particle monolayers under lateral pressure at the octane/aqueous surfactant solution interface. *Langmuir*, Vol. 16, pp. 8820-8828.

Avranas, A. & Tasopoulos, V. (2000). Aqueous solutions of sodium deoxycholate and hydroxypropylmethylcellulose: dynamic surface tension measurements. *Journal of Colloid and Interface Science*, Vol. 221, pp. 223-229.

Bachmann, J.; Ellies, A. & Hartge, K.H. (2000). Development and application of a new sessile drop contact angle method to assess soil water repellency. *Journal of Hydrology*, Vol. 231-232, pp. 66-75.

Bezerra, E.S.; Santos, J.M.T. & Paredes, M.L.L. (2010). A new predictive model for liquid/air surface tension of mixtures: Hydrocarbon mixtures. *Fluid Phase Equilibria*, Vol. 288, pp. 55-62.

Bodour, A.A.; & Miller-Maier, R.M. (1998). Application of a modified drop-collapse technique for surfactant quantitation and screening of biosurfactant-producing microorganisms. *Journal of Microbiological Methods*, Vol. 32, pp. 273-280.

Buckton, G. (1988). The assessment, and pharmaceutical importance, of the solid/liquid and the solid/vapour interface: A review with respect to powders. *International Journal of Pharmaceutics*, Vol. 44, pp. 1-8.

Buckton, G. (1993). Assessment of the wettability of pharmaceutical powders. *Journal of Adhesion Science and Technology*, Vol. 7, pp. 205-219.

Buckton, G.; Darcy, P. & McCarthy, D. (1995). The extent of errors associated with contact angles, 3. The influence of surface roughness effects on angles measured using a

Wilhelmy plate technique for powders. *Colloids and Surfaces A: Physicochemical and Engineering Aspects*, Vol. 95, pp. 27-35.

Chamarthy, S.P.; Pinal, R. & Carvajal, M.T. (2009). Elucidating raw material variability – importance of surface properties and functionalities in pharmaceutical powders. *AAPS PharmSciTech*, Vol. 10, pp. 780–788.

Chang, C.-H.; Coltharp, K.A.; Park, S.Y. & Franses, E.I. (1996). Surface tension measurements with the pulsating bubble method. *Colloids and Surfaces A: Physicochemical and Engineering Aspects*, Vol. 114, pp. 185 197.

Chang, C.-H. & Franses, E.I. (1995). Adsorption dynamics of surfactants at the air/water interface: a critical review of mathematical models, data, and mechanisms. *Colloids and Surfaces A: Physicochemical and Engineering Aspects*, Vol. 100, pp. 1-45.

Chen, P.; Policova, Z.; Pace-Asciak, C.R. & Neumann, A.W. (1999). Study of molecular interactions between lipids and proteins using dynamic surface tension measurements: A review. *Colloids and Surfaces B: Biointerfaces*, Vol.15, pp. 313–324.

Christov, N.C.; Danov, K.D.; Kralchevsky, P.A.; Ananthapadmanabhan, K.P. & Lips, A. (2006). Maximum bubble pressure method: Universal surface age and transport mechanisms in surfactant solutions. *Langmuir*, Vol. 22, pp. 7528-7542.

Cicuta, P. & Hipkinson, I. (2004). Recent developments of surface light scattering as a tool for optical-rheology of polymers monolayers. *Colloids and Surfaces A: Physicochemical Engineering Aspects*, Vol. 233, pp. 97-107.

Coltharp, K.A. & Franses, E.I. (1996). Equilibrium and dynamic surface tension behavior of aqueous soaps: Sodium octanoate and sodium dodecanoate (sodium laurate). *Colloids and Surfaces Physicochemical and Engineering Aspects*, Vol. 108, pp. 225 242

Cuenot, S.; Fétigny, C.; Demoustier-Champagne, S. & Nysten, B. (2004). Surface tension effect on the mechanical properties of nanomaterials measured by atomic force microscopy. *Physical Review B*, Vol. 69, pp. 1-5.

Currie, P.K. & van Nieuwkoop, J. (1982). Buoyancy effects in the spinning-drop interfacial tensiometer. *Journal of Colloid Interface Science*, Vol. 87, pp. 301-316.

Davis, H.T. (1975). Statistical mechanics of interfacial properties of polyatomic fluids. 1. Surface tension. *Journal of Chemical Physics*, Vol. 62, pp. 3412–3415.

de la Maza, A.; Coderch, L.; Gonzalez, P. & Parra, J.L. (1998). Subsolubilizing alterations caused by alkyl glucosides in phosphatidylcholine liposomes. *Journal of Controlled Release*, Vol. 52, pp. 159-168.

Defay, R. & Hommelen, J.R. (1958). I. Measurement of dynamic surface tensions of aqueous solutions by the oscillating jet method. *Journal of Colloid Science*, Vol.13, pp. 553-564.

Defay, R. & Pétré, G. (1962). Correcting surface tension data obtained by the oscillating jet method. *Journal of Colloid Science*, Vol. 17, pp. 565-569.

Deo, N.; Somasundaran, T. & Somasundaran, P. (2004). Solution properties of amitriptyline and its partitioning into lipid bilayers. *Colloids and Surfaces B: Biointerfaces*, Vol. 34, pp. 155–159.

Dingle, N.M. & Harris, M.T. (2005). A robust algorithm for the simultaneous parameter estimationof interfacial tension and contact angle from sessile drop profiles. *Journal of Colloid and Interface Science*, Vol. 286, pp. 670–680.

Drelich, J.; Fang, C. & White, C.L. (2002). Measurment of interfacial tension in fluid-fluid systems, in: *Encyclopedia of Surface and Colloid Science*, Hubbard AT, pp. 3152-3166, Marcel Dekker, ISBN: 9780824707965, New York.

Dreu, R.; Šircab, J.; Pintye-Hodi, K.; Burjan, T.; Planinšek, O. & Srčič, S. (2005). Physicochemical properties of granulating liquids and their influence on microcrystalline cellulose pellets obtained by extrusion-spheronisation technology. *International Journal of Pharmaceutics*, Vol. 291, pp. 99–111.

Dupres, V.; Camesano, T.; Langevin, D.; Checco, A. & Guenoun, P. (2004). Atomic force microscopy imaging of hair: Correlations between surface potential and wetting at the nanometer scale. *Journal of Colloid and Interface Science*, Vol. 269, pp. 329–335.

Eberhart, J.G. (1966). Surface tension of binary liquid mixtures. *Journal of Physical Chemistry*, Vol. 70, pp. 1183–1186.

Edwardson, J.M. & Henderson, R.M. (2004). Atomic force microscopy and drug discovery. *Drug Discovery Today*, Vol. 9, pp. 64-71.

El-Aasser, M.S.; Lack, C.D.; Choi, Y.T.; Min, T.I.; Vanderhoff, J.W. & Fowkes, F.M. (1984). Interfacial aspects of miniemulsions and miniemulsion polymers. *Colloids and Surfaces*, Vol. 12, pp. 79-97.

Escobedo, J. & Mansoori, G.A. (1996). Surface tension prediction for pure fluids, *AIChE Journal*, Vol. 42, pp. 1425-1433.

Escobedo, J. & Mansoori, G.A. (1998). Surface tension prediction for liquid mixtures. *AIChE Journal*, Vol. 44, pp. 2324-2332.

Fainerman, V.B.; Mys, V.D.; Makievski, A.V. & Miller, R. (2006). Application of the maximum bubble pressure technique for dynamic surface tension studies of surfactant solutions using the Sugden two-capillary method. *Journal of Colloid and Interface Science*, Vol. 304, pp. 222–225.

Fleming, P.D. & Vinatieri, J.E. (1979). Quantitative interpretation of phase volume behaviour of multicomponent systems near critical points. *AIChE Journal*, Vol. 25, pp. 493–502.

Fu, J.; Li, B. & Wang, Z. (1986). Estimation of fluid-fluid interfacial tension of multicomponent mixtures. *Chemical Engineering Science*, Vol. 41, pp. 2673–2679.

Galet, L.; Patry, S. & Dodds, J. (2010). Determination of the wettability of powders by the Washburn capillary rise method with bed preparation by a centrifugal packing technique. *Journal of Colloid and Interface Science*, Vol. 346, pp. 470–475.

Guggenheim, E.A. (1945). The principle of corresponding states. *Journal of Chemical Physics*, Vol. 13, pp. 253-261.

Gunde, R;. Kumar, A.; Lehnert-Batar, S.; Mäder, R. & Windhab E.J., (2001). Measurement of the surface and interfacial tension from maximum volume of a pendant drop. *Journal of Colloid and Interface Science*, Vol. 244, pp. 113–122.

Hallowell, C.P. & Hirt, D.E. (1994). Unusual characteristics of the maximum bubble pressure method using a Teflon capillary. *Journal of Colloid and Interface Science*, Vol. 168, pp. 281-288.

Hancock, B.C.; York, P. & Rowe, R.C. (1997). The use of solubility parameters in pharmaceutical dosage form design. *International Journal of Pharmaceutics*, Vol. 148, pp. 1- 21.

Handojo, A.; Zhai, Y.; Frankel, G. & Pascall, M.A. (2009). Measurement of adhesion strengths between various milk products on glass surfaces using contact angle measurement and atomic force microscopy. *Journal of Food Engineering*, Vol. 92, pp. 305–311.

Hernández-Baltazar, E. & Gracia-Fadrique, J. (2005). Elliptic solution to the Young–Laplace differential equation. *Journal of Colloid and Interface Science*, Vol. 287, pp. 213–216.

Hills, B. (1985). Alveolar liquid lining: Langmuir method used to measure surface tension in bovine and canine lung extracts. *Journal of Physiology*, Vol. 359, pp. 65-79.

Ho, R.; Hinder, J.; Watts, J.F.; Dilworth, S.E.; Williams, D.R. & Heng, J.Y.Y. (2010). Determination of surface heterogeneity of d-mannitol by sessile drop contact angle and finite concentration inverse gas chromatography. *International Journal of Pharmaceutics*, Vol. 387, pp. 79–86.

Hu, H.H. & Joseph, D.D. (1994). Evaluation of a liquid drop in a spinning drop tensiometer. *Journal of Colloid and Interface Science*, Vol. 162, pp. 331-339.

Huang, Y.-X. (1997). Laser light scattering studies on thermodynamics of C8-lecithin and monovalent salt solutions. *Journal of Chemical Physics*, Vol. 107, pp. 9141-9145.

Ishii, F.; Takamura, A. & Ogata, H. (1988). Compatibility of intravenous fat emulsions with prodrug amino acids. *Journal of Pharmarmacy Pharmacology*, Vol. 40, pp. 89-92.

Johnson, R.E. & Dettre, R.H. (1989). An evaluation of Neumann's "surface equation of state". *Langmuir*, Vol. 5, pp. 293–295.

Jon, D.I.; Rosano, H.L. & Cummins, H.Z. (1986). Toluene/water/1-propanol interfacial tension measurements by means of pendant drop, spinning drop, and laser light-scattering methods. *Journal of Colloid and Interface Science*, Vol. 114, pp. 330-341.

Jouyban, A.; Chan, H.K.; Clark, B.J. & Acree, W.E. (2002). Mathematical representation of apparent dissociation constants in aqueous-organic solvent mixtures. *International Journal of Pharmaceutics*, Vol. 246, pp. 135-142.

Jouyban, A.; Fathi Azarbayjani, A.; Barzegar-Jalali, M. & Acree, W.E. (2004a). Correlation of surface tension of mixed solvents with solvent composition. *Pharmazie*, Vol. 59, pp. 937-941.

Jouyban, A.; Fathi-Azarbayjani, A. & Acree, W.E. (2004b). Surface tension calculation of mixed solvents with respect to solvent composition and temperature by using Jouyban-Acree model. *Chemical and Pharmaceutical Bulletin*, Vol. 52, pp. 1219-1222.

Jouyban, A.; Soltanpour, Sh. & Chan, H.K. (2004). A simple relationship between dielectric constant of mixed solvents with solvent composition and temperature. *International Journal of Pharmaceutics*, Vol. 269, pp. 353-360.

Jouyban, A.; Valaee, L.; Barzegar-Jalali, M.; Clark, B.J. & Acree, W.E. (1999). Comparison of various cosolvency models for calculating solute solubility in water-cosolvent mixtures. *International Journal of Pharmaceutics*, Vol. 177, pp. 93-101.

Kauffman, G.W. & Jurs, P.C. (2001). Prediction of surface tension, viscosity, and thermal conductivity for common organic solvents using quantitative structure–property relationships. *Journal of Chemical Information and Computer Science*, Vol. 41, pp. 408–418.

Kazakov, V.N.; Vozianov, A.F.; Sinyachenko, O.V.; Trukhin, D.V.; Kovalchuk, V.I. & Pison, U. (2000). Studies on the application of dynamic surface tensiometry of serum and cerebrospinal liquid for diagnostics and monitoring of treatment in patients who have rheumatic, neurological or oncological diseases. *Advances in Colloid and Interface Science*, Vol. 86, pp.1-38.

Ketelson, H.A.; Meadows, D.L. & Stone, R.P. (2005). Dynamic wettability properties of a soft contact lens hydrogel. *Colloids and Surfaces B: Biointerfaces*, Vol. 40, pp. 1–9.

Kijevcanin, M.Lj.; Ribeiro, I.S.A.; Ferreira, A.G.M. & Fonseca, I.M.A. (2004). Water + esters + methanol: Experimental data, correlation and prediction of surface and interfacial tensions at 303.15K and atmospheric pressure. *Fluid Phase Equilibria*, Vol. 218, pp. 141–148.

Krägel, J.; O'Neill, M.; Makievski, A.V.; Michel, M.; Leser, M.E. & Miller, R. (2003). Dynamics of mixed protein-/surfactant layers adsorbed at the water/air and water/oil interface. *Colloids and Surfaces B: Biointerfaces*, Vol. 31 pp. 107-114.

Krishnan, A.; Liu, Y.-H.; Cha, P.; Woodward, R.; Allara, D. & Vogler, E.A. (2005). An evaluation of methods for contact angle measurement. *Colloids and Surfaces B: Biointerfaces*, Vol. 43, pp. 95–98.

Korhonen, M.; Hirvonen, J.; Peltonen, L.; Antikainen, O.; Yrjänäinen, L. & Yliruusi, J. (2004). Formation and characterization of three-component-sorbitan monoester surfactant, oil and water-creams. *International Journal of Pharmaceutics*, Vol. 269, pp. 227–239.

Lee, L.-H. (1993). Scope and limitations of the equation of state approach for interfacial tensions. *Langmuir*, Vol. 9, pp. 1898–1905

Li, Z.B. & Lu, B.C.Y. (2001). On the prediction of surface tension for multicomponent mixtures. *Canadian Journal of Chemical Engineering*, Vol. 79, pp. 402–411.

Li, D. & Neumann, A.W. (1990). A reformulation of the equation of state for interfacial tensions. *Journal of Colloid Interface Science*, Vol. 137, pp.304-307.

Li, Z.B.; Shen, S.Q.; Shi, M.R. & Shi, J. (1990). Prediction of the surface tension of binary and multicomponent liquid mixtures by the unifac group contribution method. *Thermochimica Acta*, Vol. 169, pp. 231–238.

Lin, H.; Duan, Y.-Y. & Min, Q. (2007). Gradient theory modeling of surface tension for pure fluids and binary mixtures. *Fluid Phase Equilibria*, Vol. 254, pp. 75–90.

Luner, P.E. & Van Der Kamp, D. (2001). Wetting characteristics of media emulating gastric fluids. *International Journal of Pharmaceutics*, Vol. 212, pp. 81–91.

Lunkenheimer, K.; Serrien, G. & Joos, P. (1990). The adsorption kinetics of octanol at the air/solution interface measured with the oscillating bubble and oscillating jet methods. *Journal of Colloid and Interface Science*, Vol. 134, pp. 407-411.

Maeda, N.; Senden, T.J. & di Meglio, J.-M. (2002). Micromanipulation of phospholipid bilayers by atomic force microscopy. *Biochimica et Biophysica Acta*, Vol. 1564, pp. 165– 172.

Martin, J.D. & Velankar, S.S. (2008). Unusual behavior of PEG/PPG/Pluronic interfaces studied by a spinning drop tensiometer. *Journal of Colloid and Interface Science*, Vol. 322, pp. 669–674.

Matsuki, H.; Shimada, K.; Kaneshina, S.; Kamaya, H. & Ueda, I. (1998). Difference in surface activities between uncharged and charged local anesthetics: Correlation with their anesthetic potencies. *Colloids and Surfaces B: Biointerfaces*, Vol. 11, pp. 287–295.

Méndez-Vilas, A.; Donoso, M.G.; Gonz´alez-Carrasco, J.L. & González-Martín, M.L. (2006). Looking at the micro-topography of polished and blasted Ti-based biomaterials using atomic force microscopy and contact angle goniometry. *Colloids and Surfaces B: Biointerfaces*, Vol. 52, pp. 157–166.

Millqvist-Fureby, A.; Malmsten, M. & Bergenståhl, B. (1999). Spray-drying of trypsin-surface characterisation and activity preservation. *International Journal of Pharmaceutics*, Vol. 188, pp. 243–253.

Miqueu, C.; Mendiboure, B. ; Graciaa, C. & Lachaise, J. (2004). Modelling of the surface tension of binary and ternary mixtures with the gradient theory of fluid interfaces. *Fluid Phase Equilibria*, Vol. 218, pp. 189–203.

Mishchuk, N.A. Fainerman, V.B. Kovalchuk, V.I.R. Miller, R. Dukhin, S.S. (2000). Studies of concentrated surfactant solutions using the maximum bubble pressure method. *Colloids and Surfaces A: Colloids and Surfaces A: Physicochemical and Engineering Aspects*, Vol. 175, pp. 207–216.

Mishima, K.; Matsuyama, K.; Ezawa, M.; Taruta, Y.; Takarabe, S. & Nagatani, M. (1998). Interfacial tension of aqueous two-phase systems containing poly (ethylene glycol) and dipotassium hydrogenphosphate. *Journal of Chromatography B*, Vol. 711, pp. 313–318.

Muster, T.H. & Prestidge, C.A. (2002). Application of time-dependent sessile drop contact angles on compacts to characterise the surface energetics of sulfathiazole crystals. *International Journal of Pharmaceutics*, Vol. 234, pp. 43–54.

Noordmans, J.; Wormeester, H. & Busscher, H.J. (1999). Simultaneous monitoring of protein adsorption at the solid–liquid interface from sessile solution droplets by ellipsometry and axisymmetric drop shape analysis by profile. *Colloids and Surfaces B: Biointerfaces*, Vol. 15, pp. 227–233.

Norris, D.A.; Puri, N.; Labib, M.E. & Sinko, P.J. (1999). Determining the absolute surface hydrophobicity of microparticulates using thin layer wicking. *Journal of Controlled Release*, Vol. 59, pp. 173–185.

Ortiz, S.E.M.; Sánchez, C.C.; Rodríguez Niño, M.R.; Añon, M.C. & Rodríguez Patino, J.M. (2003). Structural characterization and surface activity of spread and adsorbed soy globulin films at equilibrium. *Colloids and Surfaces B: Biointerfaces*, Vol. 32, pp. 57-67.

Owens, D.K. & Wendt, R.C. (1969). Estimation of the surface free energy of polymers. *Journal of Applied Polymer Science*, Vol. 13, pp. 1741–1747.

Palma, S.; Lo Nostro, P.; Manzo, R. & Allemandi, D. (2002). Evaluation of the surfactant properties of ascorbyl palmitate sodium salt. *European Journal of Pharmaceutical Sciences*, Vol. 16, pp. 37–43.

Pandey, J.D.; Chandra, P.; Srivastava, T.; Soni, N.K. & Singh, A.K. (2008). Estimation of surface tension of ternary liquid systems by corresponding-states group-contributions method and Flory theory. *Fluid Phase Equilibria*, Vol. 273, pp. 44–51.

Podczek, F.; Newton, J.M. & James, M.B. (1996). The influence of physical properties of the materials in contact on the adhesion strength of particles of salmeterol base and salmeterol salts to various substrate materials. *Journal of Adhesion Science and Technology*, Vol. 10, pp. 257-268.

Puri, V.; Dantuluri, A.K.; Kumar, M.; Karar, N. & Bansal, A.K. (2010). Wettability and surface chemistry of crystalline and amorphous forms of a poorly water soluble drug. *European Journal of Pharmaceutical Sciences*, Vol. 40 pp. 84–93.

Rafati, A.A. & Ghasemian, E. (2008). Study of surface tension and surface properties of binary alcohol/n-alkyl acetate mixtures. *Journal of Colloid and Interface Science*, Vol. 328, pp. 385–390.

Ramírez-Flores, J.C.; Bachmann, J. & Marmur, A. (2010). Direct determination of contact angles of model soils in comparison with wettability characterization by capillary rise. *Journal of Hydrology*, Vol. 382, pp. 10–19.

Ramírez-Verduzco, L.F.; Romero-Martínez, A. & Trejo, A. (2006). Prediction of the surface tension, surface concentration, and the relative Gibbs adsorption isotherm of binary liquid systems. *Fluid Phase Equilibria*, Vol. 246, pp. 119–130.

Rangsansarid, J. & Fukada, K. (2007). Factors affecting the stability of O/W emulsion in BSA solution: Stabilization by electrically neutral protein at high ionic strength. *Journal of Colloid and Interface Science*, Vol. 316, pp. 779–786.

Realdon, N.; Zennaro, L.; Perin, F.; Bettero, A.; Bortoluzzi, S.; Rigo, A. & Ragazzi, E. (2003). Surface characterisation of bags for total parenteral nutrition by tensiometry and atomic force microscopy. *International Journal of Pharmaceutics*, Vol. 265, pp. 27–35.

Redlich, O. & Kister, A.T. (1948). Algebraic representation of thermodynamic properties and the classification of solutions. *Industrial and Chemistry Engineering Research*, Vol. 40, pp. 341–348.

Santos, N.C. & Castanho, M.A.R.B. (2004). An overview of the biophysical applications of atomic force microscopy. *Biophysical Chemistry*, Vol. 107, pp. 133–149.

Schoolenberg, G.E.; During, F. & Ingenbleek, G. (1998). Coalescence and interfacial tension measurements for polymer melts: experiments on a PS-PE model system. *Polymer*, Vol. 39, pp. 765-772.

Seifert, A.M. & Wendorff, J.H. (1992). Spinning drop experiments on interfacial phenomena: Theoretical background and experimental evidence. *Colloid Polymer Science*, Vol. 270, pp. 962-971.

Semmler, A. & Kohler, H.-H. (1999). Surface properties of Alkylpyridinium Chlorides and the applicability of the pendant drop technique. *Journal of Colloid and Interface Science*, Vol. 218, pp. 137–144.

Shereshefsky, J.L. (1967). A theory of surface tension of binary solutions. 1. Binary liquid mixtures of organic compounds. *Journal of Colloid and Interface Science*, Vol. 24, pp. 317–322.

Sipahi, C.; Anil, N. & Bayramli, E. (2001). The effect of acquired salivary pellicle on the surface free energy and wettability of different denture base materials. *Journal of Dentistry*, Vol. 29, pp. 197-204.

Stückrad, B.; Hiller, W.J. & Kowalewski, T.A. (1993). Measurement of dynamic surface tension by the oscillating droplet method. *Experiments in Fluids*, Vol. 15, pp. 332-340.

Sugden S., (1924). The influence of the orientation of surface molecules on the surface tension of pure liquids. *Journal of Chemical Society Transaction*, Vol. 125, pp. 1167–1177.

Tahery, R.; Modarress, H. & Satherley, J. (2005). Surface tension prediction and thermodynamic analysis of the surface for binary solutions. *Chemical Engineering Science*, Vol. 60, pp. 4935 – 4952.

Takamura, A.; Ishii, F.; Noro, S.; Tanifuji, M. & Nakajima, S. (1984). Study of intravenous hyperalimentation: effect of selected amino acids on the stability of intravenous fat emulsions. *Journal of Pharmaceutical Science*, Vol. 73, pp. 91-94.

Tan, S.N.; Fornasiero, D.; Sedev, R. & Ralston, J. (2005). Marangoni effects in aqueous polypropylene glycol foams. *Journal of Colloid and Interface Science*, Vol. 286, pp. 719–729.

Taskinen, J. & Yliruusi, J. (2003). Prediction of physicochemical properties based on neural network modeling. *Advanced Drug Delivery Reviews*, Vol. 55, pp. 1163–1183.

Thiessen, D.B. & Man, K.F. (1999). Surface tension measurements, CRC Press, Retrieved from <http://www.engnetbase.com>

Thomas, W.D.E. & Potter, L. (1975). Solution/Air Interfaces I. An oscillating jet relative method for determining dynamic surface tensions. *Journal of Colloid and Interface Science*. Vol. 50. pp. 397-412.

Trukhin, D.V.; Sinyachenko, O.V.; Kazakov, V.N.; Lylyk, S.V.; Belokon, A.M. & Pison, U. (2001). Dynamic surface tension and surface rheology of biological liquids. *Colloids and Surfaces B: Biointerfaces*, Vol. 21, pp. 231-238.

van Oss, C.J.; Good, R.J. & Chaudhury, M.K. (1986). The role of van der Waals forces and hydrogen bonds in "hydrophobic interactions" between biopolymers and low energy surfaces. *Journal of Colloid and Interface Science*, Vol. 111, pp. 378–390.

Vasir, J.K.; Tambwekar, K. & Garg, S. (2003). Bioadhesive microspheres as a controlled drug delivery system. *International Journal of Pharmaceutics*, Vol. 255, pp. 13–32.

Vejnovic, I.; Simmler, L. & Betz, G. (2010). Investigation of different formulations for drug delivery through the nail plate, *International Journal of Pharmaceutics*, Vol. 386, pp. 185-194.

Warszunski, P.; Wantke, K.-D. & Fruhner, H. (1998). Surface elasticity of oscillating spherical interfaces, *Colloids and Surfaces A*, Vol. 139, pp. 137–153.

Xue, H.T.; Fang, Z.N.; Yang, Y.; Huang, J.P. & Zhou, L.W. (2006). Contact angle determined by spontaneous dynamic capillary rises with hydrostatic effects: Experiment and theory. *Chemical Physics Letters*, Vol. 432, pp. 326–330.

Zelkó, R.; Orbán, Á.; Süvegh, K.; Riedl, Z. & Rácz, I. (2002). Effect of plasticizer on the dynamic surface tension and the free volume of Eudragit systems. *International Journal of Pharmaceutics*, Vol. 244, pp. 81-86.

Zhang, L.-H. & Zhao, G.-X. (1989). Dynamic surface tension of the aqueous solutions of cationic-anionic surfactant mixtures. *Journal of Colloid and Interface Science*, Vol. 127, pp. 353-361.

Zhou, G.; Ge, W. & Li, J. (2008). A revised surface tension model for macro-scale particle methods. *Powder Technology*, Vol. 183, pp. 21–26.

5

Prediction of Partition Coefficients and Permeability of Drug Molecules in Biological Systems with Abraham Model Solute Descriptors Derived from Measured Solubilities and Water-to-Organic Solvent Partition Coefficients

William E. Acree, Jr.[1], Laura M. Grubbs[1] and Michael H. Abraham[2]

[1]*University of North Texas,*
[2]*University College London,*
[1]*United States*
[2]*United Kingdom*

1. Introduction

Modern drug testing and design includes experimental *in vivo* and *in vitro* measurements, combined with *in silico* computations that enable prediction of the drug candidate's ADMET (adsorption, distribution, metabolism, elimination and toxicity) properties in the early stages of drug discovery. Recent estimates place the discovery and development cost of a small drug molecule close to US $1.3 billion, from the time of inception to the time when the drug finally reaches the market place. Only 20 % of conceived drug candidates proceed to clinical trial stage testing, and of the compounds that enter clinical development less than 10 % receive government approval. Reasons for the low success rate include unsatisfactory efficacy, poor solubility, poor bioavailability, unfavorable pharmacokinetic properties, toxicity concerns and drug-drug interactions, degradation and poor shelf-life stability. Unfavorable pharmacokinetic and ADME properties, toxicity and adverse side effects account for up to two-thirds of drug failures. Traditional ADME analyses relied heavily on whole animal assays and the more labor intensive biochemical studies. High throughput screening methods, fast ADMET profiling assays, and computational approaches have allowed the pharmaceutical industry to identify quickly the less promising drug candidates in the very early development stage so that time and valuable resources are not spent pursuing compounds that have little probability of reaching the general population.

Of the fore-mentioned properties, the drug's aqueous solubility will likely be one of the first properties measured. Aqueous solubility is a major indicator of the drug's solubility in physiological gastrointestinal fluids and is a major indicator of the drug's oral bioavailability. Approximately 40 % of the proposed new pharmaceutical candidates are rejected in the very early stages of drug discovery because of their poor aqueous solubility resulting in bioavailability problems (Lukyanov and Torchilin, 2004; Keck *et al.*, 2008). The number of failures due to poor solubility is likely to increase in future years because the new drug candidates generally have higher molecular weights and more complicated molecular structures than their predecessors. Moreover, drug molecules that are insoluble in water are difficult to study with existing *in vitro* biological assays, often give unreliable biological test results, and may precipitate from solution during storage or upon dilution. The importance of aqueous solubility in drug design is further evidenced by the fact that the editors of one prominent computational journal (Llinàs *et al.*, 2008) challenged readers to develop *in silico* methods to predict the intrinsic solubilities of 32 crystalline drug like molecules in water from an experimental data set of accurately measured solubilities of 100 compounds. Only a few of the more successful approaches were actually published (Wang, *et al.* 2009; Hewitt *et al.*, 2009). Similar challenges have been published regarding the prediction and measurement of the hydration free energies of functionally diverse neutral drug-like molecules (Nicholls *et al.*, 2008; Guthrie, 2009). Aqueous solubility is the reference media to predict the absorption and bioavailability of orally administered drugs. More than 85 % of the drugs sold in the US and in Europe are administered orally.

Amidon and coworkers (1995) proposed a biopharmaceutical classification scheme (BCS) to categories drugs and drug candidates into four groups based on their combined solubility and permeability properties. The classification scheme is depicted in Figure 1a. Drug candidates in Class I exhibit high solubility and high permeability, which is preferred from both a bioavailability and drug delivery standpoint. A drug candidate is considered highly soluble when the highest dose strength is soluble in 250 ml water over a pH range 1 to 7.5. A drug candidate possesses high permeability when the extent of absorption in humans is determined to be 90% of an administered dose, based on the mass balance or in comparison to an intravenous dose. Drug candidates in Class II have low solubility and high permeability, hence, the dissolution rate becomes the governing parameter for bioavailability. These drugs exhibit variable bioavailability and need enhancement in the dissolution rate for improvement in bioavailability. Drug candidates in Class III have high solubility and low permeability. Permeation through the intestinal membrane represents the rate-determining step for Class III drug candidates, with the bioavailability being independent of drug release from the dosage form. Class IV drug candidates possess both low solubility and low permeability. Drugs in this category are generally not suitable for oral drug delivery unless one employs a special drug delivery technology (such as a nano-suspension). Wu and Benet (2005) examined the biopharmaceutical classification scheme as a predictive method for assessing drug disposition. The authors found that drugs in Classes I and II of BCS were metabolized and eliminated. Drugs in the latter two classes were eliminated unchanged from the body by renal and/or biliary elimination. On the basis of these findings the authors suggested the Biopharmaceutics Drug Disposition Classification System (BDDCS) where the extent of metabolism has replaced permeability as a classification criterion (see Figure 2b). Aqueous solubility is an important consideration in both drug classification systems. Adverse drug solubility can sometimes be overcome by structural modifications (e.g., prodrugs) or by adding an organic cosolvent, surfactant, hydrophilic macromolecular and/or an inclusion host compound (such as a modified cyclodextrin) to the drug formulation or application vehicle. Knowledge of the drug's solubility in different organic solvents aids in the selection of an appropriate organic cosolvent and provides valuable information regarding drug's molecular interactions with other organic molecules.

	Solubility	Low Solubility		High Solubility	Low Solubility
High Permeability	**Class I** High Solubility High Permeability	**Class II** Low Solubility High Permeability	Extensive Metabolism	**Class I** High solubility Highly Metabolized	**Class II** Low solubility Highly Metabolized
Low Permeability	**Class III** High Solubility Low Permeability	**Class IV** Low Solubility Low Permeability	Poor Metabolism	**Class III** High solubility Poorly Metabolized	**Class IV** Low solubility Poorly Metabolized
	a)			b)	

Fig. 1. Properties used in the Biopharmaceutical Classification Scheme (a) and Biopharmaceutics Drug Disposition Classification System (b)

Lipophilicity is another of the physical properties that is measured in the early stages of drug testing to predict the transport of molecules from the gastrointestinal track into the epithelial cells that line the inner and outer surfaces of the body. Most common drugs cross cellular barriers by transcellular pathways (across epithelial cells) that require the drug to enter the outer portion of the lipid bilayer of the cell membrane. The drug then diffuses to the inner lipid layer and travels across the cell before crossing the cell membrane once again to exit. Lipophilicity was introduced to describe a compound's affinity to be in lipid-like environment. Several solvent systems have been suggested as a surrogate to represent the lipid membrane against water. For convenience and economical reasons, the partition coefficient of the drug candidate between 1-octanol and a series of aqueous buffers has become the standard measure of lipophilicity. The *intrinsic lipophilicity* (logarithm of the water-to-octanol partition coefficient, log $P_{o/w}$) describes the equilibrium distribution of molecular drug candidate (unionized form of the molecule) between water and the aqueous buffer, and is independent of pH. The *effective lipophilicity* (logarithm of the water-to-octanol distribution coefficient) reflects the concentration ratio of the neutral drug molecule plus all ionized forms that may be present in the aqueous buffered solution at the given pH. The effective lipophilicity is often quoted at the physiological pH of 7.4. The intrinsic and effective lipophilicities are equivalent if the drug candidate contains no ionizable or protonatable functional groups. Experimental techniques employed to measure water-to-octanol partition coefficients include the traditional shake-flask method, as well as several methods based on reversed-phase liquid chromatography (hplc), counter-current chromatography and centrifugal partition chromatography (Sangster, 1989; Berthod et al., 1992; Menges et al., 1990; Berthod et al., 1988; McDuffie, 1981; Veith et al., 1979). Ribeiro and coworkers (2010) recently discussed the advantages and limitations associated with using the water-to-octanol partitioning system as a surrogate for biological membranes. The authors noted that there is a considerable difference between the homogeneous macroscopic 1-octanol solvent system and the highly-ordered microscopic structure of a lipid layer. Chromatographic retention data determined using an immobilized artificial membrane (IAM) stationary phase was suggested as a more appropriate method for measuring the lipophilicity of drug candidates and for quantifying drug-membrane interactions.

Solubility and water-to-organic solvent partition coefficients are fairly easy to measure as the equilibrated solutions contain only the dissolved drug candidate and the solubilizing solvent media. Blood-to-tissue partition coefficients, plasma-to-milk partition coefficient, percentage of human intestinal absorption and the steady-state volume of distribution are much harder to measure. The analytical methodology employed to measure these latter properties must be able to distinguish and quantify the drug from all of the many other molecules present in the biological sample. It is not easy, even with today's modern instrumentation, to design chemical analysis methods that are specific to a given molecule. Moreover, measurements involving human and/or animal tissues are expensive and are subject to larger experimental uncertainties. Replicate studies involving the same animal species have shown that the measured values can depend on gender, age and eating habits. This chapter will discuss the prediction of the blood-to-tissue partition coefficients, plasma-to-milk partition coefficients, human intestinal absorption based on the Abraham solvation parameter model and solute descriptors calculated from measured solubilities and partition coefficients.

2. Abraham solvation parameter model

The Abraham general solvation model is one of the more useful approaches for the analysis and prediction of the adsorption, distribution and toxicological properties of potential drug candidates. The method relies on two linear free energy relationships (lfers), one for transfer processes occurring within condensed phases (Abraham, 1993a,b; Abraham *et al.*, 2004):

$$SP = c + e \cdot E + s \cdot S + a \cdot A + b \cdot B + v \cdot V \qquad (1)$$

and one for processes involving gas-to-condensed phase transfer

$$SP = c + e \cdot E + s \cdot S + a \cdot A + b \cdot B + l \cdot L \qquad (2)$$

The dependent variable, SP, is some property of a series of solutes in a fixed phase, which in the present study will include the logarithm of drug's water-to-organic solvent and blood-to-tissue partition coefficients, the logarithm of the drug's molar solubility in an organic solvent divided by its aqueous molar solubility, the logarithm of the drug's plasma-to-milk partition coefficient, percent human intestinal absorption and the logarithm of the kinetic constant for human intestinal absorption, and the logarithm of the human skin permeability coefficient. The independent variables, or descriptors, are solute properties as follows: E and S refer to the excess molar refraction and dipolarity/polarizability descriptors of the solute, respectively, A and B are measures of the solute hydrogen-bond acidity and basicity, V is the McGowan volume of the solute and L is the logarithm of the solute gas phase dimensionless Ostwald partition coefficient into hexadecane at 298 K. The first four descriptors can be regarded as measures of the tendency of the given solute to undergo various solute-solvent interactions. The latter two descriptors, V and L, are both measures of solute size, and so will be measures of the solvent cavity term that will accommodate the dissolved solute. General dispersion interactions are also related to solute size, hence, both V and L will also describe the general solute-solvent interactions. Solute descriptors are available for more than 4,000 organic, organometallic and inorganic solutes. No single article lists all of the numerical values; however, a large compilation is available in one published review article (Abraham *et al.*, 1993a), and in the supporting material that has accompanied several of our published papers (Abraham *et al.*, 2006a; Abraham *et al.*, 2009a; Mintz *et al.*, 2007). Solute descriptors can be obtained by regression analysis using various types of experimental data, including water-to-solvent partitions, gas-to-solvent partitions, solubility data and chromatographic retention data as discussed below and elsewhere (Abraham *et al.*, 2010; Zissimos *et al.*, 2002a,b). For a number of partitions into solvents that contain large amounts of water at saturation, an alternative hydrogen bond basicity parameter, B^o, is used for specific classes of solute: alkylpyridines, alkylanilines, and sulfoxides.

Equations 1 and 2 contain the following three quantities: (a) measured solute properties; (b) calculated solute descriptors; and (c) calculated equation coefficients. Knowledge of any two quantities permits calculation of the third quantity through the solving of simultaneous equations and regression analysis. Solute descriptors are calculated from measured partition coefficient ($P_{solute,system}$), chromatographic retention factor (k') and molar solubility ($C_{solute,solvent}$) data for the solutes dissolved in partitioning systems and in organic solvents having known equation coefficients. Generally partition coefficient, chromatographic retention factor and molar solubility measurements are fairly accurate, and it is good practice to base the solute descriptor computations on observed values having minimal experimental uncertainty. The computation is depicted graphically in Figure 1 by the unidirectional arrows that indicate the direction of the calculation using the known equation coefficients that connect the measured and solute descriptors. Measured $P_{solute,system}$ and $C_{solute,solvent}$ values yield solute descriptors. The unidirectional red arrows originating from the center solute descriptor circle represent the equation coefficients that have been reported for blood-to-brain partition coefficient, blood-to-tissue partition coefficients, percentage of human intenstinal absorption, Draize eye scores, and aquatic toxicity Abraham model linear free energy relationships. Plasma-to-milk partition ratio predictions are achieved (Abraham *et al.*, 2009b) through an artificial neural network with five inputs, 14 nodes in the hidden layer and one node in the output layer. Linear analysis of the plasma-to-milk partition ratios for 179 drugs and hydrophobic environmental pollutants revealed that drug molecules preferentially partition into the aqueous and protein phases of milk. Hydrophobic environmental pollutants, on the other hand, partition into the fat phase. Prediction of the fore-mentioned ADMET and biological properties does require a prior knowledge of the Abraham solute descriptors for the drug candidate of interest. There are also commercial software packages (ADME Boxes, 2010) and several published estimation schemes (Mutelet and Rogalski, 2001; Arey *et al.*, 2005; Platts *et al.*, 1999; Abraham and McGowan, 1987) for calculating the numerical values of solute descriptors from molecular structural information if one is unable to find the necessary partition, chromatographic and/or solubility data. For any fully characterized system/process (those with calculated values for the equation coefficients) further values of SP can be estimated for solutes with known values for the solute descriptors.

The usefulness of Eqns. 1 and 2 in the characterization of solvent phases is that the coefficients *e*, *s*, *a*, *b*, *l* and *v* are not just curve-fitting constants. The coefficients reflect particular solute-solvent interactions that correspond to chemical properties of the solvent phase. The excess molar refraction, **E**, is defined from the solute refractive index, and hence the *e* coefficient gives a measure of general solute-solvent dispersion interactions. The **V** and **L** descriptors were set up as measures of the endoergic effect of disrupting solvent-solvent bonds. However, solute volume is always well correlated with polarizability and so the *v* and *l* coefficients will include not only an endoergic cavity effect but also exoergic solute-solvent effects that arise through solute polarizability. The **S** descriptor is a measure of dipolarity and polarizability and hence the *s* coefficient will reflect the ability of a solvent to undergo dipole-dipole and dipole-induced dipole interactions with the solute. The **A** descriptor is a measure of solute hydrogen bond acidity, and hence the *a* coefficient will reflect the complementary solvent hydrogen bond basicity. Similarly the *b* coefficient will be a measure of solvent hydrogen bond acidity. All this is straightforward for gas-to-solvent partitions because there are no interactions to consider in the gas phase. For partition between solvents, the coefficients in Eqn. 1 then refer to differences between the properties of the two phases.

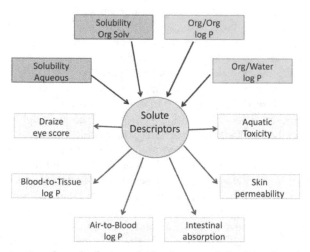

Fig. 2. Outline illustrating the calculation of Abraham model solute descriptors from experimental partition coefficient and solubility data, and then using the calculated values to estimate biological activities and partitioning, such as blood-to-tissue partition coefficients, Draize eye scores, aquatic toxicities and air-to-blood partition coefficients.

The Abraham model equation coefficients encode chemical information, and several methods have been suggested to assess the chemical similarity between different partitioning processes/systems. Abraham and Martins (2004) calculated the five-dimensional distance between the coefficients as points in five-dimensional space by straightforward geometry

$$\text{Distance} = \sqrt{(e_i - e_j)^2 + (s_i - s_j)^2 + (a_i - a_j)^2 + (b_i - b_j)^2 + (v_i - v_j)^2} \qquad (3)$$

where the subscripts "i" and "j" denote the two partitioning processes being compared. For comparison purposes, the authors suggested that for a good chemical model the calculated distance should be less than about 0.5 - 0.8. The water-to-isobutanol and water-to-octanol partitioning systems were the two chemical systems that the authors found closest to human skin permeability, with calculated distances of 1.2 and 1.9, respectively. The chemical interactions that govern skin permeability were quite different from the chemical interactions governing solute partitioning between water and isobutanol, and between water and 1-octanol. Ishiharma and Asakawa (1999) suggested a different comparison method based on calculating the cosine of the angle (cos θij) between the coefficients

$$Cos \, \Theta_{ij} = \frac{e_i e_j + s_i s_j + a_i a_j + b_i b_j + v_i v_j}{\sqrt{e_i^2 + s_i^2 + a_i^2 + b_i^2 + v_i^2} \, \sqrt{e_j^2 + s_j^2 + a_j^2 + b_j^2 + v_j^2}} \tag{4}$$

which are now regarded as lines in five-dimensional space. The angle between the two lines, Θ_{ij}, yields information regarding how the two compared processes are in terms of their chemical similarity. As Θ_{ij} approaches zero (or alternatively as cos Θ_{ij} approaches unity) the two lines coincide, and the correlation between the two partitioning processes/systems approaches unity. Analysis of the Abraham model coefficients for the solubility of gases and vapors in biological phases (blood, brain, fat, heart, kidney, liver, lung and muscle) and organic solvents (alcohols, amides, olive oil, chloroform, diethyl ether, butanone), and equation coefficients for biological activity (nasal pungency thresholds, eye irritation thresholds, odor detection and anesthesia) using Eqns. 3 and 4 (along with Principal Component Analysis) found N-methylformamide to be an excellent model for both eye irritation thresholds in humans and nasal pungency thresholds in humans (Abraham et al., 2009a). The receptor site controlling both biological responses must be protein-like in character. The study further showed that no organic solvent is a suitable model (or surrogate) for blood, brain, heart, kidney, liver, lung and muscle. Two relatively nonpolar solvents (olive oil and chloroform) were found to be suitable models for fat, which is not too surprising given that fat is about 80 % lipid.

3. Experimental methods for measuring thermodynamic and kinetic solubilities

Recent advances in automated chemical synthesis and combinatorial chemistry have generated large numbers of new chemical compounds that need to be screened for possible biological activity and desired ADMET properties. The conventional experimental methods that were once used in the pharmaceutical industry to measure solubility and water-to-organic solvent partition coefficients are inadequate to handle large numbers of new compound because of low throughput capacity and the amount of compound required for the experimental determination. Large quantities of highly purified compounds are not usually available in the initial stages of drug discovery and drug testing. To meet the demands imposed by the increased compound numbers, the pharmaceutical industry has developed miniaturized and automated sample preparation platforms, combined with rapid chemical analysis methods based on nephelometric, uv/visible absorption and/or chromatographic measurements. The experimental protocol used depends on whether one needs to measure the kinetic or thermodynamic solubility.

High throughput kinetic aqueous solubility assays are based on the detection of precipitation of compounds in aqueous or aqueous buffered solutions. Typically, small known aliquots of the stock solution are added incrementally to the aqueous (or aqueous buffered solution) at predetermined time intervals until the solubility limit is reached. The resulting precipitation can be detected optically by nephlometric or laser monitoring methods, and the kinetic solubility is defined as the solute concentration immediately preceding the point at which precipitation was first detected. Kinetic solubility thus represents the maximum solubility of the fastest precipitation species of the given compound into the desired solubilizing solvent media. Numerous modifications of kinetic assays have been suggested in recent years. The suggested modifications differ in the dilution and detection method. For example, Lipinski et al. (2001) added small aliquots of a stock solution of the drug (dissolved in dimethyl sulfoxide, DMSO) to the aqueous solvent media every minute until precipitation occurred. The DMSO in solution did increase with each added aliquot and may result in a higher measured aqueous solubility. Dimethyl sulfoxide is known to increase the solubility by helping to solvate the more lipophilic drug compounds. Solubility enhancement by dimethyl sulfoxide can be reduced if the samples are first serially diluted in dimethyl sulfoxide before the aliquots are added to the aqueous solvent system. Special 96-well plates have been designed to facilitate high throughput solubility measurements. The method depicted in Figure 3 allows one to quickly measure the aqueous solubility and aqueous-buffered solubility of 12 different drug candidates. The eight DMSO-diluted concentrations (1 mM to 100 mM) of each drug candidate are placed in the specified well of the drug's respective column. In the 12 x 9 cell matrix, the drug is identified by column number and the concentration is identified by row number. A predetermined aliquot volume from each of the DMSO diluted sample wells is transferred to the corresponding cell in the aqueous plate and aqueous-buffered plate. The volume of DMSO-diluted sample is the same for each transferred aliquot. Each cell in the aqueous plate and aqueous-buffered plate contains an identical volume of solvent. The cell contents are examined for precipitation immediately after the passage of the defined time interview, or alternatively, one can remove the solid and determine the concentration of dissolved drug by standard spectroscopic and/or chromatographic methods.

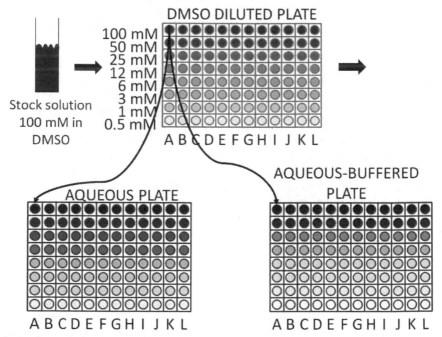

Fig. 3. Outline of a high throughput method for measuring drug solubility in water and in an aqueous-buffered solution using a 96-well plate.

Kinetic methods often overestimate the thermodynamic drug solubility because of the increased solubilization effect caused by the presence of dimethyl sulfoxide in the aqueous solvent and by the fact that one has not allowed sufficient time for equilibrium to be achieved. Thermodynamic solubility is defined as the concentration in solution of a compound in equilibrium with an excess of solid material being present in solution at the conclusion of the dissolution process. Thermodynamic solubility is considered the "true" solubility of a compound. Experimental methods for determining thermodynamic solubility may be grouped into categories, one that extends the experimental protocols of exiting kinetic solubility determinations to longer "equilibration times" and the other that conducts solubility studies on solid compounds obtained from dried stock solutions to remove the enhancement effects caused by having the added dimethyl sulfoxide present in the final equilibrated solution. The rationale behind the longer equilibration times is that sufficient time will now be afforded for the first-precipitated crystalline phase to convert to the more thermodynamically stable crystalline phase. Sugano and coworkers (2006) reported a significant decrease in solubility with equilibration time for more than half of the 26 model compounds studied.

The preceding discussion focused on aqueous kinetic and thermodynamic solubility measurements. There is no reason that the basic high throughput experimental methodologies cannot be applied to organic solvents and to aqueous-organic solvent mixtures. Measured drug solubility in organic solvents, in combination with the Abraham general solvation model, provides valuable information in regarding the molecule's hydrogen-bonding character and dipolarity. Solubility ratios are substituted into Eqns. 1 and 2 to give the following mathematical correlations:

$$\log \left(C_{A,organic} / C_{A,water} \right) = c + e \cdot E + s \cdot S + a \cdot A + b \cdot B + v \cdot V \tag{5}$$

$$\log \left(C_{A,organic} / C_{A,gas} \right) = c + e \cdot E + s \cdot S + a \cdot A + b \cdot B + l \cdot L \tag{6}$$

where $C_{A,organic}$ and $C_{A,water}$ denote the molar solubility of the solute (component A) in the anhydrous "dry" organic solvent and in water, respectively, and $C_{A,gas}$ is the molar gas phase concentration of the solute above the crystalline phase at the system temperature. This later quantity is calculable as $C_{A,gas} = P_A^o V/RT$, from the solute's vapor pressure above the crystalline phase, P_A^o.

The solubility ratio in Eqn. 5 represents a hypothetical partitioning process for transferring the solute from water to the anhydrous organic solvent as depicted in Figure 4. Also depicted in Figure 4 are the gas-to-water and gas-to-organic solvent partitioning processes, along with their respective concentration ratios. The hypothetical water-to-organic solvent partitioning process should not be confused with the direct practical organic solvent/water partitioning system that corresponds to the equilibrium solute partitioning between a water-saturated organic phase and an aqueous phase saturated with the organic solvent. For solvents that are partially miscible with water, such as 1-butanol and ethyl acetate, partition coefficients calculated as the ratio of the molar solute solubilities in the organic solvent and water are not the same as those obtained from direct partition between water (saturated with the organic solvent) and organic solvent (saturated with water). Solubility ratios and practical partition coefficients, however, are nearly identical for solvents like linear alkanes, cycloalkanes, chloroform, carbon tetrachloride and dichloromethane, which are almost "completely" immiscible with water. Tables 1 and 2 give the equation coefficients for the Abraham model solubility ratio correlations (Eqns. 5 and 6) for the different organic solvents that have been reported to date.

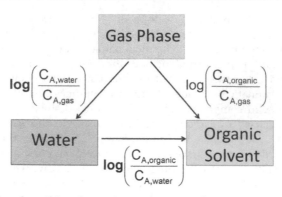

Fig. 4. Solubility ratios describing the various solute transfer processes.

Dry Solvent	c	e	s	a	b	v
Olely alcohol	-0.096	0.148	-0.841	-0.438	-4.040	4.125
Dichloromethane	0.319	0.102	-0.187	-3.058	-4.090	4.324
Trichloromethane	0.191	0.105	-0.403	-3.112	-3.514	4.395
Tetrachloromethane	0.199	0.523	-1.159	-3.560	-4.594	4.618
1,2-Dichloroethane	0.183	0.294	-0.134	-2.801	-4.291	4.180
1-Chlorobutane	0.222	0.273	-0.569	-2.918	-4.883	4.456
Butane	0.297	-0.005	-1.584	-3.188	-4.567	4.562
Pentane	0.369	0.386	-1.568	-3.535	-5.215	4.514
Hexane	0.361	0.579	-1.723	-3.599	-4.764	4.344
Heptane	0.325	0.670	-2.061	-3.317	-4.733	4.543
Octane	0.223	0.642	-1.647	-3.480	-5.067	4.526
Nonane	0.240	0.619	-1.713	-3.532	-4.921	4.482
Decane	0.160	0.585	-1.734	-3.435	-5.078	4.582
Undecane	0.058	0.603	-1.661	-3.421	-5.120	4.619
Dodecane	0.114	0.668	-1.664	-3.545	-5.006	4.459
Hexadecane	0.087	0.667	-1.617	-3.587	-4.869	4.433
Cyclohexane	0.159	0.784	-1.678	-3.740	-4.929	4.577
Methylcyclohexane	0.246	0.782	-1.982	-3.517	-4.293	4.528
Isooctane	0.318	0.555	-1.737	-3.677	-4.864	4.417
Benzene	0.142	0.464	-0.588	-3.099	-4.625	4.491
Toluene	0.143	0.527	-0.720	-3.010	-4.824	4.545
Fluorobenzene	0.139	0.152	-0.374	-3.030	-4.601	4.540
Chlorobenzene	0.065	0.381	-0.521	-3.183	-4.700	4.614
Bromobenzene	-0.017	0.436	-0.424	-3.174	-4.558	4.445
Iodobenzene	-0.192	0.298	-0.308	-3.213	-4.653	4.588
Nitrobenzene	-0.152	0.525	0.081	-2.332	-4.494	4.187
Benzonitrile	0.155	0.337	-0.036	-1.544	-4.614	3.990
Olive oil	-0.035	0.574	-0.798	-1.422	-4.984	4.210
Carbon disulfide	0.047	0.686	-0.943	-3.603	-5.818	4.921
Isopropyl myristate	-0.605	0.930	-1.153	-1.682	-4.093	4.249
Triolein	0.385	0.983	-2.083	-2.007	-3.452	4.072

Dry Solvent	c	e	s	a	b	v
Methanol	0.276	0.334	-0.714	0.243	-3.320	3.549
Ethanol	0.222	0.471	-1.035	0.326	-3.596	3.857
Propan-1-ol	0.139	0.405	-1.029	0.247	-3.767	3.986
Butan-1-ol	0.165	0.401	-1.011	0.056	-3.958	4.044
Pentan-1-ol	0.150	0.536	-1.229	0.141	-3.864	4.077
Hexan-1-ol	0.115	0.492	-1.164	0.054	-3.978	4.131
Heptan-1-ol	0.035	0.398	-1.063	0.002	-4.343	4.317
Octan-1-ol	-0.034	0.489	-1.044	-0.024	-4.235	4.218
Decan-1-ol	-0.058	0.616	-1.319	0.026	-4.153	4.279
Propan-2-ol	0.099	0.343	-1.049	0.406	-3.827	4.033
Isobutanol	0.127	0.253	-0.976	0.158	-3.882	4.114
sec-Butanol	0.188	0.354	-1.127	0.016	-3.568	3.968
tert-Butanol	0.211	0.171	-0.947	0.331	-4.085	4.109
3-Methyl-1-butanol	0.073	0.360	-1.273	0.090	-3.770	4.273
Pentan-2-ol	0.115	0.455	-1.331	0.206	-3.745	4.201
Ethylene glycol	-0.270	0.578	-0.511	0.715	-2.619	2.729
2,2,2 -Trifluoroethanol	0.395	-0.094	-0.594	-1.280	-1.274	3.088
Diethyl ether	0.350	0.358	-0.820	-0.588	-4.956	4.350
Tetrahydrofuran	0.207	0.372	-0.392	-0.236	-4.934	4.447
1,4-Dioxane	0.098	0.350	-0.083	-0.556	-4.826	4.172
Dibutyl ether	0.176	0.394	-0.985	-1.414	-5.357	4.524
Methyl tert-butyl ether	0.341	0.307	-0.817	-0.618	-5.097	4.425
Methyl acetate	0.351	0.223	-0.150	-1.035	-4.527	3.972
Ethyl acetate	0.328	0.369	-0.446	-0.700	-4.904	4.150
Butyl acetate	0.248	0.356	-0.501	-0.867	-4.973	4.281
Propanone	0.313	0.312	-0.121	-0.608	-4.753	3.942
Butanone	0.246	0.256	-0.080	-0.767	-4.855	4.148
Cyclohexanone	0.038	0.225	0.058	-0.976	-4.842	4.315
Dimethylformamide	-0.305	-0.058	0.343	0.358	-4.865	4.486
Dimethylacetamide	-0.271	0.084	0.209	0.915	-5.003	4.557
Diethylacetamide	0.213	0.034	0.089	1.342	-5.084	4.088
Dibutylformamide	0.332	0.302	-0.436	0.358	-4.902	3.952
N-Methylpyrolidinone	0.147	0.532	0.225	0.840	-4.794	3.674
N-Methyl-2-piperidone	0.056	0.332	0.257	1.556	-5.035	3.983
N-Formylmorpholine	-0.032	0.696	-0.062	0.014	-4.092	3.405
N-Methylformamide	0.114	0.407	-0.287	0.542	-4.085	3.471
N-Ethylformamide	0.220	0.034	-0.166	0.935	-4.589	3.730
N-Methylacetamide	0.090	0.205	-0.172	1.305	-4.589	3.833
N-Ethylacetamide	0.284	0.128	-0.442	1.180	-4.728	3.856
Formamide	-0.171	0.070	0.308	0.589	-3.152	2.432
Acetonitrile	0.413	0.077	0.326	-1.566	4.391	3.364
Nitromethane	0.023	-0.091	0.793	-1.463	-4.364	3.460
Dimethylsulfoxide	-0.194	0.327	0.791	-1.260	-4.540	3.361
Tributylphosphate	0.327	0.570	-0.837	-1.069	-4.333	3.919

Dry Solvent	c	e	s	a	b	v
Propylene carbonate	0.004	0.168	0.504	-1.283	-4.407	3.421
Gas-water	-0.994	0.577	2.549	3.813	4.841	-0.869

Table 1. Coefficients in Eqn. 5 for Correlating Solute Solubility in Dry Organic Solvents at 298 K

Dry Solvent	c	e	s	a	b	l
Olely alcohol	-0.268	-0.392	0.800	3.117	0.978	0.918
Dichloromethane	0.192	-0.572	1.492	0.460	0.847	0.965
Trichloromethane	0.157	-0.560	1.259	0.374	1.333	0.976
Tetrachloromethane	0.217	-0.435	0.554	0.000	0.000	1.069
1,2-Dichloroethane	0.017	-0.337	1.600	0.774	0.637	0.921
1-Chlorobutane	0.130	-0.581	1.114	0.724	0.000	1.016
Butane	0.291	-0.360	0.091	0.000	0.000	0.959
Pentane	0.335	-0.276	0.000	0.000	0.000	0.968
Hexane	0.292	-0.169	0.000	0.000	0.000	0.979
Heptane	0.275	-0.162	0.000	0.000	0.000	0.983
Octane	0.215	-0.049	0.000	0.000	0.000	0.967
Nonane	0.200	-0.145	0.000	0.000	0.000	0.980
Decane	0.156	-0.143	0.000	0.000	0.000	0.989
Undecane	0.113	0.000	0.000	0.000	0.000	0.971
Dodecane	0.053	0.000	0.000	0.000	0.000	0.986
Hexadecane	0.000	0.000	0.000	0.000	0.000	1.000
Cyclohexane	0.163	-0.110	0.000	0.000	0.000	1.013
Methylcyclohexane	0.319	-0.215	0.000	0.000	0.000	1.012
Isooctane	0.264	-0.230	0.000	0.000	0.000	0.975
Benzene	0.107	-0.313	1.053	0.457	0.169	1.020
Toluene	0.121	-0.222	0.938	0.467	0.099	1.012
Fluorobenzene	0.181	-0.621	1.432	0.647	0.000	0.986
Chlorobenzene	0.064	-0.399	1.151	0.313	0.171	1.032
Bromobenzene	-0.064	-0.326	1.261	0.323	0.292	1.002
Iodobenzene	-0.171	-0.192	1.197	0.245	0.245	1.002
Nitrobenzene	-0.275	0.001	1.861	1.119	0.000	0.925
Benzonitrile	-0.062	-0.402	1.939	2.007	0.000	0.880
Olive oil	-0.159	-0.277	0.904	1.695	-0.090	0.876
Carbon disulfide	0.101	0.251	0.177	0.027	0.095	1.068
Triolein	0.147	0.254	-0.246	1.520	1.473	0.918
Methanol	-0.039	-0.338	1.317	3.836	1.396	0.773
Ethanol	0.017	-0.232	0.867	3.894	1.192	0.846
Propan-1-ol	-0.042	-0.246	0.749	3.888	1.078	0.874
Butan-1-ol	-0.004	-0.285	0.768	3.705	0.879	0.890
Pentan-1-ol	-0.002	-0.161	0.535	3.778	0.960	0.900
Hexan-1-ol	-0.014	-0.205	0.583	3.621	0.891	0.913

Dry Solvent	c	e	s	a	b	l
Heptan-1-ol	-0.056	-0.216	0.554	3.596	0.803	0.933
Octan-1-ol	-0.147	-0.214	0.561	3.507	0.749	0.943
Decan-1-ol	-0.139	-0.090	0.356	3.547	0.727	0.958
Propan-2-ol	-0.048	-0.324	0.713	4.036	1.055	0.884
Isobutanol	-0.034	-0.387	0.719	3.736	1.088	0.905
sec-Butanol	-0.003	-0.357	0.699	3.595	1.247	0.881
tert-Butanol	0.053	-0.443	0.699	4.026	0.882	0.907
3-Methyl-1-butanol	-0.052	-0.430	0.628	3.661	0.932	0.937
Pentan-2-ol	-0.031	-0.325	0.496	3.792	1.024	0.934
Ethylene glycol	-0.887	0.132	1.657	4.457	2.355	0.565
2,2,2-Trifluoroethanol	-0.092	-0.547	1.339	2.213	3.807	0.645
Diethyl ether	0.288	-0.379	0.904	2.937	0.000	0.963
Tetrahydrofuran	0.189	-0.347	1.238	3.289	0.000	0.982
1,4-Dioxane	-0.034	-0.354	1.674	3.021	0.000	0.919
Dibutyl ether	0.153	-0.406	0.758	2.152	-0.610	1.008
Methyl tert-butyl ether	0.231	-0.536	0.890	2.623	0.000	0.999
Methyl acetate	0.129	-0.447	1.675	2.625	0.213	0.874
Ethyl acetate	0.182	-0.352	1.316	2.891	0.000	0.916
Butyl acetate	0.147	-0.414	1.212	2.623	0.000	0.954
Propanone	0.127	-0.387	1.733	3.060	0.000	0.866
Butanone	0.112	-0.474	1.671	2.878	0.000	0.916
Cyclohexanone	-0.086	-0.441	1.725	2.786	0.000	0.957
Dimethylformamide	-0.391	-0.869	2.107	3.774	0.000	1.011
Dimethylacetamide	-0.308	-0.736	1.802	4.361	0.000	1.028
Diethylacetamide	-0.075	-0.434	1.911	4.801	0.000	0.899
Dibutylformamide	-0.002	-0.239	1.402	4.029	0.000	0.900
N-Methylpyrolidinone	-0.128	-0.029	2.217	4.429	0.000	0.777
N-Methyl-2-piperidone	-0.264	-0.171	2.086	5.056	0.000	0.883
N-Formylmorpholine	-0.437	0.024	2.631	4.318	0.000	0.712
N-Methylformamide	-0.249	-0.142	1.661	4.147	0.817	0.739
N-Ethylformamide	-0.220	-0.302	1.743	4.498	0.480	0.824
N-Methylacetamide	-0.197	-0.175	1.608	4.867	0.375	0.837
N-Ethylacetamide	-0.018	-0.157	1.352	4.588	0.357	0.824
Formamide	-0.800	0.310	2.292	4.130	1.933	0.442
Acetonitrile	-0.007	-0.595	2.461	2.085	0.418	0.934
Nitromethane	-0.340	-0.297	2.689	2.193	0.514	0.728
Dimethylsulfoxide	-0.556	-0.223	2.903	5.036	0.000	0.719
Tributylphosphate	0.097	-0.098	1.103	2.411	0.588	0.844
Propylene carbonate	-0.356	-0.413	2.587	2.207	0.455	0.719
Gas-water	-1.271	0.822	2.743	3.904	4.814	-0.213

Table 2. Coefficients in Eqn. 6 for Correlating Solute Solubility in Dry Organic Solvents at 298 K

Three specific conditions must be met in order to use the Abraham solvation parameter model to predict saturation solubilities. First, the same solid phase must be in equilibrium with the saturation solutions in the organic solvent and in water (i.e., there should be no solvate or hydrate formation). Second, the secondary medium activity coefficient of the solid in the saturated solutions must be unity (or near unity). This condition generally restricts the method to those solutes that are sparingly soluble in water and nonaqueous solvents. Finally, for solutes that are ionized in aqueous solution, $C_{A,water}$, refers to the solubility of the neutral form. The second restriction may not be as important as initially believed. The Abraham solvation parameter model has shown remarkable success in correlating the solubility of several very soluble crystalline solutes. For example, Eqns 5 and 6 described the molar solubility of benzil in 24 organic solvents to within overall standard deviations of 0.124 and 0.109 log units, respectively. Standard deviations for acetylsalicylic acid dissolved in 13 alcohols, 4 ethers and ethyl acetate were 0.123 and 0.138 log units. Benzil (Acree and Abraham, 2002) and acetylsalicylic acid (Charlton et al., 2003) exhibited solubilities exceeding 1Molar in several of the organic solvents studied. In the case of acetylsalicylic acid it could be argued that the model's success relates back to when the equation coefficients were originally calculated for the dry solvents. The databases used in the regression analyses contained very few carboxylic acid solutes (benzoic acid, 2-hydroxybenzoic acid and 4-hydroxybenzoic acid). Most of the experimental data for carboxylic acids and other very acidic solutes was in the form of saturation solubilities, which were also in the 1 to 3 Molar range. Such arguments do not explain why equations (5) and (6) described the measured benzil solubility data. The benzil solubilities were measured after most of the equation coefficients were first determined.

4. High throughput experimental methods for measuring water-to-octanol partition coefficients

Each administered drug has to pass several membrane barriers in order to be delivered to the desired target site for therapeutic action. Orally administered drugs have to be absorbed into the intestine. Transdermally administered drugs need to penetrate human skin. Drugs intended to act in the central nervous system must cross the blood-brain brain barrier (BBB). This barrier is formed by the endothelial cells of the cerebral capillaries and restricts the transport of many compounds into the brain from the blood stream. The cellular architecture of the human intestine, human skin and human brain are quite different; however, the principle of transcellular absorption is the same. The dissolved drug must be transferred from an aqueous environment into the membrane phase, must diffuse across the membrane, and afterwards must partition back into an aqueous-phase compartment. The water-to-octanol partition coefficient, $P_{o/w}$, is widely regarded in the pharmaceutical industry as a quantitative measure for assessing a drug molecule's affinity for the membrane phase. Considerable attention has been afforded to developing high throughput experimental methodologies that either directly measure $P_{o/w}$ values, or that enable accurate estimation of $P_{o/w}$ from other conveniently measured properties. Poole and Poole (2003) reviewed the direct and indirect separation for obtaining water-to-octanol partition coefficients, with emphasis on the high throughput methods.

As selected examples of experimental methods that have been developed in recent years, Faller and coworkers (2005) designed a rather novel high throughput method to measure lipophilicity based on the diffusion of organic compounds between to aqueous phase compartments separated by a thin 1-octanol liquid layer coated on a polycarbonate filter. The apparatus is shown in Figure 5. The molar concentration of the compound in the aqueous acceptor compartment, $C_{acceptor,end}$ is measured at the end of the defined time endpoint, tend. The apparent membrane permeability, P_{app}, is calculated from $C_{acceptor,end}$ by

$$P_{app} = -(\frac{V_{acceptor} V_{donor}}{V_{acceptor} + V_{donor}})(\frac{1}{A t_{end}})\ln(1 - \frac{C_{acceptor,end}}{C_{equ}}) \tag{7}$$

$$C_{equ} = (\frac{V_{donor}}{V_{donor} + V_{acceptor}}) C_{donor,initial} \tag{8}$$

where $V_{acceptor}$ and V_{donor} denote the aqueous phase volumes in the acceptor and donor compartments, respectively, $C_{donor,initial}$ refers to the initial compound concentration in the donor phase, and A is the membrane accessible surface area times porosity. The water-to-octanol partition coefficient, $P_{o/w}$, is derived from the measured apparent permeability using a calibration curve constructed from measured permeabilities of standard compounds of known $P_{o/w}$ values. The assay has been used to measure water-to-hexadecane partition coefficients (Wohnsland and Faller, 2001) and can be performed using 96-well microtiter plates.

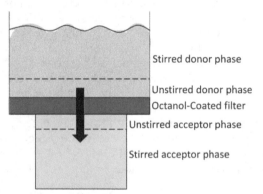

Fig. 5. High throughput experimental method for measuring water-to- octanol partition coefficients based on the diffusion of a solute betweentwo aqueous phase compartments.

Gao *et al.* (2005) developed a miniaturized method involving the dispersion of colloidal stable porous silica-encapsulated magnetic nanoparticles into water and/or an aqueous-buffered solution. Prior to dispersion, the nanoparticles are preloaded with a known amount of 1-octanol. Equilibrium is quickly established between the drug dissolved in the aqueous (or aqueous-buffered) solution and the small octanol droplets on the nanoparticles. The paramagnetic properties of the nanoparticles facilitate magnetic-induced phase separation. Once the magnetic particles are removed, the uv/visible absorbance of the solution is recorded. The log $P_{o/w}$ (or log Do/w in the case of an ionic solute) is calculated as

$$\log P_{o/w} = \log [(\frac{Abs_{before} - Abs_{after}}{Abs_{after}})(\frac{V_{aqueous}}{V_{oc\tan ol}})] \tag{9}$$

where Abs_{before} and Abs_{after} refer to the measured uv/visible absorbance of the aqueous solution prior and after partitioning, respectively, and $V_{aqueous}/V_{octanol}$ is the ratio of the aqueous phase volume divided by the volume of the octanol phase.

Henchoz and coworkers (2010) determined the water-to-octanol partition coefficients of 21 acidic and 29 basic pharmaceutical compounds using microemulsion electrokinetic capillary chromatography (MEEKC) coupled with uv absorption and mass spectrometric detection. The method involves measuring the retention factor of the investigated compound

$$k_{solute} = \frac{(t_{r,solute} - t_{r,eof})}{(1 - \frac{t_{r,solute}}{t_{r,mc}})t_{r,eof}} \tag{10}$$

where $t_{r,solute}$, $t_{r,eof}$ and $t_{r,mc}$ are the retention/migration times of the investigated drug compound, a highly hydrophilic neutral marker (such as dimethyl sulfoxide) and a highly lipophilic pseudostationary phase marker (such as dodecanophenone or 1-phenyldodecane). The migration times of the two markers define the migration window. The log $P_{o/w}$ of the drug molecules are obtained from a calibration curve

$$\log k_{solute} = slope \cdot \log P_{o/w} + intercept \tag{11}$$

established with the measured retention factors of standard compounds with known log $P_{o/w}$ values. The proposed method was validated using a set of 35 well-balanced reference compounds that contained neutral, acidic ($pK_a > 3.6$) or basic ($pK_a < 5.5$) compounds with log $P_{o/w}$ values ranging from 0.7 to 4.8. The acidic compounds were analyzed at a pH = 2, while the neutral and basic compounds were analyzed at pH = 10. The authors found that the log $P_{o/w}$ values based on MEEKC method differed by less than 0.5 log units from the log $P_{o/w}$ values determined by the more traditional shake-flask method. The method allowed log $P_{o/w}$ measurement in less than 20 minutes, which is acceptable for quick screening methods. The authors further noted that the MEEKC method could be easily automated, consumed very little sample and solvent, and did not require a highly purified drug sample. Logarithms of the water-to-organic solvent partition coefficients represent another solute property that has been successfully correlated by Eqn. 12 of the Abraham solvation parameter model.

$$\text{Log } P = c + e \cdot E + s \cdot S + a \cdot A + b \cdot B + v \cdot V \tag{12}$$

In Table 3 we have compiled the equation coefficients that have been reported describing the various water-to-organic solvent partitioning systems that have been studied. In the case of the alkane and chloroalkane (dichloromethane, trichloromethane, tetrachloromethane, 1,2-dichloroethane and 1-chlorobutane) solvents, one will note that the equation coefficients for describing log P are identical to the coefficients for correlating the log molar solubility ratios, log ($C_{A,organic}/C_{A,water}$) values. As noted previous the molar solubility ratios describe a "hypothetic partitioning" processes for solute transfer to an anhydrous "dry" organic solvent. Solubility ratios and practical partition coefficients are nearly identical for solvents that are almost "completely" immiscible with water.

Water-organic solvent based biphasic systems are widely used in liquid-liquid extraction and in calculating Abraham model solute descriptors in accordance with Eqn. 12. For compounds that react with water, or for compounds that have very low aqueous solubilities, water-based

Wet Solvent	c	e	s	a	b	v
Butan-1-ol[a]	0.376	0.434	-0.718	-0.097	-2.350	2.682
Pentan-1-ol[a]	0.185	0.367	-0.732	0.105	-3.100	3.395
Hexan-1-ol[a]	-0.006	0.460	-0.940	0.142	-3.284	3.792
Heptan-1-ol[a]	0.041	0.497	-0.976	0.030	-3.438	3.859
Octan-1-ol[a]	0.088	0.562	-1.054	0.034	-3.460	3.814
Nonan-1-ol[a]	-0.041	0.562	-1.103	0.090	-3.540	3.922
Decan-1-ol[a]	-0.136	0.542	-0.989	0.046	-3.722	3.996
Isobutanol[a]	0.249	0.480	-0.639	-0.050	-2.284	2.758
Olely alcohol [a]	-0.096	0.148	-0.841	-0.438	-4.040	4.125
Dichloromethane	0.319	0.102	-0.187	-3.058	-4.090	4.324
Trichloromethane	0.191	0.105	-0.403	-3.112	-3.514	4.395
Tetrachloromethane	0.199	0.523	-1.159	-3.560	-4.594	4.618
1,2-Dichloroethane	0.183	0.294	-0.134	-2.801	-4.291	4.180
1-Chlorobutane	0.222	0.273	-0.569	-2.918	-4.883	4.456
Butane	0.297	-0.005	-1.584	-3.188	-4.567	4.562
Pentane	0.369	0.386	-1.568	-3.535	-5.215	4.514
Hexane	0.361	0.579	-1.723	-3.599	-4.764	4.344
Heptane	0.325	0.670	-2.061	-3.317	-4.733	4.543
Octane	0.223	0.642	-1.647	-3.480	-5.067	4.526
Nonane	0.240	0.619	-1.713	-3.532	-4.921	4.482
Decane	0.160	0.585	-1.734	-3.435	-5.078	4.582
Undecane	0.058	0.603	-1.661	-3.421	-5.120	4.619
Dodecane	0.114	0.668	-1.664	-3.545	-5.006	4.459
Hexadecane	0.087	0.667	-1.617	-3.587	-4.869	4.433
Cyclohexane	0.159	0.784	-1.678	-3.740	-4.929	4.577
Methylcyclohexane	0.246	0.782	-1.982	-3.517	-4.293	4.528
Isooctane	0.318	0.555	-1.737	-3.677	-4.864	4.417
Benzene	0.142	0.464	-0.588	-3.099	-4.625	4.491
Toluene	0.143	0.527	-0.720	-3.010	-4.824	4.545
Fluorobenzene	0.139	0.152	-0.374	-3.030	-4.601	4.540
Chlorobenzene	0.065	0.381	-0.521	-3.183	-4.700	4.614
Bromobenzene	-0.017	0.436	-0.424	-3.174	-4.558	4.445
Iodobenzene	-0.192	0.298	-0.308	-3.213	-4.653	4.588
Nitrobenzene	-0.152	0.525	0.081	-2.332	-4.494	4.187
Diethyl ether[a]	0.248	0.561	-1.016	-0.226	-4.553	4.075
Diisopropyl ether[a]	0.472	0.413	-0.745	-0.632	-5.251	4.059
Dibutyl ether	0.252	0.677	-1.506	-0.807	-5.249	4.815
o-Nitrophenyl octyl ether	0.121	0.600	-0.459	-2.246	-3.879	3.574
Ethyl acetate[a]	0.441	0.591	-0.699	-0.325	-4.261	3.666
Butyl acetate[a]	-0.475	0.428	-0.094	-0.241	-4.151	4.046
PGDP[b]	0.256	0.501	-0.828	-1.022	-4.640	4.033
Methyl isobutyl ketone	0.383	0.801	-0.831	-0.121	-4.441	3.876
Olive oil	-0.035	0.574	-0.798	-1.422	-4.984	4.210

Carbon disulfide	0.047	0.686	-0.943	-3.603	-5.818	4.921
Isopropyl myristate	-0.605	0.930	-1.153	-1.682	-4.093	4.249
Triolein	0.385	0.983	-2.083	-2.007	-3.452	4.072

[a] Correlation uses the Bo solute descriptor.
[b] Propylene glycol dipelargonate.

Table 3. Coefficients in Eqn. 12 for Correlating Solute Water-to-Organic Solvent log P values at 298 K

Wet Solvent	c	e	s	a	b	l
Butan-1-ol	-0.095	0.262	1.396	3.405	2.565	0.523
Pentan-1-ol	-0.107	-0.001	1.188	3.614	1.671	0.721
Hexan-1-ol	-0.302	-0.046	0.880	3.609	1.785	0.824
Heptan-1-ol	-0.159	0.018	0.825	3.539	1.425	0.830
Octan-1-ol	-0.198	0.002	0.709	3.519	1.429	0.858
Nonan-1-ol	-0.197	0.141	0.694	3.616	1.299	0.827
Decan-1-ol	-0.302	0.233	0.741	3.531	1.177	0.835
Isobutanol	-0.095	0.262	1.396	3.405	2.565	0.523
Olely alcohol	-0.268	-0.392	0.800	3.117	0.978	0.918
Dichloromethane	0.192	-0.572	1.492	0.460	0.847	0.965
Trichloromethane	0.157	-0.560	1.259	0.374	1.333	0.976
Tetrachloromethane	0.217	-0.435	0.554	0.000	0.000	1.069
1,2-Dichloroethane	0.017	-0.337	1.600	0.774	0.637	0.921
1-Chlorobutane	0.130	-0.581	1.114	0.724	0.000	1.016
Butane	0.291	-0.360	0.091	0.000	0.000	0.959
Pentane	0.335	-0.276	0.000	0.000	0.000	0.968
Hexane	0.292	-0.169	0.000	0.000	0.000	0.979
Heptane	0.275	-0.162	0.000	0.000	0.000	0.983
Octane	0.215	-0.049	0.000	0.000	0.000	0.967
Nonane	0.200	-0.145	0.000	0.000	0.000	0.980
Decane	0.156	-0.143	0.000	0.000	0.000	0.989
Undecane	0.113	0.000	0.000	0.000	0.000	0.971
Dodecane	0.017	0.000	0.000	0.000	0.000	0.989
Hexadecane	0.000	0.000	0.000	0.000	0.000	1.000
Cyclohexane	0.163	-0.110	0.000	0.000	0.000	1.013
Methylcyclohexane	0.318	-0.215	0.000	0.000	0.000	1.012
Isooctane	0.264	-0.230	0.000	0.000	0.000	0.975
Benzene	0.107	-0.313	1.053	0.457	0.169	1.020
Toluene	0.121	-0.222	0.938	0.467	0.099	1.012
Fluorobenzene	0.181	-0.621	1.432	0.647	0.000	0.986
Chlorobenzene	0.064	-0.399	1.151	0.313	0.171	1.032
Bromobenzene	-0.064	-0.326	1.261	0.323	0.292	1.002
Iodobenzene	-0.171	-0.192	1.197	0.245	0.245	1.002
Nitrobenzene	-0.296	0.092	1.707	1.147	0.443	0.912
Benzonitrile	-0.067	-0.257	1.848	2.009	0.227	0.870

Diethyl ether	0.206	-0.169	0.873	3.402	0.000	0.882
Dipropyl ether	0.065	-0.202	0.776	3.074	0.000	0.948
Diisopropyl ether	0.114	-0.032	0.685	3.108	0.000	0.941
Dibutyl ether	0.369	-0.216	0.026	2.626	-0.499	1.124
Ethyl acetate	0.130	0.031	1.202	3.199	0.463	0.828
Butyl acetate	-0.664	0.061	1.671	3.373	0.824	0.832
Methyl isobutyl ketone	0.244	0.183	0.987	3.418	0.323	0.854
Olive oil	-0.156	-0.254	0.859	1.656	0.000	0.873
Carbon disulfide	0.101	0.251	0.177	0.027	0.095	1.068
Triolein	0.147	0.254	-0.246	1.520	1.473	0.918

Table 4. Coefficients in Eqn. 2 for Correlating Solute Gas-to-Organic Solvent log K values at 298 K

partitioning systems may not be appropriate. Poole and coworkers (Karunasekara and Poole, 2010; Qian and Poole, 2007; Ahmed and Poole, 2006a,b) have reported Abraham model correlations for several totally organic biphasic systems, such as heptane + formamide, hexane + acetonitrile, heptane + methanol, heptane + N,N-dimethylformamide, heptane + 2,2,2-trifluoroethanol, and heptane + 1,1,1,3,3,3-hexafluoroisopropanol. The organic-based biphasic systems allow one to calculate solute descriptors for compounds that might not otherwise be possible with water-based partitioning systems. For example, the biphasic hexane + acetonitrile, heptane + N,N-dimethylformamide, and heptane + 2,2,2-trifluoroethanol systems were used, in combination with chromatographic retention factors, to determine a complete set of descriptors for organosilicon compounds (Atapattu and Poole, 2009; Ahmed et al., 2007), many of which react with water. Abraham model equation coefficients are tabulated in Table 5 for seven organic solvent-to-organic solvent partitioning systems.

Partitioning system	c	e	s	a	b	v
Formamide-to-heptane	0.083	0.559	-2.244	-3.250	-1.614	2.384
N,N-Dimethylformamide-to-heptane	0.065	0.030	-1.405	-2.039	-0.806	0.721
2,2,2-Trifluoroethanol-to-heptane	0.160	0.856	-1.538	-1.325	-2.965	1.190
1,1,1,3,3,3-Hexafluoroisopropanol-to-heptane	-0.225	0.720	-1.357	-0.577	-2.819	1.161
Methanol-to-heptane	-0.056	0.164	-0.620	-1.337	-0.957	0.507
Ethylene glycol-to-heptane	0.343	0.000	-1.247	3.807	-2.194	2.065
Acetonitrile-to-hexane	0.097	0.189	-1.332	-1.649	-0.966	0.773

Table 5. Coefficients in Eqn. 12 for Correlating Solute Organic Solvent-to-Organic Solvent log P values at 298 K

5. Calculation of Abraham solute descriptors from measured solubility and partition coefficient data

The application of Eqn. 1 and Eqn. 2 requires a knowledge of the descriptors (or properties) of the solutes: E, S, A, B, V and L. The descriptors E and V are quite easily obtained. V can be calculated from atom and bond contributions as outlined previously (Abraham and McGowan, 1987). The atom contributions are in Table 6; note that they are in cm^3 mol^{-1}. The bond contribution is 6.56 cm^3 mol $^{-1}$ for each bond, no matter whether single, double, or triple, to be subtracted. For complicated molecules it is time consuming to count the number of bonds, Bn, but this can be calculated from the algorithm given by Abraham (1993a)

$$Bn = Nt - 1 + R \tag{13}$$

where Nt is the total number of atoms in the molecule and R is the number of rings.

Once **V** is available, **E** can be obtained from the compound refractive index at 20°C. If the compound is not liquid at room temperature or if the refractive index is not known the latter can be calculated using the freeware software of Advanced Chemistry Development (ACD). An Excel spreadsheet for the calculation of **V** and **E** from refractive index is available from the authors. Since **E** is almost an additive property, it can also be obtained by the summation of fragments, either by hand, or through a commercial software program (ADME Boxes, 2010). There remain the descriptors **S, A, B**, and **L** to be determined.

Partition coefficients and/or solubilities can be used to obtain all the four remaining descriptors (Abraham et al., 2004). Suppose there are available solubilities for a given compound in water and a number of solvents. Then solubility ratios, log ($C_{A,organic}/C_{A,water}$), can be obtained as shown in Eqn. 5 and Eqn. 6. If three solubility ratios are available for three solvent systems shown in Table 1, we have three equations and three unknowns (**S, A,** and **B**) so that the latter can be determined. Of more practical use is a situation where several solubility ratios are known. Then if we have, say, six solubility ratios and three equations, the three unknowns can be obtained as the descriptors that give the best fit to the six equations. The Solver add-on program to Excel can be set up to carry out such a calculation automatically. However, it is possible to increase the number of equations by the stratagem of converting the water-to-solvent solubility ratios into gas to solvent solubility ratios, $C_{A,organic}/C_{A,gas}$

$$C_{A,organic}/C_{A,water} * C_{A,water}/C_{A,gas} = C_{A,organic}/C_{A,gas} \tag{14}$$

The ratio $C_{A,water}/C_{A,gas}$ is the gas-to-water partition coefficient, usually denoted as K_w. A further set of equations is available for gas-to-solvent solubility ratios, Table 2. Thus six water-to-solvent solubility ratios can be converted into six gas-to-solvent solubility ratios, leading to a set of 12 equations. If logK_w is not known, it can be used as another parameter to be determined. This increases the number of unknowns from four (**S, A, B, L**) to five (**S, A, B, L**, logK_w) but the number of equations is increased from six to twelve. In addition, two equations are available for gas to solvent partitions themselves, see the last entries in Tables 1 and 2, making for the present case no fewer than fourteen equations.

As an example, we use data on solubilities of trimethoprim in eight solvents (Li et al., 2008) converted from mol fraction to mol dm^{-3}. The solubility in water was not given, but is known to be 2.09* 10^{-3} in mol dm^{-3} (Howard and Meylan, 1997). The eight observed solubility ratios, $C_{A,organic}/C_{A,water}$, are in Table 7, as log (ratio). We took log K_w as another parameter to be determined, leading to no less than 18 equations: the eight original equations from solubilities in the eight solvents that led to $C_{A,organic}/C_{A,water}$, the corresponding eight equations for $C_{A,organic}/C_{A,gas}$, and two equations for $C_{A,water}/C_{A,gas}$ (ie K_w). With **E** fixed at 1.892 and **V** fixed at 2.1813, the best fit values of the descriptors were **S** = 2.52, **A** = 0.44, **B** = 1.69, **L** = 11.81 and log K_w = 14.49; these yielded the calculated log (ratios) in Table 7. For all 18 values, the Average Error = -0.002, the Absolute Average Error = 0.092, the RMSE = 0.107, and the SD = 0.110 log unit. Not only do the original solubilities allow the derivation of descriptors for trimethoprim, but the latter, in turn, allow the prediction of solubility ratios and hence actual solubilities in all the solvents listed in Table 1.

Exactly the same procedure is adopted if actual partition coefficients are experimentally available, rather than solubilities. The relevant equations are now those in Table 3 and Table 4. Of course if both solubilities and actual partition coefficients have both been experimentally determined, a combination of equations from Tables 1 and 2 and from Tables 3 and 4 can be used. Even though partition coefficients refer to partition into wet solvents, descriptors obtained from partition coefficients using equations in Table 3 and Table 4 can still be used to predict solubility ratios and solubilities in dry solvents for all the solvents listed in Table 1.

C	16.35	N	14.39	O	12.43
Si	26.83	P	24.87	S	22.91
Ge	31.02	As	29.42	Se	27.81
Sn	39.35	Sb	37.74	Te	36.14
Pb	43.44	Bi	42.19		
H	8.71	He	6.76	B	18.32
F	10.48	Ne	8.51	Hg	34.00
Cl	20.95	A	1.90		
Br	26.21	Kr	2.46		
I	34.53	Xe	3.29		
		Rn	3.84		

Table 6. Atom contributions to the McGowan volume, in $cm^3 \ mol^{-1}$

Water-to-solvent	calc	obs
Methanol	1.35	1.48
Ethanol	0.98	0.94
Propanol	0.75	0.80
Butanol	0.53	0.68
2-Propanol	0.61	0.51
2-Butanol	0.65	0.62
Tetrahydrofuran	1.18	1.02
Propanone	0.90	0.94
Gas to water	14.48	14.49
Gas-to-solvent	calc	obs
Methanol	15.81	15.97
Ethanol	15.48	15.43
Propanol	15.23	15.29
Butanol	15.02	15.18
2-Propanol	15.14	15.01
2-Butanol	15.18	15.11
Tetrahydrofuran	15.70	15.51
Propanone	15.34	15.43
Gas to water	14.53	14.49

Table 7. Solubility ratios for trimethoprim, as log (ratio)

Although we have set out the determination of descriptors from experimental measurements, it is still very helpful to use the ACD software (ADME Boxes, 2010) to calculate the descriptors at the same time. Occasionally there may be erroneous solubility measurements, or solubilities may be affected through solvate formation, and the calculated descriptors afford a useful check on the obtained descriptors from experiment measurements.

6. Abraham solvation parameter model: prediction of blood-to-brain and blood-to-iissue partition coefficient

Successful drug development requires efficient delivery of the drug to the target site. The drug must cross various cellular barriers by passive and/or transporter-mediated uptake. Drug delivery to the brain is particularly challenging as there are two physiologically barriers – the blood-brain barrier (BBB) and the blood-cerebrospinal fluid barrier (BCSFB) – separating the brain from its blood supply controlling the transport of chemical compounds. The BBB is a continuous layer of microvessel endothelial cells, connected by highly-developed tight junctions, which effectively restrict paracellular transport of molecules irrespective of their molecular size. Tight junctions provide significant transendothelial electrical resistance to the brain microvessel endothelial cells and serves to further impede the penetration of the BBB. The electrical resistance between the endothelial cells is on the order of 1500 – 2000 Ω/cm^2, as compared to and electrical resistance of 3.33 Ω/cm^2 found in other body tissues (Alam et al., 2010). Under normal conditions the BBB acts as a barrier to toxic agents and safeguards the integrity of the brain. A compound may circumvent the BBB and gain access to the brain by the nose-to-brain route. The compound is transported to the brain via an olfactory pathway following absorption across the nasal mucosa.

Alternatively, compounds may permeate from the blood into the cerebrospinal fluid and permeate into the brain interstitial fluid. The BCSFB separates the blood from the cerebrospinal fluid (CSF) that runs in the subarachnoid space surrounding the brain. The BCSFB is located at the choroid plexus, and it is composed of epithelial cells held together at their apices by tight junctions, which limit paracellular flux. Hence compounds penetrate the barrier transcellularly. The CSF-facing surface of the epithelial cells, which secrete CSF into the ventricles, is increased by the presence of microvilli. The capillaries in the choroid plexus allow free movement of molecules via fenestractions and intracellular gaps. Transport across the BCSFB is not an accurate measure of transport across the BBB as the two barriers are anatomically different. However, as Begley et al. (2000) point out, for many compounds there is a permanently maintained concentration gradient between brain interstitial fluid and the CSF.

The transport of compounds into the brain can take place through 'passive' transport or 'active' transport. Nearly all the calculational models for transport into the brain deal with passive transport, although it is now known that many compounds are prevented from crossing the BBB through efflux mechanisms especially involving P-glycoprotein. The use of wildtype mice and knockout mice (the latter deficient in Pgp) has shown conclusively that for a number of drugs the brain to plasma distribution is much lower for the wildtype mice than for knockout mice. We will focus on passive transport, but it must be appreciated that any analysis might well include compounds that are actually subject to active transport and will appear as outliers in the analyses.

The steady-state distribution of a compound between the blood (or plasma) and brain, and the rate of permeation of a compound from blood (or from an aqueous saline solution) through the blood brain barrier, are two quantitative measures of drug uptake in the brain.

The logarithm of the blood-to-brain concentration ratio, log BB, is a thermodynamic quantity defining the extent of blood penetration. The log BB is mathematically given by

$$\log BB = (\frac{C_{solute,brain}}{C_{solute,blood}}) \qquad (15)$$

the ratio of the solute concentration in brain tissue divided by the solute's concentration in blood (or serum or plasma) at steady-state conditions. The blood/brain distribution ratio can be experimentally determined by intravenous administration of a single injection of ^{14}C-radioactive isotope labeled test substance in rats. The animal is sacrificed at a specified time endpoint after equilibrium is achieved. The brain and blood are immediately harvested, and the concentration in each biological sample is quantified from the measured radioactivity. Isotopic labeling provides a convenient means to distinguish the injected test substance from all other chemicals that might be present in the body. Radioactive counting methods do not distinguish between the radioactive isotope in the injected test substance and any degradation products that might have been formed before the animal was sacrificed. The distribution experiments are usually carried out over a long time scale, possibly hours, and concentrations in blood and brain obtained as a function of time. The ratio, as Eq. 15, will change with time and only if it reaches a constant value can the ratio be taken as an equilibrium value. This is very time consuming indeed, as only one measurement can be made with each rat. Despite these shortcomings, radioactive labeling is one of the more popular methods for not only determining the blood-to-brain distribution coefficient, but other blood-to-tissue partition coefficients as well.

Blood-to-brain and blood-to-tissue partition coefficients have also been measured for volatile organic compounds using the *in vitro* vial method (see Figure 6). A known amount of animal sample is placed in a glass vial of known volume. The vial is then sealed and a minute known quantity of the volatile organic compound (VOC) is introduced by syringe through the rubber septum. After equilibration a sample of the headspace vapor phase is withdrawn from the glass vial for gas chromatographic analysis. The gas-to-tissue partition coefficient is computed from mass balance considerations as the total amount of solute added, the concentration of the vapor phase, the headspace volume and amount of tissue sample are all known. The blood-to-tissue partition coefficient, $P_{tissue/blood}$, is calculated as

$$P_{tissue/blood} = P_{tissue/air} x P_{air/blood} = (\frac{C_{solute,tissue}}{C_{solute,air}}) x (\frac{C_{solute,air}}{C_{solute,blood}}) \qquad (16)$$

the product of the measured air-to-tissue partition coefficient, $P_{tissue/air}$, times the measured blood-to-air partition coefficient, $P_{air/blood}$. The *in vitro* partition coefficient data are important and are used as required input parameters in pharmacokinetic models developed to determine the disposition of volatile organic compounds that individuals inhale in the workplace and in the environment.

Abraham and coworkers (2006a) reported correlation models for the air-to-brain ($P_{brain/air}$) and blood-to-brain ($P_{brain/blood}$) partition coefficients for VOCs in humans and rats

$$\text{Log } P_{brain/air} (in\ vitro) = -0.987 + 0.263E + 0.411S + 3.358A + 2.025B + 0.591L$$
$$\left(N = 81,\ R^2 = 0.923,\ SD = 0.346,\ RMSE = 0.333,\ F = 179.0 \right) \qquad (17)$$

$$\text{Log BB} = \text{Log P}_{\text{brain/blood}}\,(in\ vitro) = -0.057 + 0.017\mathbf{E} - 0.536\mathbf{S} - 0.323\mathbf{A} - 0.335\mathbf{B} + 0.731\mathbf{V}$$
$$\left(\text{N} = 78,\ \text{R}^2 = 0.725,\ \text{SD} = 0.203,\ \text{RMSE} = 0.196,\ \text{F} = 37.9\right)$$
(18)

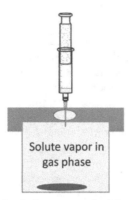

Solute vapor in
gas phase

Fig. 6. Equilibrium vial technique depicting removal of the equilibrated headspace vapor above the animal/human tissue

In Eqns. 17 and 18, N is the number of data points in the regression analysis, R^2 represents the squared correlation coefficient, SD denotes the standard deviation and RMSE corresponds to the root mean square error. Note that in a multiple linear regression equation, the denominator in the definition of SD is N – P – 1 and in the definition of RMSE it is N – P, where P is the number of independent variables in the equation. The derived correlations provided a reasonably accurate mathematical description of the observed partition coefficient data as evidenced by the high squared correlation coefficients and reasonably small standard deviations. Both correlations were validated using training set and test set analyses. In comparing calculated biological data to observed values one must remember that the measured values do have larger experimental uncertainties. A reasonable estimated uncertainty for the measured log $P_{\text{brain/air}}$ would be about 0.2 log units based on independent values from different laboratories. Rat and human partition coefficient data for each given VOC were averaged (if both values were available), and the average values were combined into a single regression analysis. In a comparison of experimental human and rat partition coefficient data for 17 common compounds, the authors had shown that the two sets of data (human versus rat) differed by only 0.062 log units, which is likely less than the experimental uncertainty associated with the measured experimental values. For the compounds studied, human and rat partition coefficient data were identical for all practical purposes. The authors also showed that blood-to-brain and plasma-to-brain partition coefficients were sufficiently close and could be combined into a single Abraham model correlation

$$\log P_{\text{brain/(blood,plasma)}} = -0.028 + 0.003\ \mathbf{E} - 0.485\ \mathbf{S} - 0.117\ \mathbf{A} - 0.408\ \mathbf{B} + 0.703\ \mathbf{V}$$
$$\left(\text{N} = 99,\ \text{R}^2 = 0.703,\ \text{SD} = 0.197,\ \text{RMSE} = 0.191,\ \text{F} = 44.1\right)$$
(19)

Eqs. (18) and (19), are not substantially different, and the statistics are almost the same. It is a moot point as to whether further values of blood to brain partition coefficients should best be predicted through Eqn. 18 or 19. We recommend that Eqn. 18 be used to predict blood-to-brain partition coefficients of VOC because it refers specifically to blood rather than to blood or plasma.

A follow-up study (Abraham et al., 2006b) considered the partitioning behavior of drugs and drug candidates (measured by in vivo experimental methods), as well as the VOC in vitro partition coefficient data discussed above. The Abraham model correlation for the in vivo log $P_{\text{brain/blood}}$ data

$$\log BB = \log P_{\text{brain/blood}}(in\ vivo) = 0.547 + 0.221\mathbf{E} - 0.604\mathbf{S} - 0.641\mathbf{A} - 0.681\mathbf{B} + 0.635\mathbf{V} - 1.216\mathbf{Ic}$$

$$\left(N = 233, R^2 = 0.75, SD = 0.33, F = 113\right)$$

(20)

differs from the correlation equation for the VOCs (see Eqn. 18). In particular, the c-coefficients differ appreciably 0.547 (SD = 0.078) as against -0.024 (SD=0.069), which suggests that there is a systematic difference between the in vivo and in vitro distributions. The authors went on to show that the difference resulted in part because the two sets of compounds (drugs versus VOCs) inhabit different areas in chemical space. The in vivo drug compounds had much larger solute descriptors, and included compounds having a carboxylic acid functional group. The independent variable $\mathbf{Ic}$ was needed as an indicator descriptor for carboxylic acids ($\mathbf{Ic} = 1$ for carboxylic acids, $\mathbf{Ic} = 0$ for noncarboxylic acid solutes).

The blood-to-brain partition coefficient provides valuable information regarding a compound's ability to penetrate the blood-brain barrier. Cruciani et al. (2000) noted that compounds having log BB values greater than 0.0 (concentration in the brain exceeds concentration in the blood) should cross the barrier, whereas compounds having log BB less than -0.3 tended not to cross the barrier. Li and coworkers (2005) used a slightly different classification scheme (see Figure 7) of dividing compounds into BBB-penetrating (BBB+) or BBB-non-penetrating (BBB-) according to whether the log BB value was ≥ -1 or ≤ -1, respectively. Many times an actual numerical log BB is not needed in the decision making process, and in such cases, an indication of BBB+ or BBB- is often sufficient. Zhao et al. (2007) proposed a fairly simple decision tree for classifying drug candidates as BBB+ or BBB- based on their Abraham solute descriptors (See Figure 7). Solute acidity and solute basicity were the two most important properties governing BBB penetration, with solute excess molar refraction playing a much smaller role. The proposed classification scheme correctly predicted the BBB penetration of 90 % of the 1093 compounds considered.

As noted above permeation of a compound from blood (or from an aqueous saline solution) through the blood brain barrier can be used to indicate drug uptake in the brain. The membrane permeability-surface area product, PS, is a kinetic parameter used in describing initial rate of unidirectional transfer

$$k_{in} = F\left(1 - e^{-PS/F}\right)$$

(21)

where k_{in} is the measured transfer constant and F is the perfusion fluid flow expressed in milliliters per second per gram. For solutes that bind rapidly and reversibly to plasma proteins, Eqn. 21 is modified as follows

$$k_{in} = F\left(1 - e^{-fu\,PS/F}\right)$$

(22)

assuming that the unbound and bound forms of the drug are in equilibrium in the fluid. In Eqn. 22, fu is the fraction of the unbound drug in the perfusion fluid. In a typical experiment, the drug (dissolved in blood or in an aqueous saline solution) is perfused into the internal carotid artery and the rate of drug uptake is determined by a radioisotope assay method. The animals are sacrificed at various time intervals. The time scale needed to perform the perfusion study is very short – typically no more than a few minutes. Because of the small time scale, perfusion measurements are less subject to degradation effects than are log BB measurements, although the same difficulties over passive and active transport still exist.

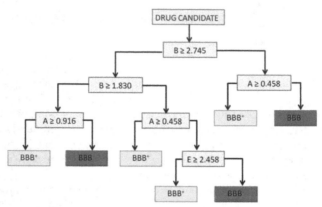

Fig. 7. Decision tree for predicting whether drugs pass through the BBB based on their Abraham solute descriptors. BBB+ indicates BBB penetrating whereas BBB- denotes BBB non-penetration. The right-handside of any decision branch is no penetration (red box), and the left-handside is yes penetration (green box). (The right-hand side of any decision branch is yes, and the left-hand side is no.)

Abraham (2004) derived the following mathematical correlation

$$\log PS = -0.716 - 0.974S - 1.802A - 1.603B + 1.893V$$
$$\left(N = 30, R^2 = 0.868, SD = 0.52, F = 42\right) \tag{23}$$

by regression analysis of the experimental log PS data for 30 neutral compounds from protein-free saline solution buffered at pH of 7.4. The contribution of the e · E term was not significant and was removed from Eqn. 23. The negative equation coefficients in Eqn. 23 indicate that an increase in compound polarity of any kind, that is dipolarity/polarizability, hydrogen-bonding acidity or hydrogen-bonding basicity, results in a decrease in the rate of permeation. Increased solute size (V solute descriptor), on the other hand, results in a greater permeation rate.

The Abraham model correlations that have been presented thus far pertain to neutral molecules. The basic model has been extended to include processes between condensed phases involving ions and ionic species

$$SP = c + e \cdot E + s \cdot S + a \cdot A + b \cdot B + v \cdot V + j_+ \cdot J^+ + j_- \cdot J^- \tag{24}$$

by adding one new term for cations and one new term for anions. J^+ is used whenever a cation is the solute, J^- whenever an anion is the solute, and neither is used whenever the solute is a nonelectrolyte. It is very important to note that the two new ionic descriptors are used together with the descriptors originally chosen for nonelectrolytes. This ensures that values of **S**, **A** and **B** for ions and ionic species are on the same scale as those for nonelectrolytes. Solute descriptors have been reported for many simple cations and anions, for carboxylates, for phenoxides, and for protonated amines and protonated pyridines. The j_+ and j_- equation coefficients have been determined (Abraham and Acree, 2010a,b,c,d) for several of the organic solvents listed in Table 1. Abraham (2011) recently reanalyzed the published log PS data in terms of Eqn. 24 to yield the following correlation model

$$\log PS = -1.268 - 0.047\mathbf{E} - 0.876\mathbf{S} - 0.719\mathbf{A} - 1.571\mathbf{B} + 1.767\mathbf{V} + 0.469\mathbf{J}^+ + 1.663\mathbf{J}^-$$
$$\left(N = 88, R^2 = 0.810, SD = 0.534, F = 48.8\right) \tag{25}$$

The 88 log PS values in Eqn. 25 were for compounds that existed in the saline perfusate entirely (or almost entirely) as neutral molecules or entirely (or almost entirely) as charged species, and which underwent perfusion by a passive process. Abraham showed that log PS values for carboxylate anions are about two log units less than those for the neutral carboxylic acids, and that log PS values for protonated base cations are about one log unit less than those for the neutral bases.

7. Abraham solvation parameter model: prediction of blood-to-tissue and gas-to-tissue partition coefficients

Air-to-blood partitioning is a major determinant governing the uptake of chemical vapors into the blood and their subsequent elimination from blood to exhaled air. Air partitioning processes are becoming increasing more important in the pharmaceutical industry given the large numbers of drugs and vaccines that are now administered by inhalation aerosols and nasal delivery devices. Inhalation drug delivery is appealing given the large surface area for drug absorption, the high blood flow to and from the lung, and the absence of first pass metabolism that is characteristic of the lung. Inhalation drug delivery results in both a rapid clearance action and a rapid onset of therapeutic action, and a reduction in the number of undesired side effects. Eixarch and coworkers (2010) proposed the development of a pulmonary biopharmaceutical classification system (pBCS) that would classify drugs according to their ability to reside in the lung or to be transferred to the bloodstream. The classification scheme would need to consider factors associated with the lung's biology (metabolism, efflux transporters, clearance) and with the drug formulation/physicochemical properties (solubility, lipophilicity, protein binding, particle size, aerosol physics). Blood-to-tissue partitionings govern the distribution throughout the rest of the body once the drug has entered the bloodstream.

Abraham model correlations have been developed to describe the air-to-tissue and blood-to-tissue partition coefficients of drugs and volatile organic compounds (VOCs). The derived mathematical equations include:

Muscle (Abraham *et al.*, 2006c):

$$\log K_{muscle/air}\left(in\ vitro\right) = -1.039 + 0.207\mathbf{E} + 0.723\mathbf{S} + 3.242\mathbf{A} + 2.469\mathbf{B} + 0.463\mathbf{L}$$
$$(N = 114, R^2 = 0.944, SD = 0.267, F = 363) \tag{26}$$

$$\log P_{\text{muscle/blood}} (in\ vitro) = -0.185 - 0.209E - 0.593S - 0.081A - 0.168B + 0.741V$$
$$\left(N = 110, R^2 = 0.537, SD = 0.207, F = 24 \right)$$
(27)

$$\log P_{\text{muscle/blood}} (in\ vivo)\ 0.082 - 0.059E + 0.010S - 0.248A + 0.028\ B + 0.110V - 1.022Ic$$
$$\left(N = 60, R^2 = 0.745, SD = 0.253, F = 25.9 \right)$$
(28)

Fat (Abraham and Ibrahim, 2006):

$$\log K_{\text{fat/air}} (in\ vitro) = -0.052 + 0.051E + 0.728S + 1.783A + 0.332B + 0.743L$$
$$\left(N = 129, R^2 = 0.958, SD = 0.194, F = 562.8 \right)$$
(29)

$$\log P_{\text{fat/blood}} (in\ vitro) = 0.474 + 0.016E - 0.005S - 1.577A - 2.246B + 1.560V$$
$$\left(N = 126, R^2 = 0.847, SD = 0.304, F = 132.7 \right)$$
(30)

$$\log P_{\text{fat/blood}} (in\ vivo) = 0.077 + 0.249E - 0.215\ S - 0.902A - 1.523B + 1.234V - 1.013Ic$$
$$\left(N = 50, R^2 = 0.811, SD = 0.33\ F = 30.7 \right)$$
(31)

Liver (Abraham *et al.*, 2007a):

$$\log K_{\text{liver/air}} (in\ vitro) = -0.943 + 0.836S + 2.836A + 2.081B + 0.561L$$
$$\left(N = 124, R^2 = 0.927, SD = 0.256, F = 376.8 \right)$$
(32)

$$\log P_{\text{liver/blood}} (in\ vitro) = -0.095 - 0.366S - 0.357A - 0.180B + 0.730V$$
$$\left(N = 125, R^2 = 0.583, SD = 0.228, F = 41.9 \right)$$
(33)

$$\log P_{\text{liver/blood}} (in\ vivo) = 0.292 - 0.296S - 0.334A + 0.181B + 0.337V - 0.597Ic$$
$$\left(N = 85, R^2 = 0.522, SD = 0.420, F = 17.3 \right)$$
(34)

Lung (Abraham *et al.*, 2008a):

$$\log K_{\text{lung/air}} (in\ vitro) = -1.250 + 0.639E + 1.038S + 3.661A + 3.041B + 0.420L$$
$$\left(N = 44, R^2 = 0.968, SD = 0.250, F = 231.8 \right)$$
(35)

$$\log P_{\text{lung/blood}} (in\ vitro) = -0.143 - 0.383B + 0.308V$$
$$\left(N = 43, R^2 = 0.264, SD = 0.190, F = 7.2 \right)$$
(36)

Correlations obtained by regression analysis of experimental drug partition coefficient data are denoted as *"in vivo"*, and correlations pertaining to volatile organic compound partitioning are indicated as *"in vitro"*. Human and rat partition coefficient data were combined into data set used in the regression analyses. The independent variable **Ic** was needed as an indicator descriptor for carboxylic acids (Ic = 1 for carboxylic acids, Ic = 0 for noncarboxylic acid solutes) for the *in vivo* correlations involving drug molecules. The *in vivo* data sets included partition coefficient data for drug molecules such as nalidixic acid and valproic acid. No carboxylic acid solutes were contained in the *in vitro* data sets. The poor R^2 statistics noted in several of the blood-to-tissue correlations are due, at least in part, to the small spread in the log P values and the increased experimental uncertainties as noted below. Each derived correlation was validated by training set and test set analyses. Based on the validation computations the derived correlations are expected to predict the log $K_{tissue/air}$ and log $P_{tissue/blood}$ values of additional compounds to within about 0.2 to 0.3 log units.

As an informational note, the experimental data sets for the *in vitro* Abraham model correlations were determined using the equilibrium vial method. The gas-to-tissue partition coefficient of the VOC was calculated from the measured vapor phase composition in the headspace above the given tissue. The measured *in vitro* gas-to-tissue partition coefficients were converted to the corresponding blood-to-tissue values, $P_{tissue/blood}$ values, through Eqn. 16. The $P_{tissue/blood}$ include the experimental uncertainty in both the $K_{tissue/air}$ and $P_{blood/air}$ values. Should the *in vitro* experimental air-to-blood partitioning data not be available for the conversion, one can estimate the needed $P_{blood/air}$ values from the three correlation models

$$\log K_{blood/air}(\text{human}) = -1.18 + 0.39E + 0.97S + 3.80A + 2.69B + 0.41L$$
$$\left(N = 155, R^2 = 0.34, RSME = 0.332, F = 474\right) \tag{37}$$

$$\log K_{blood/air}(\text{rat}) = -0.75 + 0.56E + 1.06S + 3.64A + 2.41B + 0.29L$$
$$\left(N - 127, R^2 = 0.91, SD = 0.29, RMSE = 0.286, F = 242\right) \tag{38}$$

$$\log K_{blood/air}(\text{human or rat}) = -1.069 + 0.456E + 1.083S + 3.738A + 2.580B + 0.376L$$
$$\left(N = 196. R^2 = 0.938, SD = 0.324, RMSE = 0.319, F = 572.8\right) \tag{39}$$

reported by Abraham and coworkers (2005). For any fully characterized system/process (those with calculated values for the equation coefficients) further values of SP (see Eqns. 1 and 2) can be estimated for solutes with known values for the solute descriptors. Solute descriptors can be obtained by regression analysis of measured drug solubilities in organic solvents and measured water-to-solvent and organic solvent-to-organic solvent partition coefficients as discussed above.

8. Abraham solvation parameter model: prediction of water-to-skin and blood-to-skin partition coefficients and skin permeability coefficients

Human skin is an important permeation barrier that controls the entry of chemicals into the body. The barrier properties of skin depend primarily on the outer skin cells, which are called the stratum corneum. The stratum corneum consists of multiple non-living layers of densely packed keratin-filled cells embedded in a lipid-rich extracellular matrix containing a mixture of ceramides, fatty acids, cholesterol and triglycerides (Monteiro-Riviere *et al.*, 2001). The multiple layers are 7 – 16 micrometers in total thickness in most regions of the human body; however, in the palms of the hands and soles of the feet a much total layer thickness of 400 – 600 micrometers is found (Holbrook and Odland, 1974) For a chemical to be absorbed into the body after dermal exposure, it must first dissolve in the stratum corneum and then diffuse through the remaining epidermis sub-layers and into the dermis layer, from where it will eventually enter the blood stream. Passive diffusion is the mechanism by which chemicals move through the stratum corneum. Passage through the remaining sub-layers of the skin is more rapid.

Penetration of a compound into the skin is controlled by the compound's chemical structure and physicochemical properties. Lipophilicity and hydrogen-bonding character play a major role in a compound's skin absorption profile. In general, substances possessing the greater lipophilicity are more readily absorbed by the skin than compounds with lesser lipophilicity. Dermal absorption generally increases with increasing water-to-octanol partition coefficient from $\log P_{OtOH/water} = -1$ to $\log P_{OtOH/water} = 3.5$. Highly lipophilic compounds (those with $\log P_{OtOH/water} > 5$) pass easily through the stratum corneum, but are generally too water-insoluble to pass through the remaining epidermis sub-layers to enter the blood stream. There has been increasing experimental evidence that ionized species can contribute to transdermal absorption (Netzlaff et al., 2006; Abraham and Martins, 2004; Michaels et al., 1975). When the penetrating compound can exist in both ionized and unionized forms, it is the unionized form that penetrates faster through the lipid regions. Some contribution of the ionized form to the overall permeability, however, is expected. The solubilizing vehicle and formulation ingredients can alter the skin penetration of a compound by affecting the barrier properties of the skin by a range of mechanisms including hydration, delipidization, fluidization and desmosome disruption in the stratum corneum, or by changing the partitioning of the compound into the stratum corneum.

Skin partitioning is important in the pharmaceutical industry as many medications are applied topically to the skin in ointments, in creams, in lotions and gels, and in skin patches. Once applied, the medication often needs to find its way into the blood system for delivery to the desired target site. Abraham and Martins (2004) developed a mathematical correlation between the water-to-skin partition coefficient, K_{sc}, and the Abraham solute descriptors

$$\text{Log } K_{sc} = 0.341 + 0.341\mathbf{E} - 0.206\mathbf{S} - 0.024\mathbf{A} - 2.178\mathbf{B} + 1.850\mathbf{V}$$
$$\left(N = 45, \text{ SD} = 0.216, R^2 = 0.926, F = 97\right) \tag{40}$$

based on an experimental database containing 45 solutes, including several linear alcohols (e.g. methanol through 1-decanol) and several fairly large steroidal molecules (e.g. testosterone, progesterone, hydrocortisone, corticosterone, and aldosterone) and steroid esters (e.g. hydrocortisone-21 acetate, hydrocortisone-21 pentanoate, cortisone-21 acetate, cortisone-21 octanoate). Careful examination of Eqn. 40 reveals that the water-to-skin partition coefficient increases with increasing solute size, and decreasing with increasing solute polarity and solute hydrogen-bonding character.

Abraham and Ibrahim (2007) compiled experimental data on the distribution coefficients of drugs from blood or plasma to rat skin and rabbit skin. The authors analyzed the experimental $\log P_{skin}$ data in accordance with Eqn. 1 of the Abraham model

$$\log P_{skin} = -0.253 - 0.189\mathbf{A} - 0.620\mathbf{B} + 0.713\mathbf{V} - 0.683\mathbf{I}_{acid} + 0.059\mathbf{I}_{rabbit}$$
$$\left(N = 59, \text{ SD} = 0.26, R^2 = 0.733, F = 29\right) \tag{41}$$

The $e \cdot E$ and $s \cdot S$ terms were not statistically significant and were eliminated from the final derived correlation model. The poor R^2 statistics for Eqn. 41 is due, at least in part, to the small spread in the values of log P_{skin}, from log P_{skin} = -0.82 to log P_{skin} = 1.61, for a range of only 2.43 log units. Carboxylic acids were found to be systematically retained in blood or plasma more than calculated. An indicator descriptor, I_{acid}, was needed to describe the log Pskin data of solutes containing a carboxylic acid functional group. The I_{acid} descriptor equals unity for carboxylic acid solutes, and takes the value of I_{acid} = 0 for all other compounds. The second indicator descriptor in Eqn. 41 was needed to combine the rat skin (I_{rabbit} = 0) and rabbit skin (I_{rabbit}) partitioning data into a single correlation model. The 0.059 I_{rabbit} term amounts to a 0.059 log unit offset, which is likely less than the experimental uncertainty in the measured log P_{skin} data. If the 0.059 I_{rabbit} term is omitted, the squared correlation coefficient decreases to R^2 = 0.608.

Theoretical models of passive diffusion are based on Fick's law of diffusion and the conversation of particle numbers. Fick's law of diffusion states that a chemical diffuses from a region of higher concentration to a region of lower concentration with a magnitude that is directly proportional to the chemical's concentration gradient. When applied to trans-stratum corneum diffusion, the amount of chemical passing through a unit area of the stratum corneum per unit time (J) is given by

$$J = -\frac{K_{p,sc}D\Delta C}{h} \tag{42}$$

where $K_{p,sc}$ is the chemical's solvent-to-stratum corneum partition coefficient, D represents the chemical's diffusivity in the stratum corneum lipid matrix and h is the apparent skin thickness (*i.e.*, the diffusion pathlength). Under the assumption of constant donor concentration and sink conditions (zero receptor phase concentration) Eqn. 42 simplifies to

$$J_{SS} = \frac{K_{p,sc}DC_{donor}}{h} \tag{43}$$

The permeability coefficient, k_p, is the coefficient of proportionality between the steady-state flux J_{SS} and the donor concentration, C_{donor}.

Skin permeability experiments are generally performed *in vitro* using a Franz diffusion cell (shown in Figure 8). A freshly excised skin sample is mounted on the receptor compartment of the Franz cell with the stratum corneum facing upwards into the donor compartment and the dermis facing the receptor compartment. The latter compartment is filled with the receptor solution (often a phosphate saline solution buffered at pH of 7.4), and maintained at a constant temperature of 37 °C with a water jacketed cell under constant stirring. The donor compartment is filled with the vehicle solution containing the dissolved chemical of interest. At appropriate time intervals, aliquots of the receptor medium are withdrawn for analysis, and immediately replaced with an equal volume of fresh medium. Alternative diffusion cell designs and mathematical procedures for calculating the drug's diffusivity and permeability coefficient from the experimental permeation results are described in greater detail elsewhere (Friend, 1992; Hathout *et al.*, 2010). For *in vitro* skin penetration studies, the skin retention of a drug can be assessed by the use of radiolabeled drugs (usually carbon-14 or tritium labeled). Skin samples should be exposed to the drug for no more than a maximum of 24 hours because of deterioration of skin integrity with time.

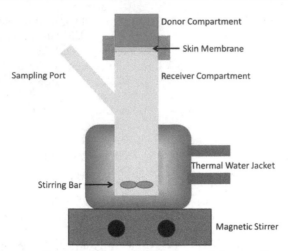

Fig. 8. Franz diffusion cell used to measure skin permeability coefficients

The parallel artificial membrane permeability assay (PAMPA) has been suggested as a high throughput screening method for rapid determination of passive transport permeability in connection with gastrointestinal (GI) absorption (Sugano *et al.*, 2002), blood-brain barrier penetration (Mensch *et al.*, 2010 and skin permeation (Ottaviani *et al.*, 2006). In the PAMPA method a 96-well filter plate coated with a liquid membrane is used to separate the donor and receptor compartments. Artificial membrane selection depends on the transport property to be determined. Ottaviani *et al.* (2006) found a reasonably accurate mathematical correlation between human skin permeability coefficient, k_p, and the effective permeability coefficient, k_{eff}, for a set of 31 compounds

$$\log k_p = 1.34 \log k_{eff} + 0.28$$
$$(N = 31, SD = 0.42, R^2 = 0.81, F = 31) \tag{44}$$

tested through an artificial membrane consisting of 70 % silicone and 30 % isopropyl myristate. The authors further noted that presence of isopropyl myristate as only a hydrogen-bond acceptor group in the artificial membrane was in accord with previous results demonstrating that stratum corneum lipids were better hydrogen-bond acceptors than hydrogen-bond donors.

Abraham and Martins (2004) reported an Abraham model correlation for human skin permeability coefficients from aqueous solution, k_p,

$$\text{Log } k_p(cm/s) = -5.426 - 0.106E - 0.473E - 0.473A - 3.000B + 2.296V$$
$$\left(N = 119, SD = 0.461, R^2 = 0.832, F = 112\right) \tag{45}$$

based on a database containing 119 experimental values at a common temperature of 37 °C. The authors adjusted the experimental data for ionization by assuming that the measured permeability coefficient was a simple addition of terms in Eqn. 46

$$k_p = f_{neutral} k_{p,neutral} + f_{ionic} k_{p,ionic} \tag{46}$$

where, k_p, $k_{p,ionic}$ and $k_{p,neutral}$ represent the overall permeation coefficient, that due to the ionic species, and that due to the neutral species; f_{ionic} and $f_{neutral}$ denote the fraction of ionic and neutral species at a given pH. For ionizable acids the skin permeability coefficient of the neutral molecule, $k_{p,neutral}$, was so much larger than the skin permeability coefficient of the ionic form, $k_{p,ionic}$, that the experimental unadjusted values of k_p was adjusted to give $k_{p,neutral}$ from the fraction of the neutral form present under the experimental conditions of pH. For ionizable bases the ratio of $k_{p,neutral}$ to $k_{p,ionic}$ was assumed to be 17.5, and this value was used to obtain $k_{p,neutral}$ values from experimental unadjusted values of k_p. If the experimental pH is near to the basic pK_a, such an adjustment will be very close to the adjustment that assumes negligible permeation of ionizable species. But as the difference in $(pH - pK_a)$ becomes larger, the adjustment will be smaller than that of negligible permeation of ionic species. To account for the temperature differences, the authors adjusted experimental log k_p values by 0.20 units from 32 °C to 37 °C, and by 0.48 units from 25 °C to 37 °C. The main factors that influence log k_p are hydrogen bond basicity (b · B term) that decreases log k_p, and solute volume (v · V term) that increases log k_p. Solute dipolarity/polarizability (s · S term) and hydrogen bond acidity (a · A term) make minor contributions, both in the sense of lowering log k_p.

9. Conclusion

The Abraham solvation parameter model provides an in silico method for estimating ADMET properties of potential drug molecules in the early stages of drug discovery. To date mathematical expressions have been reported for predicting water-to-organic solvent partition coefficients and solubilities in more than 70 organic solvents, air-to-tissue and blood-to-tissue partition coefficients for 5 human and rat tissues, water-to-human skin and blood-to-rat/rabbit skin partitions, human skin permeability coefficients, and rat (Zhao et al., 2003) and human (Zhao et al., 2002) intestinal absorption. Expressions are also available for estimating Draize rabbit eye test scores for pure liquids and eye irritation thresholds in humans (Abraham et al., 2003), odor detection thresholds and nasal pungency of volatile organic compounds (VOCs) (Abraham et al., 2007b), and the minimum alveolar concentration (MAC) for inhalation anesthetics in rats (Abraham et al., 2008b). The number of derived Abraham model correlations is expected in future years as more experimental data becomes available. Predictive applications require as input parameters the numerical values of the drug candidate's solute descriptors, which are easily calculable from measured solubility and partition coefficient data.

10. References

Abraham, M. H. & McGowan, J. C. (1987) The use of characteristic volumes to measure cavity terms in reversed phase liquid chromatography. *Chromatographia* 23 (4) 243–246.

Abraham, M. H. (1993a) Scales of solute hydrogen-bonding: their construction and application to physicochemical and biochemical processes. *Chemical Society Reviews* 22 (2),73-83.

Abraham, M. H. (1993b) Application of solvation equations to chemical and biochemical processes. *Pure and Applied Chemistry* 65 (12), 2503-2512.

Abraham, M. H.; Hassanisadi, M.; Jalali-Heravi, M.; Ghafourian, T.; Cain, W. S. & Cometto-Muniz, J. E. (2003) Draize rabbit eye test compatibility with eye irritation thresholds in humans: a quantitative structure-activity relationship analysis. *Toxicological Sciences* 76 (2), 384-391.

Abraham, M. H. (2004) The factors that influence permeation across the blood-brain barrier. *European Journal of Medicinal Chemistry* 39 (3), 235-240.

Abraham, M. H.; Ibrahim, A. & Zissimos, A. M. (2004) Determination of sets of solute descriptors from chromatographic measurements. *Journal of Chromatography, A* 1037 (1-2), 29-47.

Abraham, M. H. & Martins, F. (2004) Human skin permeation and partition: General linear free-energy relationship analyses. *Journal of Pharmaceutical Sciences* 93 (6), 1508-1523.

Abraham, M. H.; Ibrahim, A. & Acree, W. E. Jr., (2005) Air-to-blood distribution of volatile organic compounds: a linear free energy analysis. *Chemical Research in Toxicology* 18 (5), 904-911.

Abraham, M. H. & Ibrahim, A. (2006) Air to fat and blood to fat distribution of volatile organic compounds and drugs: Linear free energy analyses. *European Journal of Medicinal Chemistry* 41 (12), 1430-1438.

Abraham, M. H.; Ibrahim, A. & Acree, W. E (2006a) Air to brain, blood to brain and plasma to brain distribution of volatile organic compounds: linear free energy analyses. *European Journal of Medicinal Chemistry* 41 (4), 494-502.

Abraham, M. H.; Ibrahim, A.; Zhao, Y. & Acree, W. E., Jr. (2006b) A data base for partition of volatile organic compounds and drugs from blood/plasma/serum to brain, and an LFER analysis of the data. *Journal of Pharmaceutical Sciences* 95 (10), 2091-2100.

Abraham, M. H.; Ibrahim, A. & Acree, W. E., Jr. (2006c) Air to muscle and blood/plasma to muscle distribution of volatile organic compounds and drugs: linear free energy analyses. *Chemical Research in Toxicology* 19 (6), 801-808.

Abraham, M. H. & Ibrahim, A. (2007) Blood or plasma to skin distribution of drugs: a linear free energy analysis. *International Journal of Pharmaceutics* 329 (1-2) 129-134.

Abraham, M. H.; Ibrahim, A. & Acree, W. E., Jr. (2007a) Air to liver partition coefficients for volatile organic compounds and blood to liver partition coefficients for volatile organic compounds and drugs. *European Journal of Medicinal Chemistry* 42 (6), 743-751.

Abraham, M. H.; Sanchez-Moreno, R.; Cometto-Muniz, J. E. & Cain, W. S. (2007b) A quantitative structure-activity analysis on the relative sensitivity of the olfactory and the nasal trigeminal chemosensory systems. *Chemical Senses* 32 (7), 711-719.

Abraham, M. H.; Ibrahim, A. & Acree, W. E, Jr. (2008a) Air to lung partition coefficients for volatile organic compounds and blood to lung partition coefficients for volatile organic compounds and drug. *European Journal of Medicinal Chemistry* 43 (3), 478-485.

Abraham, M. H.; Acree, W. E., Jr.; Mintz, C. & Payne, S. (2008b) Effect of anesthetic structure on inhalation anesthesia: implications for the mechanism. *Journal of Pharmaceutical Sciences* 97 (6), 2373-2384.

Abraham, M. H.; Acree, W. E., Jr. & Cometto-Muniz, J. E. (2009a) Partition of compounds from water and from air into amides. *New Journal of Chemistry* 33 (10), 2034-2043.

Abraham, M. H.; Gil-Lostes, J. & Fatemi, M. (2009b) Prediction of milk/plasma concentration ratios of drugs and environmental pollutants. *European Journal of Medicinal Chemistry* 44 (6), 2452-2458.

Abraham, M. H. & Acree, W. E., Jr. (2010a) Equations for the transfer of neutral molecules and ionic species from water to organic phases. *Journal of Organic Chemistry* 75 (4), 1006-1015.

Abraham, M. H. & Acree, W. E., Jr. (2010b) Solute descriptors for phenoxide anions and their use to establish correlations of rates of reaction of anions with iodomethane. *Journal of Organic Chemistry* 75 (9), 3021-3026.

Abraham, M. H. & Acree, W. E., Jr. (2010c) The transfer of neutral molecules, ions and ionic species from water to ethylene glycol and to propylene carbonate; descriptors for pyridinium cations. *New Journal of Chemistry* 34 (10), 2298-2305.

Abraham, M. H. & Acree, W. E., Jr. (2010d) The transfer of neutral molecules, ions and ionic species from water to wet octanol. *Physical Chemistry Chemical Physics* 12 (40), 13182-13188.

Abraham, M. H.; Smith, R. E.; Luchtefeld, R.; Boorem, A. J.; Luo, R. & Acree, W. E., Jr. (2010) Prediction of solubility of drugs and other compounds in organic solvents. *Journal of Pharmaceutical Sciences* 99 (3), 1500-1515.

Abraham, M. H. (2011) The permeation of neutral molecules, ions and ionic species: brain permeation as an example. *Journal of Pharmaceutical Sciences*, 100, (5), 1690-1701.

Acree, W. E., Jr. & Abraham, M. H. (2002) Solubility of crystalline nonelectrolyte solutes in organic solvents: mathematical correlation of benzil solubilities with the Abraham general solvation model. *Journal of Solution Chemistry* 31 (4), 293-303

ADME Boxes, version*, Advanced Chemistry Development, 110 Yonge Street, 14th Floor, Toronto, Ontario, M5C 1T4, Canada.

Ahmed, H.; Poole, C. F. & Kozerski, G. E. (2007) Determination of descriptors for organo-silicon compounds by gas chromatography and non-aqueous liquid-liquid partitioning. *Journal of Chromatography, A* 1169 (1-2), 179-192.

Ahmed, H. & Poole, C. F. (2006a) Distribution of neutral organic compounds between n-heptane and methanol or N,N-dimethylformamide. *Journal of Separation Science* 29 (14), 2158-2165.

Ahmed, Hamid & Poole, Colin F. (2006b) Model for the distribution of neutral organic compounds between n-hexane and acetonitrile. *Journal of Chromatography, A* 1104 (1-2), 82-90.

Alam, M. I.; Beg, S.; Samad, A.; Baboota, S.; Hohli, K.; Ali, J.; Ahuja, A. & Akbar, M. (2010) Strategy for effective brain drug delivery. *European Journal of Pharmaceutical Science* 40 (5), 385-403.

Amidon, G. L.; Lennenas, H.; Shah, V. P. & Crison, J. R. (1995) A theoretical basis for a biopharmaceutic drug classification: the correlation in vitro drug product dissolution and in vivo bioavailability. *Pharmaceutical Research* 12 (3), 413-420.

Arey, J. S.; Green, W. H., Jr. & Gschwend, P. M. (2005) The electrostatic origin of Abraham's solute polarity parameter. *Journal of Physical Chemistry B* 109 (15), 7564-7573.

Atapattu, S. N. & Poole, C. F. (2009) Determination of descriptors for semivolatile organosilicon compounds by gas chromatography and non-aqueous liquid-liquid partition. *Journal of Chromatography, A* 1216 (45), 7882-7888.

Begley, D. J.; Khan, E. U.; Rollinson, C. & Abbott, J. (2000) in 'The blood-brain barrier and drug delivery to the CNS, Ed by Befley, D.J.; Bradbury, M. W. & Kreuter, J., Marcel Dekker, New York, 2000.

Berthod, A.; Han, Y. Il. & Armstrong, D. W. (1988) Centrifugal partition chromatography. V. Octanol-water partition coefficients, direct and indirect determination. *Journal of Liquid Chromatography* 11 (7), 1441-1456.

Berthod, A.; Menges, R. A. & Armstrong, D. W. (1992) Direct octanol-water partition coefficient determination using co-current chromatography. *Journal of Liquid Chromatography* 15 (15-16), 2769-2785.

Charlton, A. K.; Daniels, C. R.; Acree, W. E., Jr. & Abraham, M. H. (2003) Solubility of crystalline nonelectrolyte solutes in organic solvents: mathematical correlation of acetylsalicylic acid solubilities with the Abraham general solvation model. *Journal of Solution Chemistry* 32 (12), 1087-1102.

Cruciani, G.; Pastor, M. & Guba, W. (2000) VolSurf: a new tool for the pharmacokinetic optimization of lead compounds. *European Journal of Pharmaceutical Sciences* 11 (Suppl. 2), S29-S39.

Eixarch, H.; Haltner-Ukomadu, E.; Beisswenger, C. & Bock, U. (2010) Drug delivery to the lung: permeability and physicochemical characteristics of drugs as the basis for a pulmonary Biopharmaceutical Classification System (pBCS). *Journal of Epithelial Biology and Pharmacology* 3, 1-14.

Faller, B.; Grimm, H. P.; Loeuillet-Ritzler, F.; Arnold, S. & Briand, X. (2005) High-throughput lipophilicity measurement with immobilized artificial membranes. *Journal of Medicinal Chemistry* 48 (7), 2571-2576.

Friend, D. R. (1992) *In vitro* skin permeation techniques. *Journal of Controlled Release* 18, 235-248.

Gao, X.; Yu, C. H.; Tam, K. Y. & Tsang, S. C. (2005) New magnetic nano-absorbent for the determination of n-octanol/water partition coefficients. *Journal of Pharmaceutical and Biomedical Analysis* 38 (2), 197-203.

Guthrie J. P. (2009) A blind challenge for computational solvation free energies: introduction and overview. *Journal of Physical Chemistry B* 113 (14) 4501-4507.

Hathout, R. M.; Woodman, T. J.; Mansour, S.; Mortada, N. D.; Geneidi, A. S. & Guy, R. H. (2010) Microemulsion formulations for the transdermal delivery of testosterone. *European Journal of Pharmaceutical Sciences* 40 (3), 188-196.

Henchoz, Y.; Romand, S.; Schuppler, J.; Rudaz, S.; Veathey, J.-L. & Carrupt, P. A. (2010) High-throughput log P determination by MEEKC coupled with UV and MS detections. *Electrophoresis*, 31 (5), 952-964.

Hewitt, M.; Cronin, M. T. D.; Enoch, S. J.; Madden, J. C.; Roberts, D. W. & Dearden, J. C. (2009) In silico prediction of aqueous solubility: the solubility challenge. *Journal of Chemical Information and Modeling* 49 (11), 2572–2587.

Holbrook K A. & Odland G F. (1974) Regional differences in the thickness (cell layers) of the human stratum corneum: an ultrastructural analysis. *The Journal of Investigative Dermatology* 62 (4), 415-422.

Howard, P. H. & Meylan, W. M. (1997) Handbook of Physical properties of Organic Chemicals, CRC Press, Boca Raton, 1997.

Ishihama, Y. & Asakawa, N. (1999) Characterization of the lipophilicity scales using vectors from solvation energy descriptors. *Journal of Pharmaceutical Sciences* 88 (12), 1305-1312.

Karunasekara, T. & Poole, C. F. (2010) Model for the partition of neutral compounds between n-heptane and formamide. *Journal of Separation Science* 33 (8), 1167-1173.

Keck, C.; Kobierski, S.; Mauludin, R. & Muller, R. H. (2008) Second generation of drug nanocrystals for delivery of poorly soluble drugs: smartcrystal technology. *Dosis*, 2 (24), 124-128 .

Li, H.; Yap, C. W.; Ung, C. Y.; Xue, Y.; Cao, Z. W. & Chen, Y. Z. (2005) Effect of selection of molecular descriptors on the prediction of blood-brain barrier penetrating and nonpenetrating agents by statistical learning methods. *Journal of Chemical Information and Modeling* 45 (5) 1376-1384.

Li, Q.-S.; Li, Z. & Wang, S. (2008) Solubility of trimethoprim (TMP) in different organic solvents from (278 to 333) K. *Journal of Chemical and Engineering Data* 53 (1), 286-287.

Lipinski, C. A.; Lombardo, F.; Dominy, B. W. & Feeney, P. J. (2001) Experimental and computational approaches to estimate solubility and permeability in drug discovery and development settings. *Advances in Drug Delivery Reviews* 46 (1-3), 3-26.

Llinàs, A.; Glen, R. C. & Goodman, J. M. (2008) Solubility challenge: can you predict solubilities of 32 molecules using a database of 100 reliable measurements. *Journal of Chemical Information and Modeling* 48 (7), 1289–1303.

Lukyanov, A. N. & Torchilin, V. P. (2004) Micelles from lipid derivatives of water-soluble polymers as delivery systems for poorly soluble drugs. *Advanced Drug Delivery Reviews* 56 (9), 1273-1289.

McDuffie, B. (1981) Estimation of octanol/water partition coefficients for organic pollutants using reverse-phase HPLC *Chemosphere* 10 (1), 73-83.

Menges, R. A.; Bertrand, G. L. & Armstrong, D. W. (1990) Direct measurement of octanolwater partition coefficients using centrifugal partition chromatography with a back-flushing technique. *Journal of Liquid Chromatography* 13 (15), 3061-3077.

Mensch, J.; Jaroskova, L.; Anderson, W.; Mells, A.; Mackle, C.; Verreck, G.; Brewster, M. E. & Augustinjns, P. (2010) Application of PAMPA-models to predict BBB permeability including efflux ratio, plasma protein binding and physicochemical parameters. *International Journal of Pharmaceutics* 395, 182-197.

Michaels A. S, Chandrasekaran S. K, & Shaw J. E. (1975).Drug permeation through human skin: theory and *in vitro* experimental measurement. *AIChE Journal* 21 (5), 985–996.

Mintz, C.; Clark, M.; Acree, W. E., Jr. & Abraham, M. H. (2007) Enthalpy of solvation correlations for gaseous solutes dissolved in water and in 1-octanol based on the Abraham model. *Journal of Chemical Information and Modeling* 47 (1), 115-121.

Monteiro-Riviere, N. A.; Inman, A. O.; Mak, V.; Wertz, P. & Riviere, J. E. (2001) Effect of selective lipid extraction from different body regions on epidermal barrier function. *Pharmaceutical Research* 18 (7) 992-998.

Mutelet, F. & Rogalski, M. (2001) Experimental determination and prediction of the gas-liquid n-hexadecane partition coefficients. *Journal of Chromatography A* 923 (102), 153-163.

Netzlaff, F.; Schaefer, U. F.; Lehr, C.-M.; Meiers, P.; Stahl, J.; Kietzmann, M. & Niedorf, F. (2006) Comparison of bovine udder skin with human and porcine skin in percutaneous permeation experiments. *ATLA, Alternatives to Laboratory Animals* 34 (5), 499-513.

Nicholls, A.; Mobley, D. L.; Guthrie, J. P.; Chodera, J. D.; Bayly, C. I.; Cooper, M. D. & Pande, V. S. (2008) Predicting small-molecule solvation free energies: an informal blind test for computational chemistry. *Journal of Medical Chemistry* 51 (4) 769-779.

Ottaviani, G.; Martel, S. & Carrupt, P.-A. (2006) Parallel artificial membrane permeability assay: A new membrane for the fast prediction of passive human skin permeability. *Journal of Medicinal Chemistry* 49 (6), 3948-3954.

Platts, J. A.; Butina, D.; Abraham, M. H. & Hersey, A. (1999) Estimation of molecular linear free energy relation descriptors using a group contribution approach. *Journal of Chemical Information and Computational Science* 39 (5), 835-845.

Poole, S. K. & Poole, C. F. (2003) Separation methods for estimating octanol-water partition coefficients. *Journal of Chromatographty B* 797 (1-2), 3-19.

Qian, J. & Poole, C. F. (2007) Distribution of neutral organic compounds between n-heptane and fluorine-containing alcohols. *Journal of Chromatography, A* 1143 (1-2), 276-283.

Ribeiro, M. M. B.; Melo, M. N.; Serrano, I. D.; Santos, N. C. & Castanho, M. A. R. B. (2010) Drug-lipid interaction evaluation: why a 19th century solution? *Trends in Pharmacological Sciences* 31 (10), 449-454.

Sangster, J. (1989) Octanol-water partition coefficients of simple organic compounds. *Journalof Physical and Chemical Reference Data* 18 (3), 1111-1229.

Sugano, K.; Takata, N.; Machida, M.; Saitoh, K. & Terada, K. (2002) Prediction of passive intestinal absorption using bio-mimetic artificial membrane permeation assay and the paracellular pathway. *International Journal of Pharmaceutics* 241 (2), 241-251

Sugano, K.; Kato, T.; Suzuki, K.; Keiko, K.; Sajaku, T. & Mano, T. (2006) High throughput solubility measurement with automated polarized light microscopy analysis. *Journal of Pharmaceutical Sciences* 95 (10), 2115-2122.

Veith, G. D.; Austin, N. M. & Morris, R. T. (1979) A rapid method for estimating log P for organic chemicals. *Water Research* 13 (1), 43-47

Wang, J. M.; Hou, T. J. & Xu, X. J. (2009) Aqueous solubility prediction based on weighted atom type counts and solvent accessible surface areas. *Journal of Chemical Information and Modeling* 49 (3), 571–581.

Wohnsland, F. & Faller, B. (2001) High-throughput permeability pH profile and high-throughput alkane/water log P with artificial membranes. *Journal of Medicinal Chemistry* 44 (6), 923-930.

Wu, C. Y. & Benet, L. Z. (2005) Predicting drug disposition via application of BCS. Transportabsorption/elimination interplay and development of a biopharmaceutics drug disposition classification system. *Pharmaceutical Research* 22 (1), 11-23.

Zhao, Y. H.; Le, J.; Abraham, M. H.; Hersey, A.; Eddershaw, P. J.; Luscombe, C. N.; Butina, D.; Beck, G.; Sherborne, B.; Cooper, I. & Platts, J. A. (2002) Evaluation of human intestinal absorption data and subsequent derivation of a quantitative structure-activity relationship (QSAR) with the Abraham descriptors. *Journal of Pharmaceutical Sciences* 90 (6), 749-784

Zhao, Y. H.; Abraham, M. H.; Hersey, A. & Luscombe, C. N. (2003) Quantitative relationship between rat intestinal absorption and Abraham descriptors. *European Journal of Medicinal Chemistry* 38 (11-12), 939-947.

Zhao, Y. H.; Abraham, M. H.; Ibrahim, A.; Fish, P. V.; Cole, S.; Lewis, M. L.; de Groot, M. J. & Reynolds, D. P. (2007) Predicting penetration across the blood-brain barrier from simple descriptors and fragmentation schemes. *Journal of Chemical Information and Modeling* 47 (1), 170-175.

Zissimos, A. M.; Abraham, M. H.; Barker, M. C.; Box, K. J.; & Tam, K. Y. (2002a) Calculation of Abraham descriptors from solvent-water partition coefficients in four different systems; evaluation of different methods of calculation. *Journal of the Chemical Society, Perkin Transactions 2* (3), 470-477.

Zissimos, A. M.; Abraham, M. H.; Du, C. M.; Valko, K.; Bevan, C.; Reynolds, D.; Wood, J.; & Tam, K. Y. (2002b) Calculation of Abraham descriptors from experimental data from seven HPLC systems; evaluation of five different methods of calculation. *Journal of the Chemical Society, Perkin Transactions 2* (12), 2001-2010.

6

Drug Synergy –
Mechanisms and Methods of Analysis

Hans-Georg Breitinger
The German University in Cairo,
Egypt

1. Introduction

The term synergy is derived from the Greek *syn-ergos*, "working together". Synergies have been described in many settings and situations of life, including mechanics, technical systems, human social life, and many more. In all cases, synergy describes the fact that a system, i.e. the combination and interaction of two or more agents or forces is such that the combined effect is greater than the sum of their individual effects.

This definition implies that there are three possible ways of such an "interaction of agents or forces": these forces could simply add up, not affecting each other (no interaction), their combination could produce a greater than expected result (synergy), or the combination could lead to a result that is less than the sum of the individual effects. This "negative" summation is called antagonism.

Interactions of biologically active agents are an important aspect of pharmacology and biomedicine. In this context, interaction describes the biological activity that results from the presence of several drugs at the same time. Such situations occur in numerous clinical situations:

- combinations of cytotoxic drugs in the treatment of cancer and infections require lower doses of each drug to obtain better therapeutic effects with less side-effect toxicity.
- combinations of antibiotics likewise combine better efficiency with fewer side effects and reduced development of resistance.
- many serious clinical situations require administration of several drugs simply because of multiple therapeutic indications. Although in such a case drug combinations are not formulated to look for synergies, the interactions of these drugs need to be assessed.
- the effect of one drug may be augmented by another drug that does not produce such an effect on its own

In all these cases, multiple drugs are administered, and will show some form of interaction, synergistic, antagonistic, or none. Methods to determine and quantify drug interactions are thus an essential tool in pharmacology. Historically, extracts from plants, animals, or even soils were the first classified pharmaceuticals. These were complex mixtures rather than single agents, and some ingredients may have interacted with others. Over the years of development of pharmacy, isolation, synthesis and marketing of single drugs became the accepted standard. Whether a complex mixture or a combination of drugs is used, the biological interaction of all active substances should be known. Synergy may be observed in simple systems – two drugs that only act on one target protein can show synergism. In such a case we can study the interaction of the drugs mechanistically and determine why and how several drugs can reinforce each other (or why they do not). Synergy may also be observed in complex settings, such as patients receiving multiple medications. Usually, more than one biological target (protein, pathway, or even organ) are involved in such cases, and single mechanistic descriptions are not appropriate. Additional parameters to consider are drug absorption, tissue distribution, and clearance. It may be expected that many drugs interfere with metabolism of other drugs. Thus, a substance B that slows down clearance of an active drug A, say by blocking metabolizing enzymes or excretion, may lead to a higher effective concentration of A that remains in the body for a longer time. As a result, one would notice a greater effect of drug A when given together with B, although the two drugs have completely different modes of action. While certainly the combination of these two drugs would have a "combined effect is greater than the sum of their individual effects", their combination is synergistic in practical application, but not by the strict definition.

2. Basic models and mechanisms – Synergy on a molecular level

2.1 A simple reaction scheme for enzyme inhibition

Drug interaction and synergy has been intensively studied for more than 100 years, and some of the numerous concepts will be briefly introduced in this chapter. The simplest model cases will be presented, leading to a molecular definition of drug synergy.

Let us assume a simple enzyme following the laws of mass action and Michaelis-Menten kinetics. In the simplest case, this enzyme has an active site, where substrate is being converted into product, and possesses one or several specific binding sites for inhibitors (Fig. 1A). A competitive inhibitor by definition binds to the active site of the enzyme, displacing the substrate. Thus, a mixture of two purely competitive inhibitors will only ever target the active site. This is known as mutually exclusive binding. If only the simplest mechanistic case is considered, one would not expect a second competitive inhibitor to have any notable effect on the first one, other than raising the total amount of inhibitory molecules.

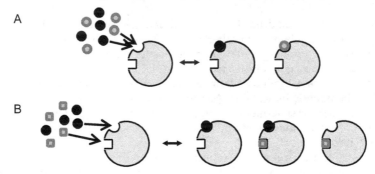

Fig. 1. Schematic representation of inhibition mechanisms (A) Competitive inhibition. Inhibitor (open circles) binds to the active site of the target protein. The agonist (solid circles) binds to the same site. By definition of competitive inhibition, all competitive inhibitors bind to the same site. Thus, binding of two competitive inhibitors must be mutually exclusive, and they cannot act synergistically on the same target protein. (B) Non-competitive inhibition. Inhibitor (open squares) binds to a site different from the active site of the target molecule. In pure non-competitive inhibition agonist binding is not affected by the inhibitor. Inhibition is due to conversion of the target protein into an inactive state.

In case of non-competitive inhibition, the inhibitor binds to a location on the enzyme different from the active site. Assuming that bound inhibitor converts the enzyme into an inactive (non product-forming) state, presence of a non-competitive inhibitor simply lowers the amount of active enzyme molecules (Fig. 1B). There are states, where both substrate and inhibitor are bound to the enzyme. The effect of several non-competitive inhibitors applied together raises the question if synergy can be observed in such a simple system. If two non-competitive inhibitors bind to the same site on their target enzyme, this inhibitory site can either be occupied by inhibitor A or B, but not by both inhibitors at the same time (Fig. 2). This would be a case of mutually exclusive binding of two inhibitors. If one inhibitor is present, and the second one added, one may observe indeed a greater extend of inhibition, but this would only be due to larger amounts of inhibitory molecules being present. At all times, we could predict the total amount of inhibition by summations. In the simplest molecular case, two inhibitors targeting the same site would produce an additive effect only.

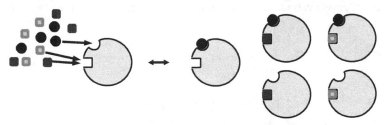

Fig. 2. Reaction scheme for two non-competitive inhibitors targeting the same site. Two non-competitive inhibitors (squares) bind to the same site on the target protein. In this case their binding is mutually exclusive. Presence of the second inhibitor increases the total amount of inhibitor causing in increased inhibitory effect. This increase is only due to simple additivity, and not synergy.

If, however, two different binding sites for non-competitive inhibitors exist on an enzyme, two inhibitors may bind simultaneously (Fig. 3). Inspection of the reaction schemes (Fig. 2, 3) shows that if two inhibitors have specific, independent sites on the enzyme, we will observe states where the enzyme indeed has two inhibitors bound (Fig. 3). These states cannot exist if both inhibitors bind to the same site (Fig. 2). Thus, if two inhibitors are able to bind simultaneously, we have a case of "mutually non-exclusive" binding. Here, presence of the second inhibitor will not only give an additive effect (increase of the number of inhibitory molecules), but will generate additional inhibited states of the enzyme. Therefore, on a molecular level we would expect a superadditive effect of two such inhibitors.

It should be noted that the considerations above are made following some basic assumptions, namely that binding of an inhibitor will convert the enzyme to an inactive state, binding of substrate and inhibitor is reversible, and binding of any compound is fully independent from all other compounds. Thus, the equilibrium binding constant for inhibitor A is the same whether A binds to the unliganded enzyme, or to the enzyme that has substrate and/or another inhibitor bound. Given these assumptions, the mechanisms for activation (Fig. 4A), and non-competitive inhibition (Fig. 4B,C) show the different states in which an enzyme exists in the presence of two non-competitive inhibitors that bind to the same site (Fig. 4B), or to different sites of the enzyme (Fig. 4B).

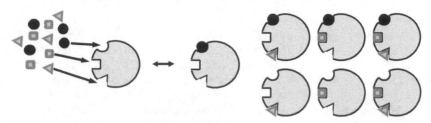

Fig. 3. Reaction scheme for two mutually non-exclusive non-competitive inhibitors. Non-competitive inhibition by two inhibitors (squares, triangles) binding to different sites on the target protein. Here, bindign of one inhibitor does not prevent binding of the other. Note that presence of the second inhibitor creates new inactive states of the target protein that are not possible if only one inhibitor is present. This applies even in the simplest theoretical case, where binding affinities of agonist and inhibitors are completely independent of each other. Thus, in the presence of two inhibitors of the same target protein that follow the rule of Bliss independence, i.e. mutually non-exclusive binding, synergy must be a necessary consequence.

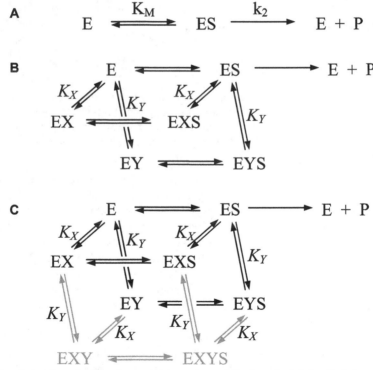

Fig. 4. Mechanism of catalysis and non-competitive inhibition of a Michaelis-Menten enzyme. (A) Mechanism for the activation of an enzyme following Michaelis-Menten kinetics. E = enzyme, S = substrate, P = product, K_M = Michaelis constant, k_2 = rate of product formation from ES. A simplified MM kinetic scheme is used, assuming no backward reaction EP → ES. (B) Inhibition of a Michaelis-Menten enzyme by two non-competitive inhibitors X and Y, which are mutually exclusive (e.g. binding to the same site). It is assumed that enzyme with

bound inhibitor is completely inactive, ie it does not form product. Either inhibitor X or Y can bind at any given time. Presence of the second inhibitor can only exert an additive effect but is not synergistic. (C) Inhibition of a Michaelis-Menten enzyme by two non-competitive inhibitors X and Y, which are mutually non-exclusive, i.e. binding to different sites on the enzyme. Here, both inhibitors may bind simultaneously, giving rise to synergistic inhibition.

2.2 Michaelis-Menten enzymes

In this section, a simple derivation of enzyme inhibition by one or two non-competitive inhibitors is given. To illustrate the consequences of mutually exclusive vs. non-exclusive binding, the simplest mechanisms are used.

From the mechanism of a Michaelis-Menten-type enzyme (Fig. 4A) and the law of mass action, we find:

$$K_M = \frac{[E][S]}{[ES]} \quad \rightarrow \quad [ES] = \frac{[E][S]}{K_M} \tag{1}$$

The enzyme E can only exist as free enzyme E, or enzyme-substrate-complex ES. The total enzyme concentration is $[E_{tot}]$, K_M is the Michaelis constant. Only ES can form product, the maximum rate of product formation is V_{max}.

$$[E_{tot}] = [E] + [ES] \tag{2}$$

$$V_{max} = k_2 [E_{tot}] \tag{3}$$

V_0, the actual rate of product formation at a given concentration of substrate depends on the fraction of ES that is present in the equilibrium. Thus V_0 can be expressed in terms of "ocupancy", or f_{ES}, the fraction of enzyme present in the enzyme-substrate complex ES.

$$f_{ES} = \frac{[ES]}{[E] + [ES]} \tag{4}$$

$$V_0 = k_2 [ES] \quad \rightarrow \quad V_0 = V_{max} \frac{[ES]}{[E_{tot}]} \quad , \quad V_0 = V_{max} \frac{[ES]}{[E] + [ES]} = V_{max} f_{ES} \tag{5}$$

Note that this equation converts readily to the common form of the Michaelis-Menten equation, if the definition of K_M (equation 1) is substituted into equation 5.

$$V_0 = V_{max} \frac{1}{1 + \frac{K_M}{S}} \tag{6}$$

In the presence of a single non-competitive inhibitor, additional enzyme species are possible (EX, EXS in Fig. 4B). By definition of an inhibitor, these do not lead to any product formation. Then f_{ES} becomes

$$f_{ES,X} = \frac{[ES]}{[E] + [ES] + [EX] + [EXS]} \tag{7}$$

The rate of product formation in presence of one non-competitive inhibitor is

$$V_{0,X} = V_{max} \frac{1}{\left(1 + \dfrac{K_M}{S}\right)\left(1 + \dfrac{X}{K_X}\right)} \tag{8}$$

For two mutually exclusive inhibitors X and Y (Fig. 4B), one obtains:

$$V_{0,X,Y} = V_{max} \frac{1}{\left(1 + \dfrac{K_M}{S}\right)\left(1 + \dfrac{X}{K_X} + \dfrac{Y}{K_Y}\right)} \tag{9}$$

And for two mutually non-exclusive inhibitors (Fig. 4C), the rate equation is

$$V_{0,X,Y} = V_{max} \frac{1}{\left(1 + \dfrac{K_M}{S}\right)\left(1 + \dfrac{X}{K_X}\right)\left(1 + \dfrac{Y}{K_Y}\right)} \tag{10}$$

There is a simple technique to determine the type of enzyme inhibition by two inhibitors, and whether their action on the enzyme is synergistic. To this end, the ratio of the initial rates in the absence (control, V_0), and in the presence of inhibitor ($V_{0,X}$) is measured. S_0 is the control signal, S_X is the signal obtained in the presence of inhibitor.

$$\frac{S_0}{S_X} = \frac{V_0}{V_{0,X}} = \frac{V_{max}\dfrac{1}{\left(1 + \dfrac{K_M}{S}\right)}}{V_{max}\dfrac{1}{\left(1 + \dfrac{K_M}{S}\right)\left(1 + \dfrac{X}{K_X}\right)}} = \left(1 + \frac{X}{K_X}\right) \tag{11}$$

Thus, a straight-line curve is obtained when S_0/S_X is plotted against [X], the (varied) concentration of inhibitor X. The slope of this line (Fig. 6) gives the inhibition constant K_X. This plot is linear over the entire range of inhibitor concentration.
In the case of two mutually exclusive inhibitors, the ratio becomes

$$\frac{S_0}{S_{X,Y}} = \frac{V_0}{V_{0,X,Y}} = \frac{V_{max}\dfrac{1}{\left(1 + \dfrac{K_M}{S}\right)}}{V_{max}\dfrac{1}{\left(1 + \dfrac{K_M}{S}\right)\left(1 + \dfrac{X}{K_X} + \dfrac{Y}{K_Y}\right)}} = \left(1 + \frac{X}{K_X} + \frac{Y}{K_Y}\right) \tag{12}$$

Presence of the second inhibitor only results in an additional term (Y/K_Y) that shifts the $S_0/S_{X,Y}$ curve upwards. This term indicates additivity of the two inhibitors, but inhibitory potency (slope of the curve) is not altered.
For two mutually non-exclusive inhibitors, the ratio is

$$\frac{S_0}{S_{X,Y}} = \frac{V_0}{V_{0,X,Y}} = \frac{V_{max}\dfrac{1}{\left(1+\dfrac{K_M}{S}\right)}}{V_{max}\dfrac{1}{\left(1+\dfrac{K_M}{S}\right)\left(1+\dfrac{X}{K_X}\right)\left(1+\dfrac{Y}{K_Y}\right)}} = \left(1+\frac{X}{K_X}\right)\left(1+\frac{Y}{K_Y}\right) \qquad (13)$$

The difference between mutually exclusive and non-exclusive inhibitors can directly be seen from an experiment where the concentration of inhibitor X is held constant, and only [Y] is varied. Equation 13 can be rearranged to:

$$\frac{S_0}{S_{X,Y}} = 1 + \frac{X}{K_X} + \frac{Y}{K_Y}\left(1+\frac{X}{K_X}\right) \qquad (14)$$

Compared to the case of mutually exclusive inhibitors, the curve of $S_0/S_{X,Y}$. Y is shifted upwards by a constant concentration of X, and the slope of the curve also increases by a factor of $(1+X/K_X)$.

The ratio method shown here applies to the simplest case of synergistic action of drugs, two substances binding to the same target. It requires some basic kinetic data to be collected and gives a simple linear graph that can be quickly inspected for a qualitative result whether two substances act on the same or on different sites on an enzyme, and thus whether these two substances can be synergistic on their target or not. It should be noted that by taking the ratios, the control signal (uninhibited case, i.e. the largest signal) is divided by a signal that becomes progressively smaller and thus carries a higher error. It is needed to detect whether two curves have the same slope (mutually exclusive binding, additive effect), or different slopes (mutually non-exclusive binding, synergy). This difference has to be clearly demonstrated from experiment and data analysis, requiring data of sufficient quality to make this distinction.

The technique provides two important pieces of information:

1. The value of K_X, the inhibition constant, is unchanged if two inhibitors are only additive, and is decreased (~ higher inhibitory potency) in the presence of the second inhibitor. Therefore, we have a clear, mechanism-derived definition of synergy on the molecular level.

2. Conversely, the method allows to determine whether two inhibitors bind to the same, or to different sites on an enzyme. This may be an important result for drug development, and is obtained without need of structural data. (Note: strictly speaking, the result only tells whether binding of two inhibitors is mutually exclusive or non-exclusive)

The method has originally been presented for ligand-gated ion channels by Karpen and Hess (Karpen, Aoshima et al. 1982; Karpen and Hess 1986), and subsequently been used for the study of action of multiple inhibitors on ion channels (Karpen, Aoshima et al. 1982; Karpen and Hess 1986; Breitinger, Geetha et al. 2001; Raafat, Breitinger et al. 2010).

The basic mechanism presented here is by far not sufficient to describe multimeric enzymes, enzynmes requiring cofactors, and various modes of inhibition. Enzymes may form multimers, binding of one inhibitor may affect binding of other others, and binding sites my overlap. More complex mechanisms of inhibition of Michaelis-Menten enzymes have been discussed, including those of several inhibitors acting on a single enzyme (Palatini 1983). Action of several inhibitors as well as antagonistic interaction of enzyme inhibitors have been studied (Asante-Appiah and Chan 1996; Schenker and Baici 2009), and a major development in drug interaction analysis was the detailed mathematical treatment of enzyme kinetics and inhibition by Chou and Talalay (Chou 1976; Chou and Talalay 1977; Chou and Talalay 1981; Chou 2006; Chou 2010), covering the mechanistic Michaelis-Menten approach as well as logistic approaches.

2.3 Ligand-gated ion channel receptors

Ligand-gated ion channels are principal mediators of rapid synaptic transmission between nerve cells and in the neuromuscular junction. Compared to Michaelis-Menten type enzymes, their mechanism of activation is more complex, requiring an additional transition (Hess 1993; Colquhoun 1998). First step of ion channel activation is binding of the activating ligand (a neurotransmitter), which is governed by the principle of mass action (Hess 1993; Colquhoun 1998). Usually, more than one ligand molecule is required; depending on receptor type, models with two or three ligands binding prior to efficient channel opening have been discussed. Ligand binding induces an conformational change, where the receptor protein converts from the closed to an open ion-conducting state (Fig. 5A) (Hess 1993; Colquhoun 1998). Only the passing ions generate an electric signal and this signal can be recorded using patch-clamp techniques. Similar to the ES complex in enzymes, only the liganded receptor can undergo the opening transition. The mechanisms of non-competitive inhibition by two inhibitors binding to the same (Fig. 5B), or different (Fig. 5C) sites have been given. A similar derivation to the one for MM-enzymes can then be made.

The signal in this case is not a rate of product formation, but an ionic current, namely the rate of ion translocation through the open channel. Assuming a constant transmembrane voltage, and only one conducting state (ie only one channel size, in reality several conductance levels have been observed for each ion channel receptor).

The observed signal S_L would then be:

$$S_L = I_L = n_{Ch} J_{ion} \tag{15}$$

where I_L is the observd current, n_{Ch} is the number of open channels, and J_{ion} is the ion translocation rate. The maximum current signal would be observed if all ion channel were open at the same time. F_{open}, the fraction of open channels, would then be equal to 1 (a theoretical value only).

$$S_{max} = I_{max} F_{open} \tag{16}$$

Assuming that only receptors with two bound ligands can undergo the opening transition (Fig. 5A), we can define the fraction of open channels as

$$F_{open} = \frac{[RL_2(open)]}{[R] + 2[RL] + [RL_2] + [RL_2(open)]} \tag{17}$$

Using the law of mass action, we can define

$$K_D = 2\frac{[R][L]}{[RL]} \tag{18}$$

$$K_D = \frac{[RL][L]}{[RL_2]} \tag{19}$$

$$\phi = \frac{[RL_2]}{[RL_2(open)]} \tag{20}$$

we can then obtain

$$S_0 = I_{max}F_{open} = I_{max}\frac{1}{\left(\frac{K_D}{L}+1\right)^2\phi+1} \tag{21}$$

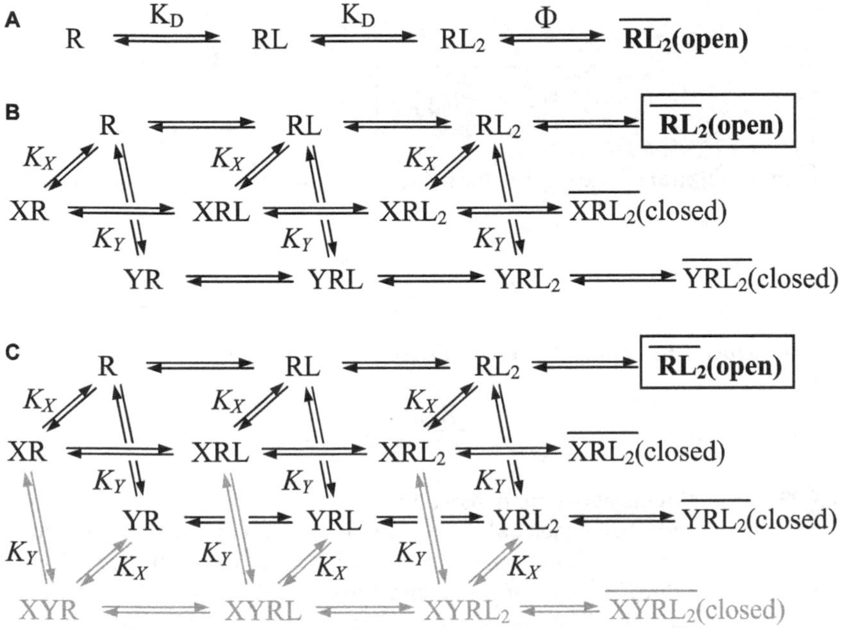

Fig. 5. Mechanisms of activation and non-competitive inhibition of ion channel receptors (A) Minimum mechanism for the activation of a ligand-gated ion channel. Note that the channel-opening reaction comprises two elementary steps, ligand binding (dissociation constant K_D) and conformational change to the open state (open-close equilibrium Φ). R = receptor, L = activating ligand. In this example binding of two ligand molecules is needed prior to channel opening. (B) Inhibition of an ion channel receptor by two non-competitive inhibitors X and Y, which are mutually exclusive (e.g. binding to the same site). Either inhibitor X or Y can bind at any given time. Presence of the second inhibitor can only exert an additive effect but is not synergistic. (C) Inhibition of an ion channel receptor by two non-competitive inhibitors X and Y, which are mutually non-exclusive, targeting different sites on the receptor. Synergism is then observed as a necessary consequence of two mutually non-exclusive inhibitors.

In the presence of one non-competitive inhibitor X, we obtain the following equation for the signal S_X:

$$S_X = I_{max} \frac{1}{\left[\left(\frac{K_D}{L}+1\right)^2 \phi + 1\right]\left(1+\frac{X}{K_X}\right)} \qquad (22)$$

where K_X is the inhibition constant, L is the concentration of activating ligand, and X the concentration of inhibitor. One can now readily compute the ratios of control current signal to signal in presence of inhibitor:

$$\frac{S_0}{S_X} = \frac{I_{max} \dfrac{1}{\left[\left(\frac{K_D}{L}+1\right)^2 \phi + 1\right]}}{I_{max} \dfrac{1}{\left[\left(\frac{K_D}{L}+1\right)^2 \phi + 1\right]\left(1+\frac{X}{K_X}\right)}} = 1 + \frac{X}{K_X} \qquad (23)$$

In case of two inhibitors binding to the same site (mutually exclusive), the ratio again becomes

$$\frac{S_0}{S_{X,Y}} = 1 + \frac{X}{K_X} + \frac{Y}{K_Y} \qquad (24)$$

For two non-exclusive inhibitors, targeting different sites on the recpetor, this ratio then is

$$\frac{S_0}{S_{X,Y}} = 1 + \frac{X}{K_X} + \frac{Y}{K_Y}\left(1+\frac{X}{K_X}\right) \qquad (25)$$

Equations 23 – 25 are identical to equations 11-14.

Similar to the treatment of Michaelis-Menten enzymes, we obtain again a system of linear equations that describes the action of one or two inhibitors of ion channel receptors. If the concentration of inhibitor X is held constant, and the concentration of the second inhibitor, Y, is varied, the ratio $S_0 / S_{X,Y}$ is shifted up by a constant amount X/K_X but the slope $(1/K_Y)$ is unchanged. The slope of the ratio curve represents the inhibitory potency, and the constant upward shift is due to the additive effect of two mutually exclusive inhibitors.

In the presence of two mutually non-exclusive inhibitors, the slope (ie inhibitory potency) is increased by a factor of $(1 + X/K_X)$. Thus, if the mechanism underlying this analysis were followed, the "amount of synergy" could be calculated as $1 + X/K_X$. Often, quality of the data does not permit this quantitation, although the qualitative demonstration of synergy (increased inhibitory potency of drug A in the presence of drug B) is statistically safe. Thus, by taking the ratios of control and inhibited signals, we arrive at an equation that becomes mechanism-independent and corresponds to the principal equations used to describe drug interactions. The ratio method results in a simple graph that describes the type of joint action of two inhibitors on a common enzyme, neurotransmitter receptor, or general target protein (Fig. 6).

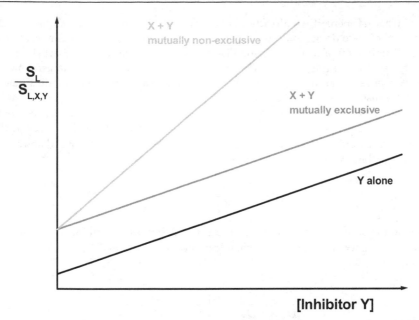

Fig. 6. Ratio method graph. Graph of signal ratio $S_0/S_{X,Y}$ vs inhibitor concentration for the case of one inhibitor (black curve), two mutually exclusive inhibitors (gray curve), and two mutually non-exclusive inhibitors (light gray curve). In case of mutually non-exclusive binding the inhibitory potency of inhibitor Y is increased in the presence of inhibitor X, as indicated by the lower value of K_Y computed from the slope of the inhibition ratio curve. Note that the formalism described here becomes mechanism-independent and applies to Michaelis-Menten type enzymes as well as to more complex mechanisms of ion channel receptor inhibition.

So far, a simple description of the action of two inhibitors on a common target has been derived. The mechanisms were based upon (i) a common binding site for two inhibitors, leading to mutually exclusive binding (Fig. 2), or (ii) two independent binding sites, leading to mutually non-exclusive binding (Fig. 3), Indeed, these simple models underlie (i) the principle of Loewe additivity (Loewe 1953; Berenbaum 1989), also referred to "similar", or "homodynamic" action of drugs. Here, the expectation value for zero interaction is just additivity. Independent inhibitor sites (Fig. 3), in contrast, correspond to Bliss independence, "dissimilar", "heterodynamic", or "independent" action of drugs (Bliss 1939; Berenbaum 1989). The combined effect of two such drugs will be more than additive, fulfilling the basic criterion of synergy. It has been recognized that these are the two limiting mechanisms for drug interaction (Bliss 1939; Finney 1942; Plackett and Hewlett 1948), and indeed both models are being used in the literature as zero interaction reference (Greco, Bravo et al. 1995).

It is intuitive, and favoured by this author to view the concept of Loewe additivity as the zero interaction reference, and noting the superadditive response from Bliss independence as synergism. This definition is widely accepted (Segel 1975; Chou and Talalay 1977; Berenbaum 1989). Furthermore, it allows for a very intuitive definition of zero interaction, proposed by Loewe: if drug A and B are the same, B being a dilution of A. Naturally, action of "both" drugs would be similar, and thus we have a perfect model of additivity.

However, what happens if we already know that drug A and B have completely different modes of action? Two drugs could be targeting different enzymes in a biochemical pathway. Of such a combination of drugs – having dissimilar action – we would expect superadditive behaviour. Can we call this synergy, or is it just expected from the mechanism and is now our zero reference? Arguments can be found for either view, and both models (and many more) are thus used and debated in the literature.

Once we move to more complicated systems, mechanism-based analysis is no longer feasible, and more general descriptions of drug interaction are needed. However, they all relate to the basic models of additivity and independence that were described above.

Equation 25 can be rearranged into the form

$$\frac{S_0}{S_{X,Y}} = 1 + \frac{X}{K_X} + \frac{Y}{K_Y} + \frac{X}{K_X}\frac{Y}{K_Y} \tag{26}$$

This equation is similar to a general equation that describes describing the joint action of two drugs on a specific target or biochemical process, presented by Greco et al. (Greco, Bravo et al. 1995).

$$1 = \frac{D_1}{ID_{X,1}} + \frac{D_2}{ID_{X,2}} + f\left(\frac{D_1}{ID_{X,1}}, \frac{D_2}{ID_{X,2}}, \alpha, p\right) \tag{27}$$

Here, D_1 and D_2 are concentrations of drug 1 and 2 in a mixture; $ID_{X,1}$ and $ID_{X,2}$ are the concentrations that produce a certain effect (corresponding to EC_{50}, or IC_{50} values); α is the synergism/antagonism parameter and p represents additional parameter(s) describing the "interaction" (joint action) of the two drugs.

The models and derivations given above are indeed the simplest approach to synergism between drugs. At this time, we do not even have a complete description of the action of every drug. It has been pointed out that under physiological conditions, it is expected that indeed presence of a drug will always result in an altered state of metabolism and thereby affect other drugs (Gessner 1974). In many patients multiple drug regimes have to be given, and the metabolism of a critically ill person may differ from a healthy "control" volunteer. Taken together, medical reality is not sufficiently described by simplified models. However, as shown above, even from simple model cases we can understand mechanisms of synergy and can derive mechanism-independent formalisms to determine the type of joint action of drug combinations.

In biomedical modelling, an alternative approach is the use of a mechanism-free description of activity, such as enzyme activity, ion channel function, the throughput of an entire biochemical pathway, or even cell survival in toxicity assays. The most common approach is the use of logistic equations that simply connect concentration of an effector (agonist or inhibitor) to the measured effect (enzyme activity, product formation, cell survival). The most comonly used formalism is that of the Hill equation.

$$E_0 = E_{max}\frac{1}{1 + \left(\frac{EC_{50}}{L}\right)^n} \tag{28}$$

Here, E_0 is the observed effect, E_{max} is the maximum signal, EC_{50} is the concentration of ligand L that produces 50 % of the maximum response, and n is a coefficient defining the steepness of the dose-response curve. The similarity to Michaelis-Menten type enzyme kinetics is obvious, yet the logistic formalism is not based on any mechanism. Indeed, complex clinical situations require use of mechanism-free models to analyze drug interactions (Chou 1976; Berenbaum 1978; Berenbaum 1980; Chou and Talalay 1981; Berenbaum 1989; Tallarida 1992; Greco, Bravo et al. 1995).

In the following section some principles and formalisms for the analysis of drug synergism are briefly reviewed. An exhaustive review of all concepts is outside the scope of this text, readers are directed to several excellent, comprehensive reviews (Berenbaum 1989; Greco, Bravo et al. 1995; Tallarida 2001; Chou 2002; Toews and Bylund 2005; Chou 2006; Tallarida 2006; Bijnsdorp, Giovannetti et al. 2011).

3. Mechanisms and techniques of synergy testing in complex biomedical settings

An example, modified from Berenbaum (Berenbaum 1989) is that of a woodcutter, able to cut 10 trees in a day. He is joined by a second woodcutter, also able to cut down 10 trees in a day. Together, they manage to cut 15 trees in one day. How do we describe this situation?

One approach is that cutter A achieves 10 trees per day, our expectation value. Addition of cutter B results in 15 trees being cut, so there is synergy. Such an approach has been proposed e.g. by Gaddum, who only considered the effect of one agent and whether it was affected by another one being added (Gaddum 1940). This formalism is not used widely, as it obviously assigns synergism to the effects of several drugs too readily.

Conversely, one would say that with two cutters, each able to cut 10 trees per day, the expectation value is 20 trees/day. If only 15 are achieved, they are antagonising each other. This is the application of additivity, and clearly, the combined effect is sub-additive, 20 trees would be just additive, and more than 20 would mean synergy.

Mechanistically, one might argue that if cutter A works on a tree, then cutter B would not work on the same tree. Their action would be mutually exclusive, and the additive result would be expected. If, however, they are willing to work at the same tree together, they will be able to cut this tree in a much shorter time. In this case, they would be able to cut more than 20 trees in a day and their action would be mutually non-exclusive, leading to synergy.

As stated above, pure mechanistic analysis is not sufficient (and not possible) for most clinical cases, so a general, mechanism-free analysis of drug interaction is needed. Berenbaum (Berenbaum 1989) has pointed out the similarity to non-parametric statistical tests that do not require information about the meaning of the values, or the distribution of populations from where the values originate. The equivalent in dose-response analysis is a logistic equation, that just describes a dose-response curve without any requirement of a mechanism. In such a setting, one would just define the desired outcome (enzyme inhibition, cell death, reduction of virus titer, ...), and then measure the effect achieved by varying doses of each drug alone, and in combination.

The mechanisms shown above illustrate just the simplest mechanistic model. In real life, the situation is more complicated, as mechanisms of enzyme or receptor acitivity are more complex. Furthermore medical intervention is not only directed at single proteins, but at entire pathways or controlling structures, such as transcription factors, that initiate or control biochemical processes. Some therapies, such as cancer chemotherapy even aim at cell destruction, i.e. they interfere with a complete living organism. In most of these situations, mechanisms of action are not known, or are too complex to work with. The additional problem is that with increasing complexity of the biological system, one finds an increasing paucity of experimental data. Even a simple dose-response curve, traditionally recorded with seven sensibly spaced concentration points, carries a significant error. By the rule of parsimony, one has to choose the simplest possible mechanism to describe experimental data. Thus, research is confronted with the dilemma of either oversimplification, or overinterpretation of results – a working compromise between these two extremes is needed. The pertinent models and methods have been extensively analyzed and reviewed in two excellent papers by Berenbaum (Berenbaum 1989), and Greco et al. (Greco, Bravo et al. 1995).

Some of the main concepts are just briefly described:
- Median effect analysis
- Interaction index, isobole method and combination index
- Response surface analysis

3.1 Median effect analysis

Chou et al. derived the median effect equation which follows from a detailed derivation of MM enzyme mechanisms (Chou 1976; Chou and Talalay 1977; Chou and Talalay 1981; Chou 2006).

$$\frac{d}{M} = \frac{E_d}{1 - E_d} \tag{29}$$

where d is the dose of a drug, E_d the effect caused by this amount of drug, M the median (dose causing 50 % effect, i.e. EC_{50} or IC_{50}). Indeed, such an equation can be derived by rearrangement of the Michaelis-Menten equation (6):

$$\frac{[S]}{K_M} = \frac{\dfrac{V_0}{V_{max}}}{1 - \dfrac{V_0}{V_{max}}} \tag{30}$$

Here, [S] is the substrate concentration that gives the observed V_0, K_M is the Michaelis constant, and V_0/V_{max} is the effect caused by [S], expressed here as the fractional velocity. The median effect equation has been proposed as a central, unified equation from which the basic equation sets of Henderson-Hasselbalch, Scatchard, Hill, and Michaelis-Menten can be derived (Chou 2006; Chou 2010). The median effect equation has been derived from MM-type enzymes from mathematical analysis. It can be extended to multiple-site systems in the form (Chou 2006)

$$\frac{E_d}{1 - E_d} = \left(\frac{d}{M}\right)^n \tag{31}$$

where n is the constant giving the slope of the dose-response curve. Note that n has often been equated with the number of binding sites, but this is an oversimplification that should be avoided since it is not valid in most cases. The value of n may be a measure of the degree of cooperativity between binding sites, but nothing more.

The equation can also be expressed in the form

$$\frac{f_A}{f_{UA}} = \left(\frac{d}{M}\right)^n \qquad (32)$$

where f_A and f_{UA} are the fractions of affected and unaffected enzyme, respectively. The importance of the median effect equation is that it is composed of ratios of effects (E_d, $(1-E_d)$, or f_A and f_{UA}) and of the dose ratio (actual dose d, median dose M). Although derived from mechanistic analysis, the median effect equation cancels out mechanism-specific constants, and just links dose and effect in dimensionless ratios. This makes it a very versatile tool for the analysis of complex systems. The median effect equation can be linearized by taking logarithms on either side, giving the Hill plot (see Berenbaum 1989) which is a straight line for the plot of $\log(f_A/f_{UA})$ vs. $\log d$.

$$\log\left[\frac{f_A}{f_{UA}}\right] = n\left(\log d - \log M\right) \qquad (33)$$

Thus the median effect equations can be seen as an extremely useful rearranged form of dose-response curves, linking ratios of drug doses to ratios of observed effects. The median equation will work with both, mechanism-based (eg Michaelis-Menten), and effect-based (eg logistic) equations, and provides a dimensionless measure for drug effects. The technique has been extensively tested and derived from mechanistic as well as purely mathematical considerations. The group of T.C. Chou have pioneered this field and developed software packages (CompuSyn ands CalcuSyn) that allow reliable testing of drug interaction parameters (Chou 2002; Chou 2006; Chou 2010). Well-founded in theory, the technique has found widespread use (Chou 2002; Chou 2006; Chou 2010; Bijnsdorp, Giovannetti et al. 2011), and the initital paper by Chou and Talalay (Chou and Talalay 1984) has been intensely cited and discussed.

3.2 Interaction index, isobole method and combination index
The interaction of two or more drugs to produce a combined effect can be described by the interaction index I (Berenbaum 1977).

$$I = \frac{D_1}{ID_{X,1}} + \frac{D_2}{ID_{X,2}} \qquad (34)$$

or written in terms of the median equations above

$$I = \frac{d_1}{M_1} + \frac{d_2}{M_2} \qquad (35)$$

where, D_1, D_2 d_1 and d_2 are concentrations of drug 1 and 2 that produce a certain effect if applied together; $ID_{X,1}$, $ID_{X,2}$, M_1 and M_2 are the concentrations that produce the same effect when given alone. For instance, if we want 50 % inhibition, then equation 34 would be:

$$I = \frac{D_1}{IC_{50,1}} + \frac{D_2}{IC_{50,2}} \qquad (36)$$

Here, $IC_{50,1}$ and $IC_{50,2}$ are the IC_{50} values of drug 1 and drug 2 alone. D_1 and D_2 are the doses of drug 1 and 2, respectively, that also produce 50 % inhibition when given together. The interaction index, proposed by Berenbaum (Berenbaum 1977), should be constant in case of zero interaction. The method has been extended by Berenbaum (Berenbaum 1985) and developed into a general method based on analysis of each drug alone and then simulating the combined action of both drugs based on Loewe additivity (see also Greco, Bravo et al. 1995).

The interaction index underlies one of the most widely used graphical representations of drug synergism and antagonism, the isobologram. Isoboles were first used by Fraser in 1870 (Fraser 1870; Fraser 1872) as simple, intuitive illustration without mathematical derivation. Here, the doses of drugs A and B give abscissa and ordinate, respectively, and the effect of drug combinations is plotted as graph (Fig. 7). In the example (Fig. 7), the effect plotted is for 50 % inhibition of an enzyme. The effects of each drug alone (i.e. IC_{50}) can be read from the axes. The isobologram shows an effect, such as IC_{50} (IC_{10} or IC_{80}, whatever effect is of interest) and which drug concentration is needed to achieve this effect.

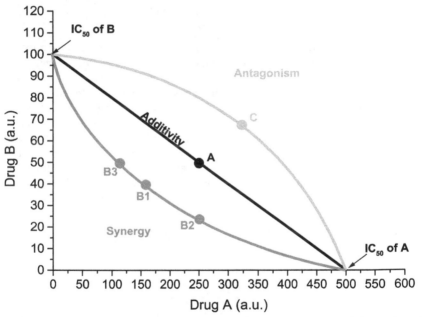

Fig. 7. Isobologram. Abscissa and ordinate units are the concentrations of drugs A and B. The solid black line connects concentrations that produce the same effect on the target protein, enzyme, or system. In this example, the IC_{50} line is given. In the simulation, drug A has an IC_{50} (concentration giving 50 % inhibition) of 500 a.u. (arbitrary units), IC_{50} of drug B is 100 a.u. From additivity (black line), the combination of 250 a.u. of A with 50 a.u. of B should also give 50 % inhibition (point A). If, 50 % inhibition are achieved at lower concentrations of the two drugs (e.g. 150 a.u. of A and 40 a.u. of B, point B1), the drugs would show synergism. If the observed inhibition by the combination was less than 50 %, drug A and B would interact in an antagonistic way (point C). Model lines of synergism (gray line) and antagonism (light gray line) are drawn. Note that in case of synergy between two drugs, the IC_{50} curve would not be a straight line but an upward concave (gray line), in case of antagonism a downward concave (light gray line). In practical application, one

would determine IC_{50} of one drug in the presence of a constant concentration of the other. IC_{50} would be found with the combination of 250 a.u. of A and 24 a.u. of B (point B2), or 110 a.u. of A and 50 a.u. of B (point B3).

Equations 34 – 36 define straight lines for two drugs that do not show any interaction (synergism or antagonism). Two drugs showing aditivity wold be expected to fall on the additivity line (Fig. 7). If the two drugs act synergistically, lower concentrations would be needed in the mixture to achieve the same effect. Their combination graph would be an upward concave (gray line in Fig. 7), following the unequality

$$\frac{D_1}{ID_{X,1}} + \frac{D_2}{ID_{X,2}} < 1 \tag{37}$$

Conversely, two antagonistic drugs would require higher doses in combination to achieve the same effect, and the resulting isobole would be an upward convex line (red line in Fig. 7), of the general (un)equation

$$\frac{D_1}{ID_{X,1}} + \frac{D_2}{ID_{X,2}} > 1 \tag{38}$$

Representing a form of median effect equationry, isoboles have become a useful tool to present complex modes of drug interaction. An excellent review by Greco et al (Greco, Bravo et al. 1995) derives isoboles as 2-D sections through three-dimensional plots of drug action data. Depending on the shapes of the dose-response curves of both drugs, isoboles do not need to be linear (Greco, Bravo et al. 1995). Also, drug combinations may be biphasic, showing concentration ranges of synergy and ranges of antagonism (Berenbaum 1989).
Equations 34 and 35 apply to the case of Loewe additivity, where the two drugs do not show synergy or antagonism. For drugs showing any type of interaction, equation 34 was extended to define a combination index (CI), indicating type and amount of interaction between two (or more) drugs with respect to the experimantal parameter being studied (Chou and Talalay 1983).

$$CI = \frac{D_1}{ID_{X,1}} + \frac{D_2}{ID_{X,2}} = \begin{array}{l} > \; 1 \; \text{for antagonism} \\ 1 \; \text{for additivity} \\ < \; 1 \; \text{for synergy} \end{array} \tag{39}$$

The CI can take values between 1 and infinity for antagonism, and runs between 0 and 1 for synergy. Chou and Chou (1988) have introduced the dose reduction index DRI (Chou and Chou 1988), which is based on the interpretation of the Combination index equation (39). Assuming that two drugs show synergy, one expects that a lower dose of each is needed to achieve the same effect. This lower concentration (D_1 and D_2 in equations 34-39) can be related to the median (IC_{50} in equation 36), to give the dose reduction index DRI.

$$CI = \frac{1}{(DRI)_1} + \frac{1}{(DRI)_2} \tag{40}$$

Both, combination index CI and DRI can be used to plot drug combination data for visualization of synergy or antagonism (Fig. 8, see (Chou 2006)).

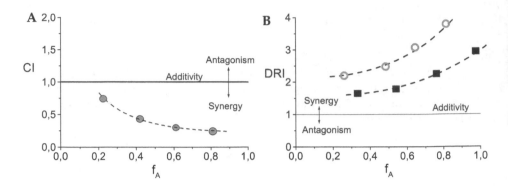

Fig. 8. Visualization of drug interaction data. (A) CI-f_A plot: The combination index CI is plotted versus f_A, the fraction of affected enzyme or biological function. (B) DRI plot: the dose reduction index DRI is plotted against f_A. See text for definitions of terms.

3.3 Response surface analysis

Response surfaces can be calculated and are a way to represent effects of drug combinations as a contour plot where drug concentrations are plotted as a horizontal x-y- plane, and the effect is plotted on the z axis. Isoboles can be seen as 2D sections through response surfaces, and the method allows graphical analysis of drug interaction data, albeit at requirement of quite some mathematical and computational effort. From the dose-response data of each drug alone, the expected response surface based on the zero interaction reference of choice, is plotted. Then actual drug combination data are entered into the plot, and similar to isobole analysis, deviations from the reference surface indicate synergism or antagonism. The technique has been applied to synergism studies (Tallarida, Stone et al. 1999), and its general use reviewed and commented in great detail (Berenbaum 1989; Greco, Bravo et al. 1995; Tallarida 2001).

3.4 Practical limitations

There is a need for a definition of synergy, antagonism, and the zero case (neither one nor the other). Sometimes, specific problems are discussed and authors feel compelled to use a unique treatment of the data. Pharmacologists, stasticians, clinicians, and representatives from other fields have different views and concepts. In various major reviews, 13 models to treat drug combination data have been proposed. The author would not encourage decisions as to right or wrong. Each model may be appropriate for a given situation, and not applicable to others. However, all models discussing synergy can be traced back to only two types of the "zero" (no interaction) case as discussed before

- Loewe Additivity
   Both drugs exert an effect but are mutually exclusive, either one or the other can be active at a given time. This corresponds to a common site of interaction in the simplest mechanistic case (Fig. 2).
- Bliss Independence
   Both drugs are mutually non-exclusive, both can be active at the same time. In the simplest case, each drug has a specific, independent interaction site (Fig. 3).

Indeed all models refer to these two basic cases. Obviously, both have a different expecation of joint action of two drugs. Loewe additivity is best described by equation 34, and any deviation from this may be considered as synergy. In case of Bliss independencs, one would expect both drugs to act independently, and therefore the zero case already includes a more than additive effect of both drugs. The author sees two problems with this definition: (i) two purely additive drugs would have to be called antagonistic, including the sham combination of a drug with itself. (ii) If two mutually non-exclusive drugs already produce a superadditive effect, and we do not yet call this synergy, how do we define "true" synergy? In terms of isoboles, the baseline (no synergy, no antagonism) is already curved, in the ratio method (Fig. 6), the slope of the inhibition curve is increased already for the zero case, and one calculates a CI of less than one. Thus, to identify synergy, one has to select a gradual increase. It may be fairly easy to identify a deviation from a straight line (isobole), but for the CI a deviation from <1 to <<1 is expected. In the ration method, the steepness of th slope may be hard to compute, as the ratio $S_X/S_{control}$ is toe be calculated from small numerical values and thus carries a large error.

Thus the definition of Loewe additivity is preferred by this author as the definition of no synergy. As shown in Fig.s 2 and 3, it can clearly be defined in mechanistic term. Dose-response analysis also follows the definition. Addtivity correctly describes the purest control experiment, sham mixtures of the same drug, and it follows the general definition of synergy, where a combination produces more thant the sum of the individual components.

It should be noted, however, that in many clinical applications, drug combinations are used that target two completely different target proteins, or pathways. In radiotherapy, the combination of radiation and drugs work together, and in combination lower doses of either are required compared to a single treatment. No baseline of Loewe additivity can be proposed for such a combination. Likewise, combinations of drugs that target completely different cellular pathways may work synergistically towards cell killing even though the two drugs are not mutually exclusive in their activity. Obviously, there is no single methodology that is appropriate for all biomedical situations.

An additional problem in interpreting drug combination data is the quality of the measured data. Biological systems invariably carry experimental error, and thus borderline cases are almost impossible to assign. For example, a combination index is calculated to be 0.9 – is this a real deviation from unity (and thus synergy), or is it experimental error?

Even with the best data, however, analysis of joint action of two drugs has another inherent problem. Two different drugs may have different dose-response characteristics. In this case, changes in effective concentrations may suggest synergy where there is none. A principal illustration of this problem is given in Fig. 9 (adapted from Chou (Chou 2006; Chou 2010)), showing that the same relative concentration change can produce quite different effects (Fig. 9 A,B). Even for a single compound, there is a marked difference whether one investigates concentrations below or around EC_{50}, or near saturation. Addition of the same drug in the concentration range around EC_{50} (ie the steepest part of the dose-response curve) gives rise to a strong increase in signal which may be misinterpreted as synergy. The shapes of isobolograms for drugs with different dose-response characteristics, and the complications resulting from this fact have been extensively studied (Berenbaum 1989; Greco, Bravo et al. 1995; Tallarida 2001; Chou 2006).

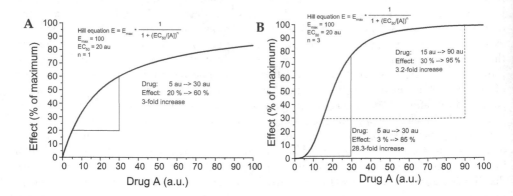

Fig. 9. Dose-effect curves of different shape. Both curves were simulated using the Hill equation and the parameters E_{max} = 100 % , EC_{50} = 20 au (arbitrary units). (A) Curve simulated for n =1 (hyperbolic curve). (B) Simulated for n = 3 (sigmoidal curve). Note the difference in curve shape, and the different effect of a change of concentration of agonist A from 5 to 30 au. In the hyperbolic case, the effect increases 3-fold, in the sigmoidal case, the increase is 28.3-fold. Effects of changes in agonist concentration are different depending on the response range where they happen. Sigmoidal dose-response curves are steepest around the median (panel B). In the example, a 6-fold raise in concentration (from 5 to 30 au) will cause a 28.3-fold increase in the observed effect. Raising the concentration from 15 to 90 au, the effect only increases 3.2-fold. Thus, if presence of a second drug B increases cooperativity of drug A, or if drug B shifts the relevant dose-response range of A towards the median by purely additive (non-synergistic) means, one would observe a higher increase in effect than expected from addition and wrongly interpret this as synergy.

4. Borderlines of synergism – Potentiation, coalism, inertism, metabolic interference

From the simplest models presented here to advanced discussions, the situations of synergy could be traced back to the simple principles of additivity vs. independence. In all those cases, both drugs were having the same effect alone or in combination. The only difference was the magnitude of the effects. Synergism can also occur with combinations of drugs or methods that have completely different modes of action. In cancer therapy a combination of radiation and cytostatica is often used. Combination of substances and environmental conditions (heat, pH, radiation) have indeed been analyzed for synergy (Johnson, Eyring et al. 1945). There are cases of one drug having no activity, but augmenting the activity of another, as observed for antinociception by acetaminophen in combination with phentolamine (Raffa, Stone et al. 2001). The extreme case would be the combination of two drugs that have no effect alone, but are effective in combination. On the othe hand, self-synergy of paracetamol has been described by Tallarida et al., who showed that the drug binds to targets in different locations and thus facilitates its own activity (Raffa, Stone et al. 2000). An interesting approach is an attempt to predict drug synergism from gene microarray data (Jin, Zhao et al. 2011).

Effect of drug combination	Both drugs have same effect individually	Only one drug is effective individually	None of the two drugs has an effect individually
Greater than zero reference	Synergy, Synergism	Synergism (potentiation)	Coalism
Equal to zero reference	Additiviy / Independence	Inertism	Inertism
Smaller than zero reference	Antagonism	Antagonism	

Table 1. The terminology of the combined action of drugs (after Greco, Bravo et al. 1995)

Another effect leading to apparent synergy or antagonism is the effect some drug may have on uptake, metabolism and clearance of other drugs. Depending on the route of administration, metabolism by first liver pass must be considered, including one of the most critical steps of drug biotransformation, namely oxygenation (thus hydrophilization) by cytochrome P450, an oxygenase that catalyzes oxygenations of substrates using NADPH and oxygen (O_2). This oxygenation R–H → R–OH is a crucial step in metabolism and eventual clearance of drugs and pharmaceuticals from the body. To date, 56 subtypes of cytochrome P450 are found in humans, some of which are critical in metabolism of endogenous substances such as medical drugs. Substances interfering with cytochrome P450 may, therefore, have an impact on drug clearance and thus on the actual concentration of a certain drug in the body (Flockhart 1995; Flockhart and Oesterheld 2000; Shin, Park et al. 2002; Takada, Arefayene et al. 2004).

Resource	Internet address	Comment
Drug interactions checker	http://www.drugs.com/drug_interactions.html	Tool to query compounds that interact with a given drug
Medscape drug interaction checker	http://reference.medscape.com/drug-interactionchecker	Tool to report on interactions between two drugs
Cytochrome P450 drug interaction table	http://medicine.iupui.edu/clinpharm/ddis/	List of drugs metabolized by cyt P450 isoforms (Flockhart 2007)
Grapefruit juice/citrus fruit juice interactions	http://www.mayoclinic.com/health/food-and-nutrition/AN00413	Short list of drugs that interact with dietary citrus fruits
Private resources	http://www.environmentaldiseases.com/article-drug-interactions.html	Website discussing case individual studies of interfering drugs

Table 2. Internet tools for drug interactions in clinical settings

There are numerous internet tools that list known drug interactions. A brief list of some such resources is given in table 2. Thus, some practical aspects have been covered, although synergisms and other interactions of drugs are not yet given enough weight in approval or recommendations of drug use. This is particularly relevant for the less well-defined field of herbal remedies. Their interaction with anticancer agents has been studied (Sparreboom, Cox et al. 2004), but our knowledge in this area is still far from comprehensive.

To date, the study of drug interaction in the biomedical field is widespread and must include the following aspects:
- mechanism of action of a single drug
- mechanisms of action of two (or more) drugs acting on the same physiological target
- interaction of two drugs through side effects, secondary targets, etc
- effects on metabolism of the primary drug
- top-down observations of the performance of drug combinations in patients

Going down this list it becomes clear that pure mechanistic studies – although essential – are not sufficient to cover all aspects of drug interaction. Clinical observation is the – equally essential – other end of the spectrum and the gap between these two positions is indeed narrowing.

5. References

Asante-Appiah, E. & W. W. Chan (1996). Analysis of the interactions between an enzyme and multiple inhibitors using combination plots. *Biochem J* Vol. 320 (Pt 1), pp. 17-26.

Berenbaum, M. C. (1977). Synergy, additivism and antagonism in immunosuppression. A critical review. *Clin Exp Immunol* Vol. 28, No. 1, pp. 1-18.

Berenbaum, M. C. (1978). A method for testing for synergy with any number of agents. *J Infect Dis* Vol. 137, No. 2, pp. 122-130.

Berenbaum, M. C. (1980). Correlations between methods for measurement of synergy. *J Infect Dis* Vol. 142, No. 3, pp. 476-480.

Berenbaum, M. C. (1985). The expected effect of a combination of agents: the general solution. *J Theor Biol* Vol. 114, No. 3, pp. 413-431.

Berenbaum, M. C. (1989). What is synergy? *Pharmacol Rev* Vol. 41, No. 2, pp. 93-141.

Bijnsdorp, I. V., E. Giovannetti & G. J. Peters (2011). Analysis of drug interactions. *Methods Mol Biol* Vol. 731, No., pp. 421-34.

Bliss, C. I. (1939). The toxicity of poisons applied jointly. *Ann Appl Biol* Vol. 26, pp. 585-615.

Breitinger, H.-G., N. Geetha & G. P. Hess (2001). Inhibition of the serotonin 5-HT3 receptor by nicotine, cocaine, and fluoxetine investigated by rapid chemical kinetic techniques. *Biochemistry* Vol. 40, No. 28, pp. 8419-8429.

Chou, T. C. (1976). Derivation and properties of Michaelis-Menten type and Hill type equations for reference ligands. *J Theor Biol* Vol. 59, No. 2, pp. 253-276.

Chou, T. C. (2002). Synergy determination issues. *J Virol* Vol. 76, No. 20, pp. 10577; author reply 10578

Chou, T. C. (2006). Theoretical basis, experimental design, and computerized simulation of synergism and antagonism in drug combination studies. *Pharmacol Rev* Vol. 58, No. 3, pp. 621-681.

Chou, T. C. (2010). Drug combination studies and their synergy quantification using the Chou-Talalay method. *Cancer Res* Vol. 70, No. 2, pp. 440-446.

Chou, T. C. & J. H. Chou (1988). Distinction between multiple ligand exclusivity and competitiveness in receptor binding topology. *FASEB J.* Vol. 2, pp. A1778.

Chou, T. C. & P. Talalay (1977). A simple generalized equation for the analysis of multiple inhibitions of Michaelis-Menten kinetic systems. *J Biol Chem* Vol. 252, No. 18, pp. 6438-6442.

Chou, T. C. & P. Talalay (1981). Generalized equations for the analysis of inhibitions of Michaelis-Menten and higher-order kinetic systems with two or more mutually exclusive and nonexclusive inhibitors. *Eur J Biochem* Vol. 115, No. 1, pp. 207-216.

Chou, T. C. & P. Talalay (1983). Analysis of combined drug effects: a new look at a very old problem. *Trends Pharmacol Sci* Vol. 4, No., pp. 450–454.

Chou, T. C. & P. Talalay (1984). Quantitative analysis of dose-effect relationships: the combined effects of multiple drugs or enzyme inhibitors. *Adv Enzyme Regul* Vol. 22, No., pp. 27-55.

Colquhoun, D. (1998). Binding, gating, affinity and efficacy: the interpretation of structure-activity relationships for agonists and of the effects of mutating receptors. *Br J Pharmacol* Vol. 125, No. 5, pp. 924-947.

Finney, D. J. (1942). The analysis of toxicity tests on mixtures of poisons. *Ann. Appl. Biol.* Vol. 29, No., pp. 82-94.

Flockhart, D. A. (1995). Drug interactions and the cytochrome P450 system. The role of cytochrome P450 2C19. *Clin Pharmacokinet* Vol. 29 Suppl 1, No., pp. 45-52.

Flockhart, D. A. (2007). Drug Interactions: Cytochrome P450 Drug Interaction Table. *Indiana University School of Medicine* . http://medicine.iupui.edu/clinpharm/ddis/

Flockhart, D. A. & J. R. Oesterheld (2000). Cytochrome P450-mediated drug interactions. *Child Adolesc Psychiatr Clin N Am* Vol. 9, No. 1, pp. 43-76.

Fraser, T. R. (1870). An experimental research on the antagonism between the actions of physostigma and atropia. *Proc. Roy. Soc. Edin.* Vol. 7, No., pp. 506-511.

Fraser, T. R. (1872). The antagonism between the actions of active substances. *Br. Med. J.* Vol. 2, No., pp. 485-487.

Gaddum, J. H. (1940). *Pharmacology*. Oxford University Press, London.

Gessner, P. K. (1974). *The isobolographic method applied to drug interactions*. In: Drug Interactions. P. L. Morselli, S. Garattini & S. N. Cohen (Eds), pp. 349-362, Raven Press, New York.

Greco, W. R., G. Bravo & J. C. Parsons (1995). The search for synergy: a critical review from a response surface perspective. *Pharmacol Rev* Vol. 47, No. 2, pp. 331-385.

Hess, G. P. (1993). Determination of the chemical mechanism of neurotransmitter receptor-mediated reactions by rapid chemical kinetic techniques. *Biochemistry* Vol. 32, No. 4, pp. 989-1000.

Jin, G., H. Zhao, X. Zhou & S. T. Wong (2011). An enhanced Petri-net model to predict synergistic effects of pairwise drug combinations from gene microarray data. *Bioinformatics* Vol. 27, No. 13, pp. i310-316.

Johnson, F. H., H. Eyring, R. Steblay, H. Chaplin, C. Huber & G. Gherardi (1945). The Nature and Control of Reactions in Bioluminescence : With Special Reference to the Mechanism of Reversible and Irreversible Inhibitions by Hydrogen and Hydroxyl Ions, Temperature, Pressure, Alcohol, Urethane, and Sulfanilamide in Bacteria. *J Gen Physiol* Vol. 28, No. 5, pp. 463-537.

Karpen, J. W., H. Aoshima, L. G. Abood & G. P. Hess (1982). Cocaine and phencyclidine inhibition of the acetylcholine receptor: analysis of the mechanisms of action based on measurements of ion flux in the millisecond-to-minute time region. *Proc Natl Acad Sci U S A* Vol. 79, No. 8, pp. 2509-2513.

Karpen, J. W. & G. P. Hess (1986). Cocaine, phencyclidine, and procaine inhibition of the acetylcholine receptor: characterization of the binding site by stopped-flow measurements of receptor-controlled ion flux in membrane vesicles. *Biochemistry* Vol. 25, No. 7, pp. 1777-1785.

Loewe, S. (1953). The problem of synergism and antagonism of combined drugs. *Arzneimittelforschung* Vol. 3, No. 6, pp. 285-290.

Palatini, P. (1983). The interaction between full and partial inhibitors acting on a single enzyme. A theoretical analysis. *Mol Pharmacol* Vol. 24, No. 1, pp. 30-41.

Plackett, R. L. & P. S. Hewlett (1948). Statistical aspects of the independent joint action of poisons, particularly insecticides; the toxicity of a mixture of poisons. *Ann Appl Biol* Vol. 35, No. 3, pp. 347-358.

Raafat, K., U. Breitinger, L. Mahran, N. Ayoub & H. G. Breitinger (2010). Synergistic inhibition of glycinergic transmission in vitro and in vivo by flavonoids and strychnine. *Toxicol Sci* Vol. 118, No. 1, pp. 171-182.

Raffa, R. B., D. J. Stone, Jr. & R. J. Tallarida (2000). Discovery of "self-synergistic" spinal/supraspinal antinociception produced by acetaminophen (paracetamol). *J Pharmacol Exp Ther* Vol. 295, No. 1, pp. 291-294.

Raffa, R. B., D. J. Stone, Jr. & R. J. Tallarida (2001). Unexpected and pronounced antinociceptive synergy between spinal acetaminophen (paracetamol) and phentolamine. *Eur J Pharmacol* Vol. 412, No. 2, pp. R1-2.

Schenker, P. & A. Baici (2009). Simultaneous interaction of enzymes with two modifiers: reappraisal of kinetic models and new paradigms. *J Theor Biol* Vol. 261, No. 2, pp. 318-329.

Segel, I. H. (1975). *Enzyme Kinetics*. John Wiley, New York.

Shin, J. G., J. Y. Park, M. J. Kim, J. H. Shon, Y. R. Yoon, I. J. Cha, S. S. Lee, S. W. Oh, S. W. Kim & D. A. Flockhart (2002). Inhibitory effects of tricyclic antidepressants (TCAs) on human cytochrome P450 enzymes in vitro: mechanism of drug interaction between TCAs and phenytoin. *Drug Metab Dispos* Vol. 30, No. 10, pp. 1102-1107.

Sparreboom, A., M. C. Cox, M. R. Acharya & W. D. Figg (2004). Herbal remedies in the United States: potential adverse interactions with anticancer agents. *J Clin Oncol* Vol. 22, No. 12, pp. 2489-2503.

Takada, K., M. Arefayene, Z. Desta, C. H. Yarboro, D. T. Boumpas, J. E. Balow, D. A. Flockhart & G. G. Illei (2004). Cytochrome P450 pharmacogenetics as a predictor of toxicity and clinical response to pulse cyclophosphamide in lupus nephritis. *Arthritis Rheum* Vol. 50, No. 7, pp. 2202-2210.

Tallarida, R. J. (1992). Statistical analysis of drug combinations for synergism. *Pain* Vol. 49, No. 1, pp. 93-97.

Tallarida, R. J. (2001). Drug synergism: its detection and applications. *J Pharmacol Exp Ther* Vol. 298, No. 3, pp. 865-872.

Tallarida, R. J. (2006). An overview of drug combination analysis with isobolograms. *J Pharmacol Exp Ther* Vol. 319, No. 1, pp. 1-7.

Tallarida, R. J., D. J. Stone, Jr., J. D. McCary & R. B. Raffa (1999). Response surface analysis of synergism between morphine and clonidine. *J Pharmacol Exp Ther* Vol. 289, No. 1, pp. 8-13.

Toews, M. L. & D. B. Bylund (2005). Pharmacologic principles for combination therapy. *Proc Am Thorac Soc* Vol. 2, No. 4, pp. 282-289; discussion 290-291.

7

Variability of Plasma Methadone Concentration in Opiate Dependent Receiving Methadone: A Personalised Approach Towards Optimizing Dose

Nasir Mohamad[1,3], Nor Hidayah Abu Bakar[2], Tan Soo Choon[3],
Sim Hann Liang[3], NIM Nazar[3], Ilya Irinaz Idrus[3] and Rusli Ismail[3]
[1]*Department of Emergency Medicine, School of Medical Sciences, Health Campus,
Universiti Sains Malaysia, Kubang Kerian, Kelantan,*
[2]*Department of Pathology, Hospital Raja Perempuan Zainab II, Kota Bharu, Kelantan,*
[3]*Pharmacogenetic Research Group,
Institute for Research in Molecular Medicine (INFORMM),
Health Campus, Universiti Sains Malaysia, Kubang Kerian, Kelantan,
Malaysia*

1. Introduction

1.1 Methadone and methadone maintenance therapy (MMT): An overview

Methadone acts on the opioid receptors and produces many of the same effects of morphine and heroin. In the treatment of opioid dependence, methadone has cross-tolerance with other opioid, including heroin and morphine and a long duration of effect. Higher doses of methadone can block the euphoric effects of heroin, morphine, and similar drugs. As a result, properly dosed methadone patients can reduce or stop altogether their use of these substances.

Methadone is a misunderstood drug and ignorance about it is common. Even professionals, physicians and pharmacists who are supposed to be the "guardians" of MMT receive very little training about the very medication that they are responsible for. To compound the issue, addiction is mostly viewed not as a disease and its care is frequently relegated to the lay public, at least until very recently. In Malaysia, addiction has solely been under the charge of "*Agensi Anti Dadah Kebangsaan*" (AADK), an agency that has mainly adopted a criminal approach to addiction. However, this has recently changed in Malaysia. Addiction is now recognized as a medical illness, under the purview of the medical professionals.

Nevertheless, many in the medical profession only have a rudimentary understanding of addiction. Most physicians, pharmacists and nurses receive very little training about addiction and much less regarding methadone. Thus, generally, both medical and other caregivers have very limited knowledge about addiction and much less about methadone. They have generally been taught to approach addiction as a character disorder and administer methadone as a substitute.

1.2 Pharmacogenetic of methadone

Methadone has variable pharmacology. It binds to the μ-opioid receptor, the NMDA ionotropic glutamate receptor to exert its effects. Its metabolism is mediated by several enzymes including CYP3A4, CYP2B6 and CYP2D6, enzymes that are polymorphic and hence exhibit great variability. It is mainly administered through the oral route and adverse effects include hypoventilation, constipation and miosis, in addition to tolerance, dependence and withdrawal difficulties.

As a full μ-opioid agonist, methadone exhibits all the opiate-like effects. Furthermore, its binding to the glutamatergic NMDA (N-methyl-D-aspartate) receptor. This makes it a receptor antagonist against glutamate which is the primary excitatory neurotransmitter in the CNS. NMDA receptors modulate long term excitation and memory formation. NMDA antagonists such as dextromethorphan (DXM), ketamine, tiletamine and ibogaine have been studied for their role in decreasing the development of tolerance to opioids and as possible for eliminating addiction /tolerance /withdrawal. Its action on the NMDA has been proposed as a mechanism by which methadone decreases craving for opioids (Xiao et al, 2001).

Methadone is a lipophilic drug and requires biotransformation for elimination. It has a slow metabolism and is longer lasting than morphine-based drugs. Typically its elimination half-life ranges from 15 to 60 hours with a mean of around 22 hours. Due to the polymorphic nature of its metabolism, its metabolism rates vary greatly between individuals, up to a factor of 100. This variability is apparently due to genetic variability in the production of the associated enzymes CYP3A4, CYP2B6 and CYP2D6. Several studies have been conducted to explain the intra- as well as inter-individual variability in methadone's pharmacokinetic and clinical response. Typically, methadone is a substrate for several CYP450 enzymes as well as P-glycoprotein (PGP). Many Single Nucleotide Polymorphisms (SNPs) have been reported to contribute to its variability. Furthermore, as it binds to μ-receptors, SNPs in *OPRM* gene that encodes for these receptors may contribute to the clinical response in MMT patients. Thus, SNPs in *OPRM* gene, *CYP* gene and *ABCB1 (MDR1)* gene may contribute to determine the clinical outcomes of the MMT (Lötsch et al, 2009).

1.3 Pharmacokinetic of methadone

The pharmacokinetic parameters of methadone were first published in 1975 (Verebely et al, 1975). Methadone is a lipophilic basic drug with a pKa of 9.2, which is administered orally in a racemic mixture. There is strong evidence that the enantiomers differ in their distribution and elimination, though the majority of the studies were carried out on the racemic mixture. It has been suggested that methadone undergoes adaptive changes during chronic use according to the administered doses.

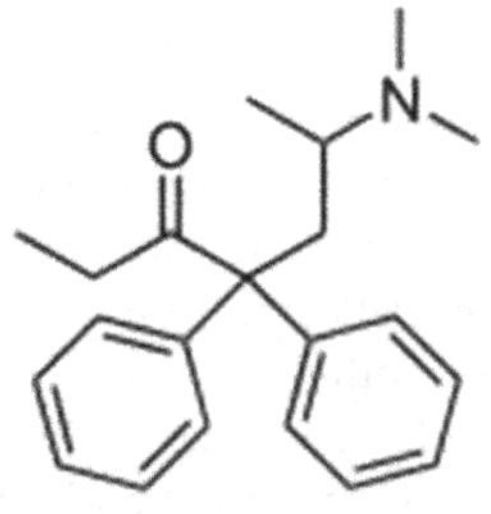

Fig. 1.1. Methadone, (RS)-6-(Dimethylamino)-4,4-diphenylheptan-3-one

Several attributes have been suggested such as clearance and *CYP3A4*. Accordingly, several pharmacokinetic studies have been carried out to investigate whether therapeutic drug monitoring (TDM) is effective as a clinical endpoint, on the one hand, and to study the methadone kinetic profile, on the other. There has been suggestive evidence to non-frequently monitor the kinetic of methadone to explain some unpredicted clinical response (Loimer and Schmid, 1992; Schmidt *et al*, 1993; Wolff and Hay, 1994; de Vos *et al*, 1996). It may be useful especially when all other measures have been taken adequately and a patient still cannot hold on methadone with high doses.

It should be noted that methadone Cp cannot be used directly to describe the clinical response, as a certain time is required for the drug to distribute adequately in the nervous system. Thus, some researchers have suggested the use of an effect-compartment or link-model to describe the effect appropriately (Ekblom *et al*, 1993). So far, only four studies have modeled methadone by this approach and only one among them for MMT patients (Dyer *et al*, 1999). It was noticed that there is an inverse relationship between plasma concentrations and withdrawal scores and pupil diameters. On the other hand, there was a direct relationship between plasma concentrations and pain threshold in the same patients. The area under the curve did not differ between those who reported withdrawal symptoms and those who did not. The study suggested that there is correlation between methadone clinical responses and changes in the plasma levels for methadone racemic mixture.

1.3.1 Absorption

The absorption of methadone following oral administration is fast and almost complete. The mean time to achieve peak concentration ranges from 2.5 - 30 hours depending on the formulation (Wolff *et al*, 1991). Oral bioavailability of methadone may range from as little as 45 percent up to 90 percent following a single dose (Meresaar *et al*, 1981). As methadone is a basic drug, acid secretions may contribute to such huge variability (Kukanich *et al*, 2005).

1.3.2 Distribution

Being a lipo-soluble drug, methadone distributes widely in body tissues such as: liver, lung, kidney, gut, brain, and muscle with different distribution coefficients (Sawe, 1986). In opioid addicts, the volume of distribution at a steady state (Vss) ranged from 0.2 to 9.2 L/kg. On the other hand, in patients with chronic pain, Vss ranged from 1.71 to 5.34 L/kg (Inturrisi *et al*, 1990), though higher doses are usually given in such situations.

Methadone pharmacokinetic is described as a two-compartment model. Although there are wide differences in the reported clearance, the reported terminal half-life was estimated to range from 23-26 hours. Half-life depends also on the volume of distribution, making the explanations much more complicated and inconclusive (Eap *et al*, 2002; Li *et al*, 2008)

Methadone binds to plasma protein to a high degree of 86 percent, predominantly to acute α-glycoprotein (AAG) (Romach *et al*, 1981; Eap *et al*, 1990). AAG is an acute phase protein that exhibits significant variations in its plasma levels according to the physiological and/or pathological situation of the patient (Fournier *et al*, 2000; Yang *et al*, 2006; Mestriner *et al*, 2007). AAG levels are significantly increased in stress, leading to very low concentrations in the free fraction (fu) of methadone in cancer patients compared to healthy participants (Abramson, 1982; Gómez *et al*, 1995). Therefore, some studies have measured the concentration of AAG itself to study the impact of their concentration on methadone concentration and / or clinical outcomes. Rowland and Tozer (1995) have stated that 'after a rapid input of methadone, a decrease in fu will be indicated by an increase in Cp, because Vss is proportional to fu. On the other hand, Cu levels remain unchanged. So, if the Cu is the pharmacologically active concentration, a decrease in fu will not modify the maximum response. Thus, it has been suggested that AAG is significantly higher in patients exhibiting abstinence syndrome compared to those who are stable (Garrido et al, 2000) and AAG may contribute to the variations in methadone plasma levels.

Other factors that may contribute to variability include age and sex. It has been suggested that these factors may explain about 33 percent of the inter-individual variations in Vss. These parameters are found to be higher in females and they are directly related to weight (Wolff et al, 2000).

Furthermore, it has also been suggested that a time-dependent increase in methadone clearance may result from auto-induction of its own metabolism by CYP3A4, and the change in Vss may be due to up or down-regulation of AAG (Rostami-Hodjegan et al, 1999). Therefore, a time-dependent decrease in Vss may be associated with the observed time-dependent increase in AAG.

1.3.3 Elimination

Generally, there is a huge inter-individual variability in methadone clearance that can reach up to 20 -100 folds in magnitude (Eap et al, 2002; Li et al, 2008). Methadone is eliminated by hepatic metabolism and renal excretion. It has been shown that at urinary pH of six and above, renal clearance accounts for four percent only. However, when urinary pH was lower than 6, the clearance of unchanged drug will be increased by 33 percent (Rostami-Hodjegan et al, 1999). It was concluded that, about 20-50 percent of the inter-individual variability can be explained by urinary excretion (KuKanich and Borum, 2008). With regard to hepatic clearance, methadone can be recognized as a drug with a low extraction ratio, 0.16 in MMT patients.

2. Objective of clinical study

2.1 General objective

To investigate factors that influence successful MMT in opiate-dependent individuals,

2.2 Specific objective

To investigate the impact of daily clinical methadone dose on plasma concentration of methadone.

3. Clinical study

The study involves opiate-dependent individuals who consented, met our study criteria and were invited to participate in the study. The study involved them taking prescribed doses of daily methadone according to Methadone Maintenance Therapy (MMT) guidelines prepared by the Malaysian Ministry of Health and be monitored regularly based on our study protocols. They were followed up for 12 months during the study period. At follow up, 5 ml of venous blood were drawn for the determination plasma methadone level using in-house methadone ELISA kit.

However, at 12th month follow up, 88 out of the 128 participants fail to meet the inclusion criteria. Thus, in order to assess the efficacy of low dose methadone on the withdrawal effect and sleeping quality, a subset of only 40 patients was further selected to participate. They were given a fixed 40 mg daily dose of methadone. Their withdrawal score and sleeping quality were assessed during the fourth week of the study.

4. Results

One hundred and twenty eight patients were enrolled for this pilot study. Their doses were titrated appropriately as tolerated. However, at 12th month follow up, 88 patients out of the 128 participants fail to meet the inclusion criteria. Thus, in order to assess the efficacy of low dose methadone on the withdrawal effect and sleeping quality, a subset of only 40 patients was further selected to participate where they were given a fixed 40 mg daily dose of methadone. Daily dose averaged 57.2 mg (SD ± 22.7) (Table 4.1) and ranged from 20 to 160 mg per day (Figure 4.1). The corresponding plasma methadone concentration averaged 281.3 ng/ml (SD ± 567.9) (Table 4.1) and ranged from 0 to 4634 ng/ml (Figure 4.2, Figure 4.3)

	Daily Dose,(mg)	Plasma Concentration, (ng/ml)
Mean	57.19828	299.842
Standard Error	2.110416	57.0856
Median	50	180.8249
Standard Deviation	22.72988	582.1612
Sample Variance	516.6473	338911.6
Kurtosis	2.263482	39.11501
Skewness	1.040586	5.905204

Table 4.1. The Summary of Statistics, Daily Methadone Dose (mg) and Plasma Methadone Concentration (ng/ml)

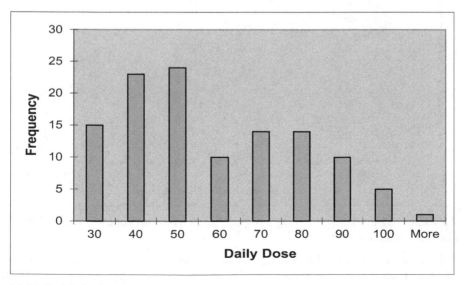

Fig. 4.1. Daily Methadone Dose in the Study Patients

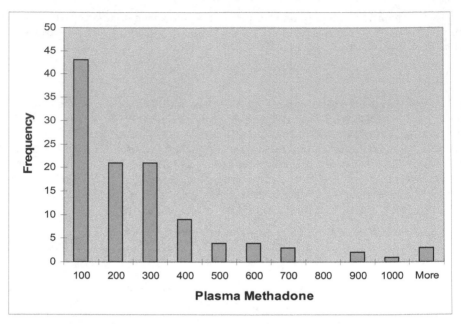

Fig. 4.2. Plasma Methadone Concentrations (ng/ml) as a function of daily methadone dose in the studied patients (outlying concentrations were removed).

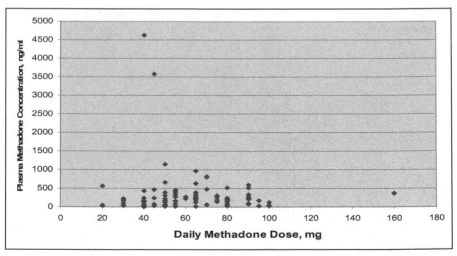

Fig. 4.3. Plasma Methadone Concentrations (ng/ml) as a Function of Daily Methadone Dose (mg) in the Studied Patients

Both the daily doses and the resulting plasma concentrations showed a non-normal distribution, more so for the plasma concentrations compared to the daily dose. Thus, although the daily dose averaged 57 mg, its median was lower at 50 mg. Similarly, although plasma concentration averaged 300 ng/ml, its median was only 181 ng/ml. A closer look revealed that 33% of patients had doses of 40 mg/day or lower, 54% received 40 – 80 mg/day dose and only 13% had doses 80 mg or more per day. In terms of plasma methadone, most, 84%, had concentrations of 400 ng/ml and 16% had 400 ng/ml and above, 400 ng/ml being the proposed minimum concentration for effectiveness. Six percent of patients on the other hand, had potentially toxic concentrations of more than 700 ng/ml. (Table 4.2 and Table 4.3)

Statistics	Day 1	Day 7	Day 14	Day 21
Mean	136.25	242.91	196.94	216.52
Standard Error	13.49	21.13	18.27	19.66
Median	135.06	194.12	162.05	190.25
Standard Deviation	80.92	126.79	109.65	117.96
Sample Variance	6548.10	16075.43	12022.56	13913.47
Skewness	0.56	1.08	2.14	2.35
Range	317.65	463.53	573.99	584.88
Minimum	14.09	92.36	60.66	81.16
Maximum	331.74	555.89	634.65	666.04

Table 4.2. Plasma Methadone Concentrations (ng/ml) on Days 1, 7, 14 and 21 While Patients Received MMT 40 mg Daily

Plasma Methadone, up to mg/ml	Day 1		Day 7		Day 14		Day 21	
	N	Cumulative %	N	Cumulative %	N	Cumulative %	N	Cumulative %
100.00	10	32.26%	2	6.06%	0	0.00%	1	3.85%
200.00	10	64.52%	16	54.55%	17	56.67%	11	46.15%
300.00	10	96.77%	7	75.76%	5	73.33%	8	76.92%
400.00	1	100.00%	3	84.85%	7	96.67%	4	92.31%
500.00	0	100.00%	1	87.88%	0	96.67%	1	96.15%
600.00	0	100.00%	4	100.00%	0	96.67%	0	96.15%
700.00	0	100.00%	0	100.00%	1	100.00%	1	100.00%
800.00	0	100.00%	0	100.00%	0	100.00%	0	100.00%

Table 4.3. Plasma Methadone Concentrations (ng/ml) on Days 1, 7, 14 and 21 While Patients Received MMT 40 mg Daily

The Subjective and Objective Withdrawal Score from patient taking MMT 40 mg daily was poorly manifested (Figure 4.4 and Figure 4.5). It showed that methadone at 40 mg a day was not adequate to suppress the withdrawal from opiate dependence.

Subjective withdrawal scores (SOW) were determined at four weeks for patients given 40 mg daily dose of methadone. Scores averaged 32 (SD ±10.4). The lowest score was 11 and the highest 51. Objective withdrawal scores (OOW) were also determined at four weeks for patients given 40 mg daily dose of methadone. Scores averaged 8.2 (SD ±1.5).

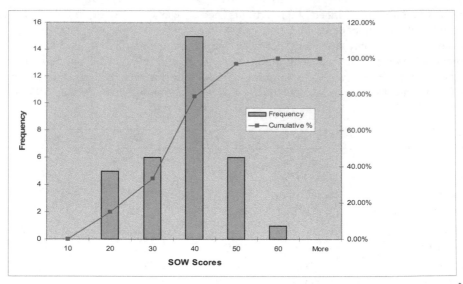

Fig. 4.4. Subjective Objective Withdrawal Scores from Patients Taking MMT 40 mg daily

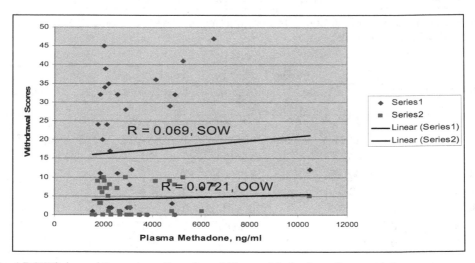

Fig. 4.5. Withdrawal Scores as a Function of Plasma Methadone Concentrations

(Series 1 = SOW; Series 2 = OOW)

5. Discussion

Methadone has a complex pharmacology. There is widespread "opiophobia" and it is frequently perceived negatively by physicians, patients and the society so much so that many just accept it as a necessary evil. The complex pharmacology and "opiophobia" present a great challenge to patients, physician and programs in terms of finding the most appropriate dose to

Variability of Plasma Methadone Concentration in Opiate Dependent Receiving Methadone: A Personalised
Approach Towards Optimizing Dose

161

achieve the desired results. This study was an attempt to comprehensively look at MMT. Among our notable findings included the variable ages of our patients, the male predominance, the variable daily methadone doses used and the importance of high daily maintenance dose, the variable plasma methadone obtained and its poor correlation with daily doses. Eighty eight patients were excluded from plasma concentration of methadone because they did not comply with the protocol. We investigated only 40 patients for the outcomes of MMT when the daily dose was fixed at 40 mg. We found that this daily dose was associated with high withdrawal scores implying failure of therapy.

In our clinical study, initially we enrolled 128 patients. They comprised of heroin/opiate dependent individuals receiving MMT in our clinics. As have been observed in many previous studies with MMT, patients enrolled in this study were mostly males with most in the productive age group. The youngest was 20, the oldest 56 years old. They were also mainly Malays. This fact underscores the importance of proper management of drug use disorder. These young and otherwise healthy males, if not successfully managed, are lost to the society and may lead a criminal life to feed their habits, given the difficulties, stigma and discrimination they face to be employed. Thus, instead of becoming the work force of the country needed to generate economic activity, these youngsters in turn add the burden of the country. There will be added burdens in terms of law enforcement costs, judiciary costs and other related costs. This would be over and above other costs like the society and health-care costs.

Of note was a high prevalence of HIV positivity at 36%. In most countries with good harm reduction programs for injecting drug users, the prevalence of HIV positivity is generally 1-2% (Central Intelligence Agency). The high prevalence seen in our cohort underscores the need for urgent effective measures. As there is no cure for HIV/ AIDS, this high prevalence would mean that many young Malay males in Malaysia would eventually succumb to the disease. This would reduce the pool of available males for population growth and if this is allowed to go on unabated, this will impact on the demography of the Malaysian population. Ethnic proportions can change and population growth in some communities may be halted. They may face troubles to obtain gainful employment and may resort to crimes to feed their habits, themselves and may be even their families. Co-morbid conditions like psychiatric illnesses and stigma and discrimination may make them dangerous to self, family and the society.

No age is however spared by the drug use disorder. The youngest of our patients was a 20 year-old. They began their drug habit as early as when they were 12 years. The oldest patient was 56 years of age and the oldest age a patient started with the habit was 32 years. Drug use disorder is a chronic relapsing disease. The duration of illness among our patients ranged from two years to 38 years and averaged 13 years. These have implications. For one, preventive measures for drug use disorder must begin early and should be continued through all ages. Patients afflicted with the disease should also have long follow ups as they evidently continue with their habits right through their golden years. The longer they continue on the habit, the greater is the chance for them to contract diseases like HIV, if they have not yet been infected. Being young and otherwise healthy, young addicts may find themselves constrained in various activities and this may lead them to many unhealthy practices.

Drug users do not live in isolation. They have sexual partners and families. Apart from transmission through the sharing of injection equipments, having the HIV reservoir, drug users can also transmit the disease to their sexual partners, through penetrative sex. Thus, what started as a concentrated epidemic among drug users is now showing evidence for a more generalized epidemic into the community through sexual transmission. In the beginning, less than one percent of HIV victims were females. Now it stands at about 20% and this clearly demonstrates the generalization of the HIV epidemic in Malaysia that began as a concentrated epidemic among drug users. Most of the afflicted females are also wives and spouses of drug users who are themselves HIV positive and not sex workers as many would have expected. There is however evidence for a growing epidemic among sex workers and this again has the potential to generalize into the community.

For the forty patients studied, their daily dose averaged 57.2 mg and ranged from 20 to 160 mg per day. Median dose was 50 mg per day. The corresponding plasma methadone averaged 281.3 ng/ml. It ranged from 0 to 4634 ng/ml. Daily methadone doses poorly predicted resulting plasma methadone concentrations, a hallmark for a drug metabolized by genetically polymorphic enzymes. Indeed when we measured plasma methadone concentrations in patients who received a fixed 40 mg daily methadone , they varied from 14 ng/ml to 331 ng/ml, a 23-fold difference. It is thus evident that no one dose fits all. As with many drugs used in the management of chronic diseases, methadone doses should be individualized to optimum outcomes that must be determined objectively.

It is also interesting to note that, despite claims by many physicians that relatively lower doses of methadone would be sufficient for our Malaysian patients, our observation of high withdrawal scores among patients who were maintained at 40 mg daily of methadone would imply this was not so. Severe withdrawal would discourage patients from remaining on treatment and by inference, they will not be retained. Indeed it has consistently been found that a sufficiently high dose of substitution therapy was required for improved outcome (Brady et al, 2005). High doses of methadone were significantly more effective in suppressing illicit heroin use and in retaining patients in the program (Family Health International; Mattick et al, 2003) and in producing optimum outcomes (Farré et al, 2002).

Inadequate doses and premature termination are the greatest threats to a successful MMT program in Malaysia. Malaysian doctors may outwardly say that they use lower methadone doses because of their fear for ethnic difference that would put their patients at higher risks for toxicity if they were to use doses as high as those recommended by the Western literature. What they may not want to admit is the fact that, inwardly, they have fears with methadone (and all opiates actually!) just for the simple reason that methadone is an opiate, just like the dreaded heroin and morphine! Indeed Malaysian doctors are not alone in this. Many doctors everywhere share the same view. Thus, despite ample evidence for the need to maintain patients at a daily dose of 80 mg to 100 mg, most patients are maintained on much less, and many are encouraged early termination.

It is probably understandable that the lay public may not understand the scientific basis for MMT and could be disparaging and become critical of it. It is however less clear why many physicians and other health care providers have the same views. Even those directly involved with MMT programs frequently fail to adhere to the basic principles of MMT. Most have actually received clear information on the pharmacologic principles underlying MMT and their claim that they want to prescribe as few medications as possible sound hollow, as they frequently easily prescribe other mood altering drugs, such as the benzodiazepines that are often prescribed with abandon and can produce psychological and physiologic dependency. Even if they claim they fear adverse effects, the adverse, physiologic effects of MMT are minimal and methadone is probably associated with the least side effects of any drug in a physician's pharmacologic armamentarium, when used appropriately. The real reason is probably more to do with the general "opiophobias" as it is known that some doctors even hesitate to use opiates even when indications are clear. Efforts should therefore be made urgently to reeducate these doctors. In their hands is the future of the nation. Their failure to prescribe adequate methadone doses will lead to therapeutic failure for MMT. This has dire consequences.

There is another problem. The expectation of the public, doctors and patients as regards treatment of addiction is to have a drug-free ending. This puts extra pressures on the doctor and patient alike and this will encourage doctors and patients to use low doses for the shortest possible time. This is despite the fact that maintenance therapy for at least two years with adequate doses is known to be associated with the maximum chance of remaining abstinent when methadone has been tapered. Many patients can thus receive less than two years of treatment with methadone with encouragements to discontinue maintenance frequently coming from health care providers working in maintenance programs. Most treating doctors also often do not try to discover reasons why patients started drug in the first place, or the existence of comorbid psychiatric illnesses. This less than holistic approach to MMT can result in increased anxiety among patients that can lead to the use of other psycho-active drugs, such as the benzodiazepines.

Notwithstanding the requirement for higher doses, as with any drugs, the dosing of methadone should be individualized (Latowsky, 2006). While low doses are associated with relapse and failure, too high a dose may lead to toxicities such as prolongation of QT interval and subsequent fatal polymorphic ventricular fibrillation (Fanoe et al, 2007). As regards plasma methadone concentrations, although we did not observe a clear correlation between plasma concentration and clinical effects, in the individual patients they may prove useful as illustrated in the cases we described above. Notwithstanding that, it is clear that a dose of 40 mg a day is generally inadequate. Subjective withdrawal scores (SOW) at four weeks for patients given 40 mg daily dose of methadone averaged 32 and the standard deviation was large at 10.4. The lowest score was 11 and the highest 51. Objective withdrawal scores (OOW) were also determined at four weeks for patients given 40 mg daily dose of methadone. Scores averaged 8.2 (SD ±1.5). It is evident that severe withdrawals occurred in patients maintained on 40 mg daily.

6. Conclusion

We concluded that the variable plasma methadone obtained was poorly correlated with daily doses of methadone and low dose methadone was inadequate to suppress opiate withdrawal.

A daily dose of 40 mg was associated with a high incidence of opiate withdrawal. Thus, prescription of methadone dose should be individualised to achieve a higher success of MMT.

7. Acknowledgement

I would like to thank USM (Universiti Sains Malaysia) RU grant 1001/PSSP/812056 for sponsoring this project.

8. References

Abramson, F.P. Methadone plasma protein binding: alterations in cancer and displacement from alpha 1-acid glycoprotein. *Clin Pharmaco Ther.* 1982. 32(5): 652-658.

Brady, T.M., Salvucci, S., Sverdlov, L.S., Male, A., Kyeyune, H., Sikali, E., DeSale, S. and Yu, P. Methadone dosage and retention: an examination of the 60 mg/day threshold. *Journal of Addictive Diseases*. 2005. 24(3): 23-47.

de Vos, J.W., Ufkes, J.G.R., van Brussel, G.H.A. & van den Brink, W. Craving despite extremely high methadone dosage. *Drug and Alcohol Dependence*. 1996. 40(3): 181-184.

Dyer, K.R., Foster, D.J.R., White, J.M., Somogyi, A.A., Menelaou, A. & Bochner, F. Steady-state pharmacokinetics and pharmacodynamics in methadone maintenance patients: Comparison of those who do and do not experience withdrawal and concentration-effect relationships[ast]. *Clin Pharmacol Ther*. 1999. 65(6): 685-694.

Eap, C.B., Buclin, T. & Baumann, P. Interindividual variability of the clinical pharmacokinetics of methadone: implications for the treatment of opioid dependence.. *Clin. Pharmacokinet*. 2002. 41(1153-1193.

Eap, C.B., Cuendet, C. & Baumann, P. Binding of d-methadone, l-methadone, and dl-methadone to proteins in plasma of healthy volunteers: role of the variants of alpha 1-acid glycoprotein. *Clin Pharmaco Ther*. 1990. 47(3): 338-346.

Ekblom, M., Hammarlund-Udenaes, M. & Paalzow, L. Modeling of tolerance development and rebound effect during different intravenous administrations of morphine to rats. *Journal of Pharmacology and Experimental Therapeutics*. 1993. 266(1): 244-252.

Family Health International. Managing opioid dependence: treatment and care for HIV-positive injecting drug users Disember 27,2009, from http://www.fhi.org/training/en/HIVAIDS/IDUModules/pdf/Module_04_Treatment_Care_for_HIV_positive_IDUs.pdf

Fanoe, S., Hvidt, C., Ege, P. and Jensen, G.B. Syncope and QT prolongation among patients treated with methadone for heroin dependence in the city of Copenhagen. *Heart*. 2007. 93(9): 1051-1055.

Farré, M., Mas, A., Torrens, M., Moreno, V. and CamI, J. Retention rate and illicit opioid use during methadone maintenance interventions: a meta-analysis. *Drug and Alcohol Dependence*. 2002. 65(3): 283-290.

Fournier, T., Medjoubi-N, N. & Porquet, D. Alpha-1-acid glycoprotein. *Biochimica et Biophysica Acta (BBA) - Protein Structure and Molecular Enzymology*. 2000. 1482(1-2): 157-171.

Garrido, M.J., Aguirre, C., Trocóniz, I.F., Marot, M., Valle, M., Zamacona, M.K. and Calvo, R. Alpha 1-acid glycoprotein (AAG) and serum protein binding of methadone in heroin addicts with abstinence syndrome. *Int J Clin pharmaco Ther*. 2000. 38(1): 35-40.

Gómez, E., Martinez-Jordá, R., Suárez, E., Garrido, M.J. & Calvo, R. Altered methadone analgesia due to changes in plasma protein binding: Role of the route of administration. *General Pharmacology: The Vascular System*. 1995. 26(6): 1273-1276.Xiao, Y., Smith, R.D., Caruso, F.S. & Kellar, K.J. Blockade of Rat α3β4 Nicotinic Receptor function by Methadone, its metabolites, and structural analogs. *JPET*. 2001. 299(1): 366-371.

Inturrisi, C.E., Portenoy, R.K., Max, M.B., Colburn, W.A. & Foley, K.M. Pharmacokinetic-pharmacodynamic relationships of methadone infusions in patients with cancer pain. *Clin Pharmaco Ther*. 1990. 47(5): 565-577.

KuKanich, B. & Borum, S.L. The disposition and behavioral effects of methadone in Greyhounds. *Veterinary Anaesthesia and Analgesia.* 2008. 35(3): 242-248.

Kukanich, B., Lascelles, B.D.X., Aman, A.M., Mealey, K.L. & Papich, M.G. The effects of inhibiting cytochrome P450 3A, p-glycoprotein, and gastric acid secretion on the oral bioavailability of methadone in dogs. *Journal of Veterinary Pharmacology and Therapeutics.* 2005. 28(5): 461-466.

Latowsky, M. Methadone death, dosage and torsade de pointes: risk-benefit policy implications. *J Psychoactive Drug.* 2006. 38(4): 513-519.

Liu, E., Liang, T., Shen, L., Zhong, H., Wang, B., Wu, Z. & Detels, R. Correlates of methadone client retention: a prospective cohort study in Guizhou province, China. *The International Journal on Drug Policy.* 2009. 20(4): 304-308.

Li, X. & Wei, W. Chinese materia medica: combinations and appication Hertfordshire: Donica Publishing. 2002. 75-76.

Li, Y., Kantelip, J.P., Gerritsen-van, S.P. & Davani, S. Interindividual variability of methadone response: impact of genetic polymorphism [Abstract]. *Mol Diagn Ther.* 2008. 12(2): 109-124.

Loimer, N. & Schmid, R. The use of plasma levels to optimize methadone maintenance treatment. *Drug and Alcohol Dependence.* 1992. 30(3): 241-246.

Lötsch, J., von Hentig, N., Freynhagen, R., Griessinger, N., Zimmermann, M., Doehring, A., Rohrbacher, M., Sittl, R. & Geisslinger, G. Cross-sectional analysis of the influence of currently known pharmacogenetic modulators on opioid therapy in outpatient pain centers. *Pharmacogenetics and Genomics.* 2009. 19(6):

Mattick, R.P., Breen, C. and Kimbler, J. Methadone maintenance therapy versus no opioid replacement therapy for opioid dependence. *Cochrane Database of Syst Rev.* 2003.

Meresaar, U., Nilsson, M.I., Holmstrand, J. & Änggård, E. Single dose pharmacokinetics and bioavailability of methadone in man studied with a stable isotope method. *European journal of clinical pharmacology.* 1981. 20(6): 473-478-478.

Mestriner, F.L.A.C., Spiller, F., Laure, H.J., Souto, F.O., Tavares-Murta, B.M., Rosa, J.C., Basile-Filho, A., Ferreira, S.H., Greene, L.J. & Cunha, F.Q. Acute-phase protein α-1-acid glycoprotein mediates neutrophil migration failure in sepsis by a nitric oxide-dependent mechanism. *Proceedings of the National Academy of Sciences.* 2007. 104(49): 19595-19600.

Romach, M.K., Piafsky, K.M., Abel, J.G., Khouw, V. & Sellers, E.M. Methadone binding to orosomucoid (alpha 1-acid glycoprotein): determinant of free fraction in plasma. *Clin Pharmaco Ther.* 1981. 29(2): 211-217.

Rostami-Hodjegan, A., Wolff, K., Hay, A.W.M., Raistrick, D., Calvert, R. & Tucker, G.T. Population pharmacokinetics of methadone in opiate users: characterization of time-dependent changes. *British Journal of Clinical Pharmacology.* 1999. 48(1): 43-52.

Rowland, M. & Tozer, T.N. Physiologic concepts and kinetics: distribution. In Rowland, M. and Tozer, T. N. (Eds.), *Clinical Pharmacokinetics. Concepts and Applications.* 3rd ed. Philadelphia: Lippincott Williams & Wilkins. 1995. 137–155.

Sawe, J. High-dose morphine and methadone in cancer patients. Clinical pharmacokinetic considerations of oral treatment. *Clin Pharmacokinet.* 1986. 11(2): 87-106.

Schmidt, N., Sittl, R., Brune, K. & Geisslinger, G. Rapid Determination of Methadone in Plasma, Cerebrospinal Fluid, and Urine by Gas Chromatography and Its

Application to Routine Drug Monitoring. *Pharmaceutical Research*. 1993. 10(3): 441-444-444.

Wolff, K. & Hay, A.W. Plasma methadone monitoring with methadone maintenance treatment. *Drug Alcohol Depend*. 1994. 36(1): 69-71.

Wolff, K., Rostami-Hodjegan, A., Hay, A.W.M., Raistrick, D. and Tucker, G. Population-based pharmacokinetic approach for methadone monitoring of opiate addicts: potential clinical utility. *Addiction*. 2000. 95(12): 1771-1783.

Wolff, K., Sanderson, M., Hay, A.W. and Raistrick, D. Methadone concentrations in plasma and their relationship to drug dosage. *Clinical Chemistry*. 1991. 37(2): 205-209.

Verebely, K., Volavka, J., Mulé, S. & Resnick, R. Methadone in man: pharmacokinetic and excretion studies in acute and chronic treatment. *Clinical Pharmacology and Therapeutics*. 1975. 18(2): 180-190.

Yang, Y., Wan, C., Li, H., Zhu, H., La, Y., Xi, Z., Chen, Y., Jiang, L., Feng, G. & He, L. Altered Levels of Acute Phase Proteins in the Plasma of Patients with Schizophrenia. *Analytical Chemistry*. 2006. 78(11): 3571-3576.

8

Herbal Medicine in the Treatment of Malaria: *Vernonia amygdalina*: An Overview of Evidence and Pharmacology

Anoka A. Njan
Department of Pharmacology and Toxicology, Faculty of Pharmaceutical Scinces,
Usmanu Danfodiyo University, Sokoto,
Nigeria

1. Introduction

Traditional medicines occupy a central place among rural communities of developing countries for the provision of health care in the absence of an efficient public health care system (WHO, 2003).

The use of traditional remedies is common in sub-Saharan Africa, and visits to traditional healers remain a mainstay of care for many people because of preference, affordability, and limited access to hospitals and modern health practitioners (Homsy et al., 1999).

It is an important part of medical care in Uganda and throughout Africa, representing first line therapy for 70% of the population, (Homsy et al., 2004). For many, traditional herbal medicines may be the only source of treatment available. The main reasons to explain this are: traditional medicines are often more accessible compared with licensed drugs; there are no records attesting the resistance to whole-plant extracts possibly due to the synergistic action of their constituents; phytotherapy, possibly produces fewer adverse effect than chemotherapy (Willcox and Bodeker, 2000).

In Africa more than 2,000 plants have been identified and use as herbal medicines. However, very few of these plants have been screened for safety in resource-constrained countries including Uganda. It is time to ask in a systematic and scientific manner how these local treatments work, what are the best means to establish their safety and can they be used as traditionally prepared? The source of antimalarial drugs such as artemisinin derivatives and quinolines currently in use today were isolated from medicinal plants. Renewed interest in traditional pharmacopoeias has meant that researchers are concerned not only with determining the scientific rationale for plants usage, but also with the discovering of novel compounds of pharmaceutical value for the treatment of malaria.

Herbals are as old as human civilization and they have provided a complete storehouse of remedies to cure acute and chronic diseases. Numerous nutraceuticals are present in medicinal herbs as key components. Scientific evaluation of herbal products has been limited, yet herbal products are the most commonly consumed health care products. Because of known pharmacological effects and potential interaction of many of these compounds with therapeutic drugs, a history of herbal intake should be considered as part of routine medical history and should be evaluated before any change in prescription drugs and before medical procedures (Schwartz et al 2000)

At present, work conducted on traditional medicine in Africa has mainly concentrated on the collection, identification, and classification of herbal products for treatment of different ailments. However, research in the areas of safety and toxicology is lacking.

Traditional medicines, like modern pharmaceuticals can do harm, but because humans have been using herbal drugs for long time, they are considered safe and non-toxic so the toxicological actions of these agents have been mostly ignored, even while the effectiveness is either already known or under study (O'Hara et al., 1998). Willcox (1999), carried out a clinical study on 'AM' (coded to protect the intellectual property right of the traditional healers), a popular antimalarial herb that has a long history of use among the people of south-western Uganda. In her result, 'AM' significantly reduced parasite count between day 1 and day 7, patients showed symptomatic improvement, but 50% of them experienced some side effects including vomiting, nausea and stomach upset. These were partly attributed to malaria itself as well as to 'AM' ingestion (Willcox, 1999).

If the origin of herbs' toxicity is not identified, the adverse effects may be wrongly associated with other environmental exposures or some traditional belief. Failure to establish the true cause of exposure also means that the patient continues taking the toxic herb. Thus, the screening of traditional remedies for safety and toxicity is recommended to protect public health. On the other hand, several plants used in Uganda traditional medicine can cause damage to genetic material and therefore have potential to cause long-term damage in patients when administered as medicinal preparations (Steenkamp, 2005).

1.1 The main groups of active principle or constituents obtained from medicinal herbs

The therapeutic effects of plant species are determined by their constituents. These affect the condition and function of the various human body organs, clear up residual symptoms or destroy the cause of the disease in most cases infectious micro-organisms. They help increase the body's resistance to disease, retard or delay the processes of natural aging or facilitate the adaptation of the organism to certain conditions (Forantisek, 2001). Over the centuries, man used medicinal plants even though he was unable to find a rational explanation for their effects. It was not until the 19th century and after the rapid development of organic chemistry and pharmacology, that man determined which active or group of principles are responsible for a given therapeutic effect. Knowledge of these substances frequently served as a model for the synthetic preparation of new medicines, enabling the drug to be modified and made more effective. It was soon discovered that a better therapeutic effect was often obtained by the particular combination of active principle naturally present in each plant that by a single, isolated substance. The most important constituents are the secondary metabolism in plants, which includes alkaloids, glycosides, essential oils, tannins and the bitter principles. Products of secondary metabolism of plants are responsible for the plants' therapeutics effects. Of greater importance for the plants themselves of course are the products of primary metabolism which are necessary for the proper function of the basic life processes in plants. Primary metabolism products are also used by man. This group includes sugars, fatty oils, organic acids, vitamins and protein. These products of primary metabolism themselves may have no therapeutic effect but may possibly increase the efficiency of the therapeutically important principles (70)

1.2 *Vernonia amygdalina*

(Aseraceae), also called bitter leaf is a popular African vegetable that grows as a shrub or small tree indigenous to Central and East Africa including Uganda (Huffman et al, 1996). It produces large mass of forage and is drought tolerant (Hutchioson and Dalziel, 1963), it is 2 – 5 m with petiolate leaf of about 6 mm diameter and elliptic shape. The leaves are green with a characteristic odour and a bitter taste. No seeds are produced and the tree has therefore to be distributed through cutting. It is known locally as Omubirizi in south-western Uganda and used traditionally for pain relief and malaria attack. Patients are instructed to soak the plant leave in hot water about (80ºC). They should then drink half a glass (about 0.25l) two times daily for 4-7 days. Smaller doses are prescribed for children according to their weight.They are used as vegetable and stimulate the digestive system in some other countries in the continent.

This plant has ethnomedical use in treating veneral diseases, gastrointestinal problems and malaria (Kambizi et al, 2001; Huffman et al, 2003; Hamill et al, 1992). Furthermore, they are used as local medicine against leech, which are transmitting bilharzias. Free living chimpanzees eat the leaves, if they have attacked by parasites (Huffman, M.A. 2003). There are reports concerning the hypoglycaemic, antineoplastic antibacterial and antioxidant properties of the plant. (Akah et al, 1992; Izevbigie et al, 2004; Taiwo et al, 1999; Iwalewa et al, 2005). Despite the varied uses of the plant, there are no information on its analgesic properties and exact toxicology on sub-chronic exposure, although some reports describe its antiplasmodial effects (Abosi et al 2005; Masaba et al 2000; Tona et al, 2004; Wilcox et al, 1999). Previous phytochemical reports have shown the presence of steroid, saponins, flavonoids.

2. Methods

2.1 Research design
Ninety traditional healers were identified through community and healers association leaders. Once identified, study staff members approached the individuals to determine eligibility. Eligibility criteria included 30 years of age and older, recognition as a traditional healer by the local community council, and having established an active practice in the community. Three districts (Kanungu/Bwindi area, Bushenyi and Mbarara) south-western Uganda were identified. With consent a taxonomist samples of antimalarial herb were obtained for this research study.

To evaluate consistency, interviews were conducted by a person specially trained in interview administration and who is fluent in the language of the participants.

The ethnographic interview included questions about common plant names, sources of products, method of preparation, purpose of use, quantity of herbs use and perceived benefit of herbs in ameliorating malaria symptoms and improving overall health. Ethical forms were used in order to assure them of the defense of their knowledge and intellectual property right was applied. Traditional healer's name, age, gender, and ethnicity tribe, were asked. We relied on the knowledge of healers and the taxonomist to select the products of greatest importance. This enabled us target products that have a high likelihood of possessing significant pharmacological activity.

A strategy was developed that respected the healers' rights to maintain propriety of unique blends of herbal medicine. Also, a memorandum of understanding was developed that disclosed our study objective, which is to characterize the pharmacologic activity and to elucidate the toxicity of these remedies in order to determine any potential adverse effect. We emphasized that we were interested in general knowledge about the remedy and not in specific formulation, and that it was not our intention to use the knowledge gained from this study for commercial profit. Rather we would report back to them in a workshop the remedy's indication and contraindication after completion of the study. We requested that all parties sign the agreement and copies were kept in a secure file. The result of the study was used to determine the most common botanical/herbal products used by the healers to treat malaria. Among the herbal products, *Vernonia amygdalina* which appeared in 80% in the interview was chosen for studies.

Fidelity level: The fidelity level (Fl) (Alexiades et al, 2000) among the healers from the same district was calculated according to the following formula:

$$Fl\,(\%) = (Np/N) \times 100$$

Np is the number of healers from one given district that claim a use of a plant species to treat a particular disease, and N is the number of healers from the same district that use the plants as a medicine to treat any given disease. The formula was applied in order to compare data from different district where the survey was performed.

2.2 Extract preparation

Leaves of *V. amygdalina* were collected from the botanical garden of the Rukararwe Traditional Medicine Health Center, a division of Rukararwe Partnership Workshop for Rural Development (RPWRD) in Bushenyi district. The plant was authenticated by Dominic Byarugaba, a botanist with the Department of Plant Biology, Mbarara University of Science and Technology (MUST), Uganda. A voucher specimen is kept in the department. The plant material was air-dried and grounded into a coarse powder. About (350g) of this powder were macerated in 2 L of distilled water for 24 h with occasional shaking (GFL 3017 Germany) and then extracted using a soxhlet extractor (Gallemkamp, England). The resultant extract was evaporated in a water bath, under controlled temperature not exceeding the one used by the healers in their plant preparation (80°C) to yield a 32.3 g of semi solid residue.

2.3 Animals

Adult Wistar rats (130 – 150g) and Swiss albino mice (18 – 26g) of either sex, maintained at Animal Facility Centre were used for the acute toxicity and 14 days sub-chronic experiments. The animals were kept in plastic cages at room temperature and moisture, under a naturally illuminated environment of 12:12 h dark/light cycle. Animals were fed the standard diet and had access to tap water *ad libitum*.

Male Wistar rats were used for the 6 week exposure studies.. At dosing, animals were 8 to 12 weeks old. All animals were clinically monitored at the time of delivery and during acclimation period, and were maintained at the Animal Facility Centre. Animals found unsuitable were excluded from the experiment. Animals were housed in plastic cages under same conditions described above; they were fed with standard diet (Mice pallet), and had access to tap water *ad libitum*. The animal experiments were conducted according to the NIH Guide on Laboratory Animals for Biomedical Research (NIH, 1978) and ethical guidelines for investigation of experimental pain in conscious animals (Zimmermann et al, 1983).

2.4 Antiplasmodial activity

The test was conducted according to the curative procedure described earlier (Saidu et al, 2000; Adzu et al, 2003). A donor mouse infected with rodent malaria (*Plasmodium berghei*) was anaesthetized with chloroform and the abdomen opened. Blood was collected through cardiac puncture with a sterile needle and syringes in such a way that 0.2 ml of the blood containing about 1×10^7 infected red cells. Twenty-five mice were inoculated i.p. with 0.2 mL each. The mice were then randomized and grouped into five (n = 5) and treated as follows on day 3 (D_3). Group 1 received normal saline, group 2 received chloroquine (CQ, 5mg/kg, i.p.); while groups 3-5 received (50, 100, and 200 mg/kg, i.p.). The treatment continued daily until day 7. Thick and thin blood smear were collected daily from tail blood, fixed with methanol, stained with 4% Giemsa at pH 7.2 for 45 min and examined microscopically (Nikon YS2-H Japan). The increase/decrease in parasitaemia, defined as the number of infected and uninfected red blood cell RBCs, were counted on five different fields, and mean survival time (within 30 days) was recorded.

2.5 Evaluate the antinociceptive activity of the selected antimalarial
2.5.1 Acetic acid-induced writhing in mice
Analgesia was assessed according to the method of Siegmund et al. (1957), as was modified by Koster et al, 1959). The mice were divided into different groups (of five mice each). They were differently pre-treated with the extract (50, 100, 200mg/kg i.p), aspirin (100mg/kg i.p) and normal saline (10ml/kg i.p). 30, 60, 90 and 120min after the treatment, 0.7% acetylsalicylic acid (ASA) (Sigma Chemicals Co) 10ml/kg i.p was administered to the mice. They were placed in a transparent cage, 5mins after administration of acetic acid, the number of abdominal constrictions (writhes) made within 10min of every mouse was counted. The results of the treatment groups were compared with those of normal saline pre-treated control. The percentage of the writhes was calculated as (test mean/control mean) × 100.

2.5.2 Formalin test
For the formalin studies, rats were injected with 0.05 ml of formalin (2.5% formaldehyde) into the sub-plantar surface of the left hind paw 30min after treatment with saline, extract or ASA. Severity of pain (for both control and test groups (n = 5)) were simultaneously observed and rated as scores using (Dubuisson et al, 1977) pain measurements. This was rated as follows: (0) rat can bear weight on injected paw; (1) light resting of the paw on floor; (2) partial elevation of the injected paw, and (3) total elevation, licking and biting of paw. These observation were recorded every minute for the first 10 min (early phase) and at every 5 min for the period between 15 and 60min (late phase).

2.5.3 Tail-flick test
This test as first described [28], and subsequently modified (Janssen et al, 1969; Asongalem et al 2004a) was used. Briefly, before treatment, the terminal (2 cm) of each rat tail was immersed in hot water contained in a 500ml beaker and maintained at $55 \pm 1^{\circ}C$ using a thermo-regulated hot plate (Ugo Basile, Socrel DS-35) and the time (in seconds) between the onset of stimulation and tail withdrawal was measured as the tail-flick latency. Twenty five rats that shows response within 0 – 4 s were selected and grouped into five (n = 5) for the study. Immediately after basal latency assessment, normal saline, reference drug (Pethidine hydrochloride; Bayer, England) or the plant extract were administered and the reaction time again recorded at 30 and 60min. after administration the extract. (50 – 200 mg/kg p.o) (Sanchez-Mateo et al, 2006).

2.6 Acute and sub-chronic toxicity of the herbs
2.6.1 Acute – toxicity test
The intraperitoneal (i.p) acute toxicity of the extract was evaluated in Swiss albino mice using a slightly modified Lorke's method (Lorke, 1998). Briefly, this method involved the determination of LD_{50} value in biphasic manner. The animals were starved of feed but allowed access to water 24 h prior to the study. In the initial investigatory step (phase 1), a range of doses of the extract producing the toxic effects was established. This was done by intraperitoneal administration of geometric doses of the extract (10, 100, 1000, 1500 mg/kg) to four groups of mice (n = 4). Based on the results obtained, a phase 2 investigatory step was done by giving more specific doses (200, 400, 600, 800 mg/kg i.p) to four other groups of mice.

The mice were observed for 24 h for such behavioral signs as, excitement, dullness, ataxia or death. The LD_{50} was estimated from the geometric mean of the dose that caused 100% mortality and the dose which caused no lethality.

The same procedure was used in rats which received (1000, 2000, 3000, 5000 mg/kg oral) in phase 1 and (1500, 3000, 4000, 5000 mg/kg oral) in the second phase.

2.6.2 Two weeks sub-chronic toxicity test
Twenty eight Wistar rats divided into four weight-matched groups, of seven rats each, (both sexes) were used for the study. Three test groups received 500, 1000, 2000 mg/kg *V. amygdalina* by gavage with biomedical needle (G 16, Length 76.2mm, diameter 3mm, Straight Harvard Apparatus) for 14 days. The control group received normal saline.

Food and water intake were measured daily while the animal's body weights were taken every other day. All animals were observed at least once daily for clinical signs (behavior such as lethargy, hyperactivity, depression and diarrhea). On day 14, immediately prior to euthanasia, all animals were anesthetized with chloroform and bled via the descending aorta for hematology and clinical chemistry determination. Organs were dissected and weighed to determine absolute and relative weight. The blood for clinical chemistry was allowed to clot in microtainer separator tubes, centrifuged and sera collected and stored at -20°C till ready for biochemical analyses. Commercial kits for Biosystem BTS-310, (Biosystem S.A Costa Brava 30, Barcelona, Spain) and Vitrous DT systems, Orthoclinical Diagnostics Johnson Company (US17) were used to analyze liver function, renal function and the electrolyte test.

The hematological tests were carried out in an ethylene diamine tetra-acetic acid (EDTA) – anticoagulated blood. Hemoglobin (Hb) concentration was analysed by the cyanmethaemoglobin method, packed cell volume (PCV) by the micro-method, and white blood cell (WBC, total and differential) and platelet counts by visual methods Dacia et al, 1991). The mean cell hemoglobin concentration (MCHC) was calculated by dividing Hb by PCV (Dioka et al, 2002).

2.6.3 Six weeks sub-chronic toxicity test
For the six-week exposure studies, twenty eight male Wistar rats were divided into four weight-matched groups of seven rats each. Three of the four test groups received 750 1500, 3000 mg/kg *V. amygdalina* by gavage with biomedical needle (G 16, Length 76.2mm, diameter 3mm, Straight Harvard Apparatus) consecutively for 43 days. The control group received distilled water vehicle only, via gavage.

Food and water intake were measured daily while the animal's body weights were taken preexposure and weekly during exposure. All animals were observed at least once daily for clinical signs (behavior such as lethargy, hyperactivity, depression and diarrhea), and once/week clinical observations were performed on each rat by removing it from its cage and examining it for changes in general health. On day 44, immediately prior to euthanasia, all animals were anesthetized with chloroform and bled via the descending aorta for hematology and clinical chemistry determination. Organs were dissected and weighed to determine absolute and relative weight. The blood for clinical chemistry was allowed to clot in microtainer separator tubes, centrifuged and sera collected and stored at -70 ^{0}C until performing the biochemical analyses. The biochemical and hematological parameter were analyzed in the (New Italian Laboratory). Mbarara University of Science and Technology (MUST).

The collected plasma samples were analyzed using a (HumanStar 180 and Humalyze 2000, Germany) autoanalyzer. Sixteen biochemical parameters were studied; plasma sodium, potassium and chloride were also assayed with (Humalyzer 17410, Germany) autoanalyzer with appropriate Human Kits.

Hematological parameters were analyzed using (Beckman and Coulter, USA) with the appropriate kit (Coulter ACT 5 diff Diluent's).

3. Results

In the study, a total of 90 healers from - sub-county from the three districts were interviewed. Most of them were members of traditional healers association in their district. Men dominate the practices of traditional medicine.

Most of the traditional healers interviewed (81 out of 90), indicated to have passed through a several routes to become healers. All of the 81 were raised in families with traditional healers, who had involved them in the healing process and they were familiar with the profession. After some time they started to practice on their own. All reported on the importance of the family environment of a traditional healer in the context of acquiring knowledge and experience by members of the family. Furthermore it was reported that, the entrance into practice through these routes is facilitated through training by an experienced healer or a family member, who decides when the apprentice is ready to become an independent healer or to take up the practice. Eight out of 81 of the traditional healers indicated to have been instructed through dreams by their ancestral spirits to take up the traditional healing practice. They were required to learn and observe traditional healing procedures as dictated by the spirits. Indeed, the ancestral spirits are considered to be supernaturally powerful and ignoring them is to invite punishment to an individual and or her family. Of the 90 healers interviewed, two indicated to be self-taught healers.

The leaves are the most frequently used plant part (56.3%), the root and fruits are used about 30% and 8.5% respectively, and the less used plant part is the bark (5.3%). The majority of the remedies are prepared in the form of decoction of fresh leaves. In our study area people do usually not store remedies for prolonged period of time. When needed they go out and collect the plant and prepare the remedy from fresh or sun dried material. Powders are prepared by pounding the fresh plant part or the crushed plant material after sun drying,

Decoction is the most frequent method way of remedy preparation (65%) followed by infusion (13%), which is used for the powders; the maceration (11%) is mostly used for the root preparation. Some remedies are prepared from a single plant species; however, in a few cases mixtures of plants or other substances are added as noted in Table 2

Most of the remedies are taken orally and by external application as body bath, steam bath, and as ointment. Fumigation is mainly used in the treatment of headache and chest pain.

For most of the remedies, the administered dose depends on the patient's age, physical and health condition, and the duration of the illness. The doses vary from a teacup (70 ml) for adults to a handful (25 ml) for a child; a lack of agreement among the healers on doses of remedies was sometimes noted. The variation of the doses from one healer to another may show that the plants have a low degree of toxicity. For pharmacological investigation the active doses of these plants may not be high since they appear to treat the patients with low doses. The duration of treatment is not given for all remedies. According to the healers duration of treatment is difficult to determine and depends on how long the patient has been ill. The patient is supposed to take the remedy until healed. The only person able to determine the end of a treatment is the patient himself since the remedy is taken at home in the absence of the healers.

The reported adverse effects for the use of these medicinal plants are vomiting and dizziness. According to the healers these effects are generally due to an overdose of the remedy. The adverse effects are generally moderate, and disappear at the end of the treatment. Also, patients are advice to drink a lot of milk, meat soup or porridge made from sorghum to help alleviate serious side effects.

Districts	Sub-County	Numbers of healers	Sex		Age range
			Males	Females	
Kanungu		5	4	1	28–76
		5	3	2	30–79
		5	5	0	42–85
		5	5	0	35–55
		5	4	1	65–85
Bushenyi	kyangyenyi	5	5	0	47–70
	Kigarama	5	5	0	38–80
		5	5	1	27–70
		5	5	0	49–104
		5	5	0	56–80
Mbarara	Nyakayojo	10	8	2	45–73
	Kinoni	10	10	0	55–62
	Rugando	10	9	1	50–61
	Bugamba	10	9	1	50-59

Table 1. An overview of the traditional healers interviewed.

3.1 Acute toxicity test
The median lethal dose LD_{50} was established to be 560 ± 1.21 mg/kg i.p. in mice and 3.32 ± 0.15 g/kg oral in rats. Adverse signs of gaiting, reduction in stereotypic activities and deaths were however seen in high doses.

3.2 Acetic acid-induced writhing in mice
The aqueous extract of *V. amygdalina* (50, 100, 200mg/kg i.p) exhibited a significant (P<0.05) antinocicetive activity against acetic acid-induced writhing in mice. 50 and 100 mg/kg oral doses exhibited a dose-dependent anti-nociception that progressively reduced over a period of 90 min post-treatment. However, at 120min the reduced anti-nociceptive activity increases again at these doses. The dose of 200 mg/kg on the other hand caused a total anti-nociception up to 120min. These results compared favorably with those of aspirin (100mg/kg i.p; Fig 1).

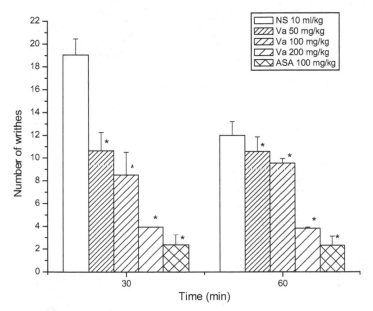

Fig. 1. Effect of aqueous extract of *V.amygdalina* leaves on acetic acid-induced writhing in mice for 5 min (NS, normal saline; Va, *V. Amygdalina*; ASA acetysalicylic acid). All data are presented as means ± S.E.M., n=5. The asterisk (*) denotes, significance (p<0.05) between treated group and NS control

3.3 Formalin and tail-flick tests
The extract at doses of 100 and 200 mg/kg induced significant (p<0.05) reduction in pain response in both phases (aphasic and tonic) of pain induced by formalin in comparison with control (Fig 2).
In all cases ASA, a positive analgesic agent demonstrated significant anti-nociceptive action with a slightly stronger pharmacological intensity than *V. amygdalina* at 200 mg/kg in the late phase. The extract exerted no significant effect on nociception in tail-flick as values

obtained correspond with those with saline. However pethidine the reference agent markedly prolonged the tail-flick reaction time in rats (Fig 3)

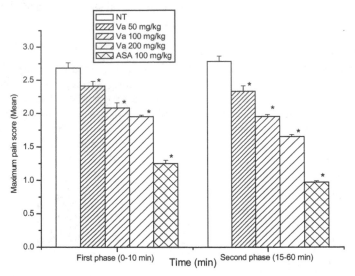

Fig. 2. Effect of aqueous extract of *V.amygdalina* leaves on formalin test in rats (NT, non treated animals; Va, *V. Amygdalina*; ASA acetyl salicilic acid). All data are presented as means ± S.E.M., n=5. The asterisk (*) denotes significance (p<0.05) between treated group and NT control

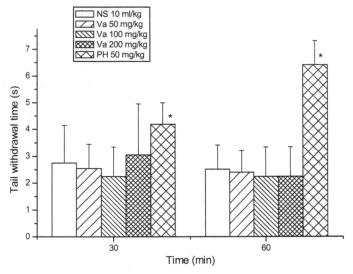

Fig. 3. Effect of aqueous extract of *V.amygdalina* leaves on thermal stimulus-induced tail-flick test in rats (NS, normal saline; Va, *V. Amygdalina*; PH, penthidine hydrochloride). All data are presented as means ± S.E.M., n=5. The asterisk (*) denotes significance difference (p<0.05).

3.4 Antiplasmodial activity

The extract caused a significant ($P < 0.05$) and dose-dependent reduction in mean parasitaemia in mice infected with Plasmodium berghei in comparison to CQ (5 mg/kg). The extract caused a parasitaemia reduction of 52% in 50 mg/kg, 64% and 73% in 100 and 200 mg/kg respectively (Table 2). One animal death was recorded in the 200 mg/kg extract groups throughout the 30 days observation period of the experiment while the remaining mice recovered fully. All mice in the saline group were lost within 15 days of the study.

Treatment	Dose (mg/kg, p.o.)	Mean prasitaemia ($D_2 - D_6$)	Inhibition (%)
NS (10ml/kg)	-	14.2 ± 0.25	-
V. amygdalina	50	$6.7 \pm 0.17*$	52.8
	100	$5.0 \pm 0.22*$	64.8
	200	$3.7 \pm 0.17*$	73.9
CQ	5	$3.1 \pm 0.25*$	78.2

Values are mean count S.E.M. (for n = 5)
*Significantly (p<0.05) different from saline control group
N.S., Normal saline

Table 2. Curative activity of the aqueous extract of V. amygdalina and CQ against Plasmodium berghei in mice.

3.5 Sub-chronic toxicity (14 days exposure)

No treatment deaths occurred and no treatment related clinical signs were noted during the study. The extract did not exert significant changes on mean body and organ weight, fluid and food intake (Table 3). All animals demonstrated a progressive increase in body weight during the exposure. The organ weights were expressed as a percentage of the body weight (% relative organ weight), rather than as absolute weights, so as to take into consideration differences in the organ weight that may solely be attributable to differences in the body weights of the respective rats. The hematology result showed a significant decrease (p<0.05) in red blood count at the dose of 2000mg/kg compared to control (Table 4). The result of the clinical chemistry parameter showed a dose-dependent increase in direct and total bilirubin, there was also an increase in uric acid at the doses of 500 and 1000mg/kg compared to control (Table 5).

3.6 Six weeks exposure

Clinical observation, Body and organ weight

At the end of the 43-day-period of drug administration, No overt signs of toxicity were seen in any of the animals during the course of the study. No statistical difference was observed between the body and organ weight of the control group and the assay group in the male rats receiving the three doses, all animals exhibited a gain in body weight. Organ weights (% relative organ weights) were similar to those of the corresponding organs from the control. (Fig 5 and 6).

Treatment (mg/kg)	Food Intake (g SEM)	Fluid Intake (mL SEM)	Initial Body	Final Body	Weight (g SEM)										
					Liver		Heart		Kidney		Lungs		Spleen		
					Absol.	Relat.	Absol.	Relat.	Absol.	Relat.	Absol.	Relat.	Absol.	Relat.	
0(Control)	131.82 7.04	155.63 11.64	147.92 7.35	178.92 6.51	7.03 0.18	3.96 0.19	0.65 0.02	0.35 0.01	1.43 .49	0.79 .02	1.42 0.12	0.80 0.07	0.84 0.05	0.48 .04	
500	131.82 10.52	148.33 19.22	161.38 14.77	181.11 14.11	6.78 0.42	3.72 0.47	0.83 0.09	0.46 0.08	1.34 0.09	0.76 .06	1.66 0.23	0.97 .20	0.76 0.62	0.43 .03	
1000	113.49 10.14	120.16 6.51	137.62 14.32	158.17 17.93	5.37 0.58	3.64 0.52	0.64 0.08	0.44 0.07	1.26 .10	0.85 .11	1.50 .10	0.99 0.11	0.63 .05	0.46 .05	
2000	129.82 12.20	147.16 12.18	134.58 9.72	156.94 6.85	6.43 0.11	4.17 0.41	0.74 0.06	0.48 0.06	1.36 .09	0.88 .07	1.33 .09	0.87 0.07	0.74 0.42	0.48 .05	

Values are expressed as mean ± S.E.M. for n = 7
Relative organs weight = Absolute Organ Weight X 100
Final Organ Weight

Table 3. Effect of *V. Amygdalina* on daily food and fluid intake, body weights and organs weight of rats. (14days exposure)

Parameter	Control	500mg/kg	1000mg/kg	2000mg/kg
Hb (g/dl)	12.17± 0.27	9.97± 0.73	11.88± 0.78	10.54±0.47
PCV (%)	36.14±0.79	29.71±2.20	35.42± 2.34	31.42± 1.41
MCHC (g/dl)	32.14±0.34	30.28±0.60	32.00±0.65	30.85±0.40
RBC (x 10¹²/L)	4.64±0.13	3.84±0.25#	4.30±0.35#	3.58±0.14#
Platelet (x 10⁹)	156.42±3.77	139.85±4.38	153.28±6.95	136.71±3.82#
WBS (x 10⁹/L)	6.57±0.43	5.57±0.87	6.68±0.51	3.47±0.89#
Neutrophil (%)	20.57±2.42	25.57±1.95*	24.00±1.77*	21.00±1.67
Lymphocyte (%)	79.28±2.53	74.42±1.95	77.4±2.47	83.28±3.48*

Values are expressed as means ± S.E.M for n = 7
* Significantly increased (P≤0.05) compared to control.
# Significantly reduced (P≤0.05) compared to control.

Table 4. Effect of *V. amygdalina* on selected hematological parameter in rats (14days Exposure)

Parameters	Control	500 mg/kg	1000 mg/kg	2000 mg/kg
AKL.Phos (iu/L)	212.1±2.21	215.5±3.77	218.8±8.11	218.7±3.45
Total Protein (g/L)	71.5± 1.11	74.3±2.69	77.0± 0.54	73.7± 2.21
Albumin (g/L)	38.3± 1.25	39.7± 1.04	40.0± 0.94	39.6± 0.76
Direct Biliru (µMol/L)	1.8± 0.82	2.5± 1.01*	3.2± 1.51*	4.0± 1.78*
Total Biliru (µMol/L)	4.2±2.65	6.28±2.63*	5.71±2.53*	6.57± 3.19*
ALT (iu/L)	32.7±5.80	34.60±10.18	35.10±11.04	33.70± 6.23
AST (iu/L)	42.28±10.27	40.43±10.68	41.29±12.32	41.14± 5.52
Chol (µMol/L)	1.23±0.32	0.92±0.33	1.25±0.34	1.10± 0.28
Trig (µMol/L)	0.51±0.04	0.86± 0.18	0.60±0.60	0.47± 0.06
HDL (iu/l)	0.44±0.39	0.44± 0.31	0.36±0.07	0.42± 0.44
LDL (µMol/L)	0.37±0.20	0.53± 0.19	0.69±0.20	0.64± 0.16
VLDL (µMol/L)	0.23±0.02	0.39±0.08	0.27±0.02	0.21± 0.03
CHO/HDL (µMol/L)	2.80±0.84	1.95±0.73	2.60±0.69	2.72± 0.80
K+ (mMol/L)	6.92±028	8.04±0.50	7.02±0.52	7.35± 0.48
Na+ (mMol/L)	139.14± 3.34	140.71± 5.84	147.43 ±2.79*	145.57 ± 1.06*
Cl⁻ (mMol/L)	107.57 ± 2.72	110.70 ± 5.32	117.40 ±4.37*	114.00 ± 1.46*
HCO₂⁻ (mMol/L)	23.71±0.91	22.28±1.32	21.14±0.39	21.14± 0.40
Uric Acid (µMol/L)	106.6± 6.74	164.6± 19.18	168.6±8.21	134.8±9.50
Urea (mMol/L)	6.80±0.44	7.31±0.39	6.82±0.72	4.60± 0.41#
Creat (mMol/L)	76.57±2.80	73.71± 8.4	70.14±2.52	76.85± 4.06

Values are expressed as means ± S.E.M. for n = 7
* Significantly increased (P≤0.05) compared to control.
# Significantly reduced (P≤0.05) compared to control.
ALT, Alanin Amino transferase
AST. Aspartate amino transferase
ALK. Phos, Alkaline Phosphatase.

Table 5. Effects of *V.Amygdalina* on Clinical Chemistry Parameter in rats. (14days exposure)

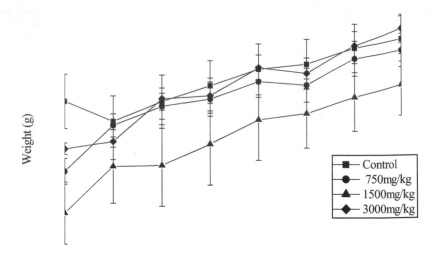

Weeks

Fig. 5. Evolution of the mean ±SE of rat body weight during the subchronic toxicity of *Vernonia amygdalina* extract.

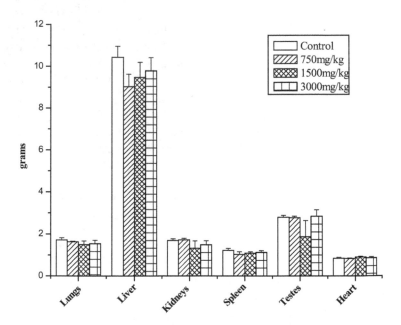

Fig. 6. Plots of the mean SE. Of the harvested organ weights during the sub-chronic toxicity study of *V.amygdalina* extract.

3.7 Hematological analysis

The mean values of the nine haematological parameters are reported in (Table 6)

Doses mg/kg	WBC (10⁹/l)	RBC (10¹²/l)	HGB (g/dl)	HCT (%)	MCV (fL)	MCH (pg)	MCHC (g/dl)	PLT (10⁹/µl)	MPV (fL)	NE (%)	LY (%)
Control	4.8±0.8	8.4±1.2	16.9±2	44±6	53±4	20±2	38±2	429±50	6.7±0.1	0.5±0.01	4.1±0.7
750mg/kg	6.6±1.0	8.7±1.1	17.2±3	45±1	52±4	19±1	38±4	464±18	6.5±1.0	1.0±0.4*	5.4±0.8
1500mg/kg	8.0±0.7*	8.2±0.6	16.7±1	43±3	53±2	20±0.3	38±3	555±43	6.5±0.1	0.7±0.1	6.9±0.6*
3000mg/kg	8.5±0.3*	8.4±0.2	17.1±0.2	44±8	52±3	20±0.3	38±3	436±161	6.7±0.3	0.7±0.1	7.3±0.3*

Values presented as mean ± standard deviation.

n = 7

WBC = White blood cell; RBC = Red blood cell; HGB = Hemoglobin; HCT = Hematocrit; MCV = Mean corpuscular volume; MCH = Mean corpuscular hemoglobin; MCHC = Mean corpuscular hemoglobin concentration; PLT = Platelets; NE = Neutrophil; LY = Lymphocyte

Statistical analysis: ANOVA, then Dunnett's test

*Mean value of group is significantly different from control at p<0.05

Table 6. Mean hematology values of rats after repeated (6 weeks) oral dosing with extract leave of *V.amygdalina.*

The WBC count presented a significant increase in the two high doses (8.47 ± 0.3 in 3000 mg/kg/d) and (8.02 ± 0.7 in 1500 mg/kg/d) versus control (4.80 ± 0.8).

There was a significant increase in the lymphocyte values in high doses (7.33 ± 0.2 in 3000 mg/kg/d) and (6.94 ± 0.6 in 1500 mg/kg/d) as compared to control (4.13 ± 0.7)

There was also a significant increase in the values of Neutrophil count (1.08 ± 0.7 in 750 mg/kg/d) versus control (0.53 ± 0.02). However, no major difference was noted between the control and assayed groups.

3.8 Biochemical analysis

Clinical chemistry analysis of the rats indicate increased ASAT and ALAT ratios in the 1500 mg/kg/d dose, compared to control values (Table 7). In addition, significant increased in HDL levels were noted in the same dose level when compared to controls.

Dose Mg/kg/d	ASAT (U/L)	ALAT (U/L)	ALB (g/dl)	TRIG (mg/dl)	UREA (mg/dl)	CALC (mg/dl)	T.PROT (g/L)	PHOS (mg/dl)	CREAT (mg/dl)	T.BIL (mg/dl)	URICAC (μmol/l)	D.BIL (mg/dl)	T.CHO (mg/dl)	HDL (mg/dl)	LDL (mg/dl)	K (mmol/l)	NA (mmol/l)	AMY (U/L)
Control	132	93	3.4	120	52	12	33	24	0.5	0.38	80	0.20	88	4.1	68	5.9	152	1196
	±26	±4	±0.1	±15	±3	±3	±10	±6	±0.3	±0.1	±30	±.02	±10	±0.7	±9	±0.2	±3	±49
750	202	94	3.5	115	56	14	39	40	0.6	0.42	81	0.12	69	3.4	55	5.7	146	1301
	±29	±9	±0.2	±13	±2	±4	±15	±11	±0.2	±0.1	±40	±.03	±10	±0.5	±7	±0.3	±5	±36
1500	373*	186*	3.7	112	56	6.4	24	28	0.6	0.80	70	0.18	83	6.7*	59	5.9	147	1219
	±77	±26	±0.2	±17	±3	±1.8	±5	±5.9	±0.2	±0.2	±25	±.02	±19	±0.7	±15	±0.4	±4	±94
3000	313	140	3.3	104	57	3.9	24	16	0.5	0.58	148	0.10	76	4.8	56	5.9	151	1267
	±63	±23	±0.1	±15	±3	±1.2	±4	±3.0	±0.02	±0.1	±19	±.02	±7	±0.6	±6	±0.4	±2.4	±63

$n = 7$, Values presented as mean ± standard deviation
ASAT = Aspartate aminotransferase; ALAT = Alanine aminotransferase; ALB = Albumin; TRIG = Triglyceride; CAL = Calcium; T.PROT = Total protein; PHOS = Phosphate; CREAT = Creatine; T. BILI = Total bilirubin ; D. BILI = Direct bilirubin; T.CHO = Total Cholesterol; HDL = High density lipoprotein; LDL = Low density lipoprotein; K = Potassium; NA = Sodium; AMY = Amylase
Statistical analysis: ANOVA, Dunnett's test
*Mean values of groups is significantly different from control at p<0.05.

Table 7. Mean clinical chemistru values of rats after repeated (6 weeks) orad dosing with aqueous extract leave of *V.amygdalina*.

4. Discussion

As herbal medicine become more popular especially in rural areas, pharmacological evidences to understand the action of these medicine and the underlying mechanisms, to support the proper and safe use of these medicine are indispensable

Our ethnopharmacology survey showed that medicinal plants are still widely used by the population in the area where the study was conducted. Several types of preparations of plants were used. The plants grow over an extended area and are used by healers separated by long distances.

In the current study, the analgesic effect of the leave extract of *Vernonia amygdalina* was assessed using three nociceptive animal models. In the writhing response model, acetic acid is injected into the peritoneal cavity of mice. The acid causes nociception in the abdomen due to the release of various substances that excite pain nerve ending (Raj, 1996). According to previous reports this assay is commonly used in mice to detect both central and peripheral analgesic efficacy of agents (Dewey, 1970; Fukawa et al 1980), *V amygdalina* showed an ability to diminish the numbers of the writhing episode in a dose-dependent manner. The results of the writhing test alone did not ascertain whether antinociceptive effects are central or peripheral.

The formalin test is considered a model for chronic pain (Duduisson and Dennis, 1977). In this test, animals present two distinct nociceptive behavior phases, which probably involve different stimuli. The first phase initiates immediately after formalin injection and lasts 3 to 5 mins, resulting from chemical stimulations of nociceptor. The second phase initiates 15 to 20 mins after formalin injection, lasts 20 to 40 mins and seems to depend on a peripheral mechanism as well as a central one. While substance P and bradykinins are involved in the first phase, histamine, 5HT, prostaglandins and bradykinin are involved in the second phase. The effect of extract was significant in both phases. Since the mechanism of the analgesic effect of *V. amygdalina* is apparent in these two models, it can however be speculated that this effect may be linked to processes in the prevention of sensitization of the nociceptor, down-regulation of the sensitized nociceptor and/or blockade of the nociceptor at peripheral and/or central levels.(Ferreira, 1990). Another possible mechanism may be that the extract blocks effect or the release of endogenous substances, including prostaglandin E_2 (PG_{E2}) and $PGF_{2\alpha}$ that excites pain nerve ending which is found in writhing response test model of mice (Deraedt, et al, 1980).

The extract fails to exhibit antinociceptive effect in the tail-flick test, as values obtain were not significantly different from control animals. Pethidine (50mg/kg p.o.) the reference drug used exhibited significant antinociceptive effect in rats. It is known that the tail-flick (thermal nociceptive) response appears to be a spinal reflex sensitive to opioid $_\mu$-agonists and non-thermal tests to opioid $_\kappa$-agonists (Abbott, 1988; Furst et al, 1988), furthermore thermally-induced pain is also mediated by $A\delta$ and C fibers. The data in the present study suggest the involvement of $_\kappa$ opioid receptors in the analgesic activity and a decrease activity of $A\delta$ and C fibers against inflammatory-induced activation but not thermally-induced activation (Puig and Sorkin, 1980).

Aqueous extracts of *V. amygdalina* were found to have *in vivo* activities against *P. berghei* in mice. At 200 mg/kg the antiplasmodial activity were comparable to CQ treated mice. Empirically, this plant is used in decoction alone, other plants may be added to reduce the side effect of nausea that result from the herb's bitter taste (15).

The acute oral toxicity results from the *V. amygdalina* extract (3.32 ± 0.15 g/kg p.o) indicate that the extract may be safe based on the chemical labeling and classification of acute systemic toxicity on oral LD_{50} values, recommended by the organization for Economic Cooperation and Development (Walum et al,1986). It has, however, been reported, that the median lethal dose is not an absolute value but is an inherently variable biologic parameter that cannot be compared to constants such as molecular weight or melting point (Oliver, 1986). The adverse signs of gaiting, reduction in stereotypic activities and deaths were however seen in high doses.

In the sub-chronic study, the hematologic parameter shows a decrease in the RBC counts and an increased neutrophil in the treated groups. The serum chemistry parameter shows an increase in the direct and total bilirubin value. In several organs, mainly heart and liver, cell damage is followed by increased levels of a number of cytoplasmic enzymes in the blood, a phenomenon that provides the basis for clinical diagnosis of heart and liver diseases . For example, liver enzymes are usually raised in acute hepatotoxicity but tend to decreased with prolonged intoxication due to damage to the liver cells (Orisakwe et al, 2004). In this study, the extract did not exert significant effects on the serum chemistry parameters, the increased in bilirubin levels were probably due to the decrease RBC values.

Since the traditional healers reported use of the drug as prophylactics against malaria, male rats were exposed to the extract for 6 weeks. No extract-related deaths occurred, the clinical condition of the animals, body weight gain, and food consumption were unaffected. Clinical pathology parameters (hematology, serum chemistry) exhibited no treatment-related effect. Organ weight changes can be sensitive indicators of target organ toxicity, and significant changes in organ weights may occur in the absence in changes in other pathology parameters (Bailey,S.A., 2004), for example, increased liver weight associated with hepatic cytochrome P450 induction is a common finding in toxicology studies. Liver weight increases of up to 20% relative to control without microscopic evidence of hepatocellular hypertrophy or changes in serum chemistries (Amacher, et al., 2000). Similarly modest dose-related changes in kidney weight commonly occur in toxicology studies without histopathologic evidence of cellular alteration (Greaves, P. 2000).

In conclusion, the results of this study showed analgesic activity of the extract with clear and significant antiplasmodial effects in mice, no indication of toxicity in rats, incidental findings below or above standard reference levels were all within control values based on historical reference ranges. This might explain the pharmacological basis for the successes in pain and malaria treatment claimed by traditional healers who use *V. amygdalina*.

5. Acknowledgments

This study received financial support from Innovation at Makerere Committee (I@mak.com) grant. The authors are grateful to Prof. F.I.B. Kayanja (Mbarara University of Science and Technology) for his valuable input. We also thank The Rukararwe Traditional Medicine Health Center in Bushenyi District for providing plant material for the study.

6. References

Abosi AO, Raseroka BH: In vivo antimalarial activity of *Vernonia amygdalina. Br J Biomed Sci* 2003;60:89–91.

Adzu B, Abbah J, Vongtau H, Gamaniel K: Study on the used of *Cassia singueana* in malaria ethnopharmacy. *J Ethnopharmacol* 2003;88:261–267.

Akah PA, Okafor CI: Hypoglycaemia effect of *Vernonia amygdalina* Del in experimental rabbits. *Plant Med Res* 1992;1:6–10.

Amacher,D.E. et al (1998) The relationship among microsomal enzyme induction, liver weight and histological change in rat toxicology studies, *Food Chem.Toxicol*. 36, 831,

Asongalem, E.A., Foyet, H.S., Ngogang, J., Folefoc, G.N., Dimo, T., Kamchouing, P. Analgesic and anti-inflammatory activities of *Ergeron floribundus*. *J Ethnopharmacol* 2004a, 91: 301-308.

Bailey, S. A., Zidell, R. H., and Perry R. W., (2004) Relationships between organ weight and body/brain weight in the rat: what is the best analytical endpoint? *Toxicl. Pathol.*, 32, 448.

Deraedt R, Jougney S, Falhout M: Release of prostaglandin E and F in an algogenic reaction and its inhibition. *Eur J Pharmacol* 1980;51:17–24.

Dewey, W.L., Harris, L.S., Howes, J.F., Nuite, J.A. The effect of various neurohumoral modulators on the activity of morphine and the narcotic antagonists in the tail-flick and phenylquinous tests. *J Pharmacol.Exp.Ther* 1970, 175: 435 – 442

Dioka C, Orisakwe OE, Afonne OJ, *et al*.: Investigation into the haematologic and hepatotoxic effects of rinbacin in rats. *J Health Sci* 2002;48:393–398.

Dubuisson, D, Dennis SG: The formalin test: a qualitative study of analgesic effects of morphine, meperidine and brain stem stimulation in rats and cats. *Pain* 1977;4:161–174.

Dubuisson, D., Dennis, S.G. The formalin test: a qualitative study of analgesic effects of morphine, meperidine and brain stem stimulation in rats and cats. *Pain* 1977, 4:161-174.

Ferreira SH: A classification of peripheral analgesics based upon their mode of action. In: *Migraine: A Spectrum of Ideas* (Sandler M, Collins GM, eds.). Oxford University Press, Oxford, 1990, pp.59–72.

Fukawa K, Kawano O, Hibi M, Misaki M, Ohba S, Hatanaka Y: A method for evaluating analgesic agents in rats. *J Pharmacol Methods* 1980;4:251–259.

Greaves,P., (2000) *Histopathology of Preclinical Toxicity studies*, 2nd ed., Elsevier, Amsterdam, chap 9

Guide for the Care and Use of Laboratory Animals, revised. NIH publication No. 83-23. National Institutes of Health, Bethesda, MD, 1978.

Hamill FA, Apio A, Mubiro NK, Mosango M, *et al*.: Traditional herbal drugs of Southern Uganda 1. *J Ethnopharmacol* 2000;70: 281-300.

Homsy J.K.E., Kabatesi D., Mubiru F., Kwamya L., Tusuba C., Kasolo S., Mwebe D., Ssentamu L., Okello M., King R., Evaluating herbal medicine for the management of

Homsy J.K.E., King R., Balaba D., Kabatesi D. Traditional health practitioners are key to scaling up comprehensive care for HIV/AIDS in sub-Saharan Africa. AIDS, 2004 18(12)1723-1725.

Huffman MA, Koshimizu K, Ohigashi H: Ethnobotany and zoopharmacognosy of *Vernonia amygdalina*, a medicinal plant used by humans and chimpanzees. In: *Compositae: Biology Utilization. Proceedings of the International Compositae Conference* (Caligary PDS, Hind DJN, eds.). The Royal Botanical Garden, Kew, UK, 1996, pp. 351–360.

Huffman MA: Animal self-medication and ethno-medicine exploration and exploitation of the medicinal properties of plant. *Proc Nutr Soc* 2003;62:371–381.

Iwalewa EO, Adewunmi CO, Omisote NO, *et al*.: Pro-and antioxidant effects and cytoprotective potentials of nine edible vegetables in southwest Nigeria. *J Med Food* 2005;4:539–544.

Izevbigie EB, Bryant JL, Walker A: A novel natural inhibitor of extracellular signal-regulated kinases and human breast cancer cell growth. *Exp Biol Med* 2004;229:163–169.

Janssen, P.A.J., Niemegeers, C.J.E., Dony, J.G.H. The inhibitory effect of fentanyl and other morphine-like analgesic on the warm water induced tail withdrawal reflex in rats. Arzneim-Forsch *Drug Res* 1963, 6: 502-507

K.Saidu, J. Onah, A. Orisadipe, A.Olusola, C. Wambebe, Kgamaniel, (2000) Antiplasmodial, analgesic, and anti-inflammatory activities of the aqueous extract of the stem bark of Erythrina senegalensis. Journal of Ethnopharmacology 71,275 – 280.

Kambizi L, Afolayan AJ: An ethnobotanical study of plants used for the treatment of sexually transmitted disease. *J Ethnopharmacol* 2001;77:5–9.

Koster, R., Anderson, N., De Beer, E. J. Acetic acid for analgesic screening. Federation Proceedings 1959, 18: 412.

Lorke D: A new approach to practical acute toxicity testing. *Arch Toxicol* 1998;5:275–289.

Masaba SC: The antimalarial activity of *Vernonia amygdalina* Del. (Compositae). *Trans R Soc Trop Med Hyg* 2000;94:694–695.

O'Hara, M; Kiefer D; Farrel K and Kemper K (1998) A review of 12 commonly used medicinal herbs. *Arch. Fam. Med.* 7: 523-536.

Oliver JA: Opportunities for using fewer animals in acute toxicity studies. In: *Chemical Testing and Animal Welfare*. The National Chemicals Inspectorate, Solna, Sweden, 1986, pp. 119-143.

Orisakwe OE, Njan AA, Afonne OJ, Akumka DD, Orish VN, Udemezue OO: Investigation into the nephrotoxicity of Nigerian bonny light crude oil in albino rats. *Int J Environ Res Public Health* 2004;2:91-95.

Raj PP: Pain mechanisms. In: *Pain Medicine, A Comprehensive Review*. Mosby-Year Book, St. Louis, 1996, pp. 12-24.

Sanchez-Mateo CC, Bonkanka CX, Hernandez-Perez M, Rabanal RM: Evaluation of analgesic and topical anti-inflammatory effects of *Hypericum reflexum* L. fil. *J Ethnopharmacol* 2006;107:1-6.

Sanchez-Mateo, C.C., Bonkanka, C.X., Hernandez-Perez, M., Rabanal, R.M. Evaluation of analgesic and topical anti-inflammatory effects of *Hypericum reflexum* L. fil. *J Ethnopharmacol* 2006, 107: 1-6.

Siegmund EA, Cadmus RA, Lu G: Screening of analgesic including aspirin-type compound based upon the antagonism of chemically induced writhing in mice. *J Pharmacol Exp Ther* 1957;119:184–186.

Taiwo O, Xu HX, Lee SF: Antibacterial activites of extracts from Nigerian chewing sticks. *Phytother Res* 1999;8:675–679.

Tona L, Cimanga RK, Mesia K, *et al.*: Antiplasmodial activity of extracts and fractions from seven medicinal plants. *J Ethnopharmacol* 2004;93:27–32.

WHO, (2003). Assessment and monitoring of antimalarial drug efficacy for the treatment of uncomplicated faciparum malaria. Geneva.

Wilcox ML: A clinical trial of 'AM', a Uganda herbal remedy for malaria. *J Public Health Med* 1999;21:318–324.

Willcox, M.L, G. Bodeker (2000). Plant-based malaria Control: research initiative on traditional antimalaria methods. *Parasitology Today* 16: 220 – 221.

Zimmermann M: Ethical guidelines for investigations of experimental pain in conscious animals. *Pain* 1983;16:109–110.

9

Experimental and Computational Methods Pertaining to Drug Solubility

Abolghasem Jouyban[1] and Mohammad A. A. Fakhree[2]
[1]Drug Applied Research Center and Faculty of Pharmacy,
[2]Liver and Gastrointestinal Diseases Research Center,
Tabriz University of Medical Sciences, Tabriz,
Iran

1. Introduction

Solubility of a drug is one of its important physico-chemical properties. More attention has been paid to the aqueous solubility since water is the unique solvent of biological systems. It is obvious that a drug should be reached to its receptors in the body through the aqueous and non-aqueous media. The chance of a low water soluble drug to be appeared in the market place is very low and nearly 40 % of the drug candidates fail to reach higher phases of the drug trials simply because of their low water solubility. The solubility in non-aqueous solvents is not too important from clinical viewpoint however these solubilities play curious roles in drug discovery and development investigations. Most of drugs are synthesized in non-aqueous media and/or extracted from natural sources using non-aqueous extracting solvents. Different polymorphs of some drugs could be produced from their crystallization using organic solvents.

There are various methods for solubility determination of drugs which is discussed in this chapter. The experimental determination is tedious and time-consuming process and sometimes there is restrictions in the availability of enough amount of a drug candidate to be used in the solubility measurements, especially in the early stages of drug discovery investigations in which only small amount of a drug is synthesized/extracted and large number of preliminary biological tests should be carried out. To cover this limitation, and in order to provide a faster and easier tool, mathematical models have been developed to correlate/predict the solubility of drugs. These models are discussed in this chapter to provide an overall view for a pharmaceutical scientist who is working in the research and development department of a company and/or a research laboratory within academia. In addition to the accurate calculations which are expected from these models, the simplicity of the required computations is another parameter which should be taken into account, since more complex computations did not attract more attention in the pharmaceutical industry.

1.1 Solubility and dissolution

When talking about solubility, there are two concepts which might be confused with each other: solubility and dissolution. The term solution (i.e. thermodynamic solution) is used to define the state which is thermodynamically stable and shows the neat result of an equilibrium between a solute (the compound which is going to be dispersed molecularly in another medium which is called solvent) and its dissolved form in the medium. The dissolving process is the migration of the molecules of the solute to the solvent medium and makes the solution which after reaching a steady state is called homogenous solution and can be represented by the following equilibrium:

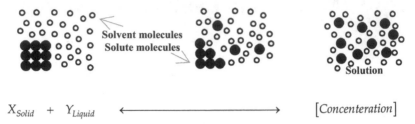

$$X_{Solid} + Y_{Liquid} \longleftrightarrow [Concenteration]$$

How much a solute is molecularly dispersed in the solvent is called solubility and the rate of dissolving is called dissolution. Hence, the solubility value is a thermodynamic property while the dissolution rate is a kinetic one. In other words, time has no effect on solubility value and is not important in its related subjects, but it is important in dissolution related subjects.

The solubility is important in stable forms including liquid formulations and dissolution is important in transient states including the release of the drug from its formulation to biological fluids and permeability (Sinko and Martin, 2006). In pharmaceutical sciences, especially in formulation, designing a stable liquid formulation requires the knowledge on the solubility value and an effective drug delivery to the body mostly depends on the dissolution rate which is affected by the solubility (Allen et al., 2006). However, they both affect each other based on Noyes-Whitney equation (Sinko and Martin, 2006):

$$\frac{dW}{dt} = \frac{DA(C_S - C)}{L} \tag{1}$$

where dW/dt is the rate of dissolution, A is the surface area of the solid which is in direct contact with the molecules of the solvents, C is the concentration of the solute in the medium (dissolved amount), C_S is the concentration of the solute in the diffusion layer, D is the diffusion coefficient, and L is the thickness of the diffusion layer.

Based on the discussed topics, solubility and dissolution are in relation with each other, but not the same. So, they must not be used in place of each other as the consequences can be awful! For example, a drug substance might be highly soluble, but dissolves slowly (or vice versa). So, in the formulation of such compounds, the difference between solubility and dissolution must be considered.

1.2 Solubility of base form of drugs

The apparent solubility (S_{App}) of a weak electrolyte is expressed by:

$$S_{App} = S_M + S_I \tag{2}$$

in which S_M is the molecular form of the drug and S_I is the ionized form of the drug in the solution. For strong electrolytes, S_I is predominant whereas for nonelectrolytes S_M is the only form of the solubilized drug in the solution. S_M is also called intrinsic solubility or S_0. In early stages of drug discovery, only small amount of the new drug is available and its purity is not assured. In this stage, the solubility determination in acidic and/or basic solutions could be used in practice. Increased apparent solubility in acidic or basic medium reveals that the new drug is a basic or an acidic solute. No increase in the solubility means that the drug is a nonelectrolyte. Increased solubility in both acidic and basic media indicates either zwitterionic or amphoteric behaviour. The intrinsic solubility of a drug could be determined from apparent solubility data at various pH values. When the purity of a drug candidate is not assured, a phase-solubility diagram, i.e. the solubility at different solute:solvent ratios, is recommended. In this diagram, the co-solute effect (self association, complexation, solubilization) increases the solubility and the common ion effect decreases the solubility and no change in the solubility might mean that drug is pure and no interaction exists.

1.3 Solubility of salt form of drugs
Salt formation of weak acidic or basic drugs is one of their solubility increasing methods since the ionized species have greater solubility in water and other polar solvents and a number of drugs are marketed as their salt forms. The most common salts used for salt formation of acidic drugs are sodium, potassium, calcium and zinc and those for basic drugs are hydrochloride, sulphate, mesylate, maleate, phosphate, tartrate, citrate and besylate (Wells, 1988). Different slats of a given drug possess various solubilities. As an example, the solubility of lamotrigine with the counterions of tartrate, saccharinate, succinate and fumarate are 2.63, 1.37, 0.61 and 0.43 millimole per liter (Galcera and Molins, 2009). The selection of the salt of a drug is mainly carried out by trial and error basis considering practical issues such as cost of raw materials, ease of crystallization, percent yield, thermal stability and hygroscopicity of the resulting salt. Black et al. (2007) investigated the salt formation of 17 salt forms of ephedrine and reported their physicochemical properties and tried to develop a relationship between these properties which was not successful. Any model representing the properties of salt forms of drugs is a highly in demand subject in the pharmaceutical industry. As an example, the relation between the dielectric constant of the solvent and the solubility of drugs in their salt form, can be mentioned (Fakhree et al., 2010).

1.4 Solubility of pharmaceutical macromolecules
Polymers and macromolecules are important parts of drug design and development. The emerging technology of proteins, peptides, DNA and RNA sequences as pharmaceutical active ingredients makes it necessary for consideration of their physicochemical properties in pharmaceutical sciences, including solubility. For the beginning, in terms of macromolecules, it is better to use dispersion versus solubility in a medium and this makes a difference between their solubility in comparison with small organic molecules. The dispersion of the macromolecules in the solution results in formation of new properties for the solution such as increase in viscosity, light scattering, molecular network formation (e.g. gel) etc (Sinko and Martin, 2006). Another important note about macromolecules, is the fact that they have been produced in an aqueous medium and have philia to watery media (not always, but in most of the cases). Hence, they are sensitive to presence of organic solvents and might be precipitated by addition of the organic solvents (unlike small organic nonelectrolyte molecules which dissolve in organic media more than aqueous solutions).

The solubility of proteins is influenced by the ratio of the hydrophobic and hydrophilic residues of amino acids and their arrangement in the final structure of the protein (Bolen, 2004). For example, globular proteins have hydrophobic residues in their core and hydrophilic residues in their surface. It is also affected by the pH and ionic strength of the water, presence of organic solvents and other polymers (Burgess, 2009). When talking about the solubility of proteins, there are different kinds of low solubility for the proteins:

1. in-vitro low solubility due to structural properties of the protein (hydrophobic residues),
2. in-vivo low solubility due to over expression of the protein in an organism (*E. coli*),
3. amyloid formation which results in aggregation of the proteins because of their hydrophobic, residue charge, and β-sheets in the structure, and
4. low solubility due to conformational changes (Trevino et al., 2008).

For increasing a protein's aqueous solubility, one of the strategies is addition of additives such as L-arginine and L-glutamic acids. Fusion of peptides and proteins is another method which is addition of a solubilizing sequence of amino acids or protein to the structure of the low soluble protein. Mutation in the hydrophobic amino acids sequences to hydrophilic ones is another strategy. However, this might not work in all of the cases (Trevino et al., 2008). Another approach is screening to find a more soluble homologue of that protein in other organisms (Waldo, 2003).

1.5 Solubility of drugs in biological fluids

For understanding the dissolution of a drug in the human body fluids, it is crucial to focus on the solubility of drugs in more realistic environment and to acquire larger amount of experimental data for simulating the solubility at different pHs, in the presence of bile salts etc which exists in the real solubilization media within human body. Solubility data of drugs in biorelevant media are increasingly required in early phases of drug discovery to predict the bioavailability of a drug after oral administration.

1.6 Solubility modifications

Solubility modification of drugs is required in separation, purification, analysis and formulation investigations and different methods are used to achieve the increased/decreased solubility values.

1.6.1 Solubility increasing

Several methods have been used to enhance the aqueous solubility of drugs including cosolvency, hydrotropism, complexation, ionisation, use of the surface active agents, crystal structure modifications and addition of ionic liquids. These methods have been discussed in details in the literature (Myrdal and Yalkowsky, 1998). Mixing a permissible non-toxic organic solvent with water, i.e. cosolvency, is the most common and feasible technique to enhance the aqueous solubility of drugs. The common cosolvents which, are used in the pharmaceutical industry are ethanol, propylene glycol, glycerine, glycofural, polyethylene glycols (mainly 200, 300 and 400), N,N-dimethyl acetamide, dimethyl sulfoxide, 2-propanol, dimethyl isosorbide, N-methyl 2-pyrrolidone (NMP) and room temperature ionic liquids (Rubino, 1990; Mizucci et al., 2008; Jouyban et al., 2010a). Their applications and possible side effects have been discussed in the literature (Spiegel and Noseworthy, 1963; Tsai et al., 1986; Patel et al., 1986; Golightly et al., 1988; Rubino, 1990). Hydrotropes are a class of amphiphilic molecules that cannot form organized structures, such as micelles, in water but they increase the aqueous solubility of drugs. Often strong synergistic effects are observed when hydrotropes are added to aqueous surfactant or polymer solutions. Caffeine and nicotinamide are well known hydrotropic agents and their ability to solubilize a wide variety of therapeutic drugs including riboflavin (Lim and Go, 2000) has been demonstrated. Complexation of drugs is another solubilization technique and there are a number of reports on complexation of drugs by cyclodextrins. Ionization is applicable for weak electrolytes and the solubility of some drugs could be increased by changing pH of the solution.

1.6.2 Solubility decreasing

In precipitation and crystallization processes as a part of extraction and purification of the pharmaceutically related compounds, lowering the solubility is desirable. Lowering the solubility for pharmaceutical compounds might include using of temperature alteration, addition of antisolvent, using of a low soluble salt or ester of the drug, and producing low soluble polymorphs (Blagden et al., 2007; Widenski et al., 2009).

Precipitation or crystallization both can be used in this regard depending on the rate of solubility decreasing. If it is happened quickly, then the solid state might be in amorphous form and the process called precipitation. If the lowering of solubility takes place in a controlled way that crystal growth can happen, then the process called crystallization. Precipitation of proteins and macromolecules such as DNA and RNA are other examples for this kind of solubility modification. In protein biosynthesis and extraction, different methods of desolubilization are used which include: salting out, isoelectric point precipitation, precipitation with organic solvents, addition of non-ionic hydrophilic polymers, flocculation by polyelectrolytes, and addition of polyvalent metallic ions (Burgess, 2009). Another reason making it desirable to precipitate macromolecules such as proteins, DNA, and RNA is pre-treatment of biological analytes before starting analyses.

Recrystallization is another process which is used in pharmaceutical sciences and means to dissolve a compound in a medium, and by modifying the physicochemical conditions made the dissolved compound to crystallize again. This technique is widely used in crystal engineering technology which can produce amorphous, different polymorphs, and psudopolymorphs of a drug (Blagden et al., 2007). This is important in modification of pharmaceutically interested physicochemical properties such as compressibility in formulation process, size of particles, dissolution rate, as well as solubility (Allen et al., 2006; Gibaldi et al., 2007).

The above mentioned processes are related to preformulation processes. In formulation of pharmaceutical active ingredients the desire for lowering solubility can be seen in designing of sustained release and depot dosage forms or drug delivery systems (Allen et al., 2006; Gibaldi et al., 2007). For making a sustained release dosage form of a drug, different formulation techniques such as use of polymeric matrix, osmotic pumps, and crystallization of a poorly water soluble compound are used. For designing a depot drug delivery system, possible solutions include: use of low soluble salts or esters of a drug (e.g. methylprednisolone acetate), addition of additives (e.g. zinc and insulin), very concentrated non-aqueous solutions of drug (e.g. Leuprolide and NMP), and depot dosage forms (e.g. implants of low soluble compounds such as sex hormones) (Strickley, 2004; Allen et al., 2006; Gibaldi et al., 2007).

Also low solubility is useful when stability of a pharmaceutical compound is low in its solubilized form (Sinko and Martin, 2006). Hence, suspension formulations (i.e. ready to use and lyophilized powder for suspension preparation) might be a useful strategy.

In the recent decade, emerging technologies such as micro-formulation, micro-encapsulation, nano-formulation, and nano-encapsulation are using solubility decreasing principals as a part of their processes. This is usually done by addition of antisolvent and fine particle stabilizers to gain a suspension with micro/nano-sized particles.

2. Experimental methods for determination of solubility

The solubility of a drug could be measured experimentally using two procedures, namely the thermodynamic and kinetic solubility methods. The thermodynamic solubility determination methods are not feasible at the early discovery stage because of the large sample requirement, low throughput and laborious sample preparation. The kinetic solubility determinations could be used as an alternative method at this stage.

2.1 Determination of thermodynamic solubility

Solubility determination of drugs in a liquid could be classified as analytical and synthetic methods. The main advantage of the analytical (shake flask) method is the possibility of measuring a large number of samples simultaneously however this method is tedious and time-consuming.

2.1.1 Shake flask method

The shake-flask method of Higuchi and Connors (1965) is the most reliable method for low soluble compounds and widely used solubility measurement method. In this method, an excess amount of drug is added to the solubility medium. The added amount should be enough to make a saturated solution in equilibrium with the solid phase. In case of acidic or basic drugs dissolved in an un-buffered solubility medium, further addition of the solid could change pH of the solution and consequently the solubility of the drug (Wang et al., 2002; Kawakami et al., 2005; Jouyban and Soltanpour, 2010). Depending on the dissolution rate and type of agitation used, the equilibration time between the dissolved drug and the excess solid could be varied. Equilibration is often achieved within 24 hours. To ensure the equilibration condition, the dissolution profile of drug should be investigated. The shortest time needed for reaching the plateau of drug concentration against time could be considered as a suitable equilibration time. Any significant variation on dissolution profile after reaching the equilibration should be inspected, since there are a number of possibilities including degradation of the drug and also its polymorphic transformation. Both these affect the solubility values of a drug dissolved in the dissolution media. Heating, vortexing or sonicating the sample prior to equilibration could shorten the equilibration time. To overcome the poor wettability of low soluble drugs, one may use small glass microspheres or sonication. Then the two phases, solid and solution phases, are separated using two common methods of filtration and/or centrifugation. Filteration is the easiest method, however, the possible sorption of the solute on the filter should be considered as a source of error in solubility determination, especially for very low soluble drugs. Pre-rinsing the filter with the saturated solution could reduce the sorption of the solute on the filter by saturating the adsorption sites. Centrifugation or ultra-centrifugation is preferred in some cases, and the higher viscosity of the saturated solutions, e.g. in mixed solvents, should be kept in mind as a limitation. A combination of filtration and centrifugation is also could be used. The UV spectrophotometric analysis is the most common and the easiest analytical method. The next is the HPLC methods both in isocratic and gradient elution modes. The HPLC analysis could also detect the possible impurities or degradation products if a highly selective method was used. X-ray diffraction (XRD) and differential scanning calorimetry (DSC) of the residual solid separated from the saturated solution confirm the possible solid phase transformations during equilibration.

2.1.2 Synthetic method

The synthetic method (Hankinson and Thompson, 1965; Ren et al., 2005; Yang et al., 2008; Yu et al., 2009) which is so called laser monitoring technique (Li et al., 2006), last crystal disappearance method (Hao et al., 2005) and dynamic method (Peisheng and Qing, 2001; Weiwei et al., 2007; Wang et al., 2008) is based on disappearance of the solid drug (from the mixture of solvent and drug) monitored by a laser beam. The history of this method backs to 1886 and first introduced by Alexejew and then modified by other research groups (Ward, 1926). The disappearance of drugs could be achieved either by changing the temperature or by addition of a known amount of the solvent. It is claimed that the synthetic method is much faster and more reliable than analytical method (Yang et al., 2008). Figure 1 illustrates a schematic representation of the most completed set up used in the synthetic method.

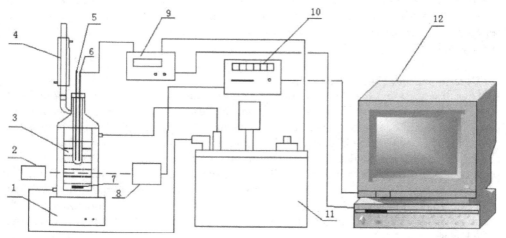

Fig. 1. Schematic representation of the synthetic method for determination of solubility of drugs; 1, magnetic stirrer; 2, laser generator; 3, jacketed glass vessel; 4, condenser pipe; 5, thermometer; 6, thermocouple; 7, rotor; 8, photoelectric transducer; 9, controller; 10, laser strength display; 11, constant temperature bath; 12, workstation. (Figure is reproduced from Ren et al., 2005).

The solubility apparatus consisted of a jacketed glass vessel (varying from 60 to 250 mL) maintained at the desired temperature by circulating water that was provided by a constant-temperature bath. The water temperature was controlled by a workstation with a temperature accuracy of (0.1 K) achieved continuous stirring, and a condenser (or a perforated rubber cover) was fitted to reduce the solvent's evaporation. A thermometer with an uncertainty of 0.01 K was used to determine the temperature of the system. A laser beam was used as a tool to observe dissolving the solid in liquid. The signal transmitted through the vessel was collected by a detector that decided the rate of temperature rise and estimated the equilibrium point of the given system on the basis of the signal change. The solute and the solvent were prepared using an electronic balance with the estimated uncertainty in the mole fraction of less than 0.001. A predetermined quantity of drug and solvent was placed into the jacketed vessel. The system was slowly heated (heating rate increase is 0.5 to 2 K·hr^{-1}) with continuous stirring. When the solute particles disappeared thoroughly, the signal approached a maximum value. The workstation judged the signal difference at 10-min intervals; if the interval was less than 10, then the workstation gave an order to stop heating and record the temperature. The temperature recorded was the liquid temperature of a given composition upon the complete dissolution of the drug (Ren et al., 2005). In another version of this set up, predetermined masses of drug and solvent were placed in the vessel and the contents were stirred continuously at a constant temperature. As the particles of the drug are dissolved, the intensity of the laser beam increased gradually and reaches to the maximum value when the drug is dissolved completely. Then an additional known mass of the drug is introduced to the vessel and the procedure is repeated until the laser beam could not return to the maximum value which means the last addition could not be dissolved. The total amount of the added drug is recorded and used to calculate the solubility value (Yang et al., 2008). The synthetic method is preferred over shake flask method for solubility determination of drugs in viscous solvents where separation of the excess solids from saturated solutions is not achievable (Grant and Abougela, 1983).

2.2 Determination of kinetic solubility

In drug discovery and development, one of the rationalized methods is high-throughput screening (HTS) which includes the design and synthesis of a large set(s) of chemicals to find hit compounds based on specific physicochemical properties (PCPs) and to develop lead compound. One of the important PCPs in determination of hit and lead compounds is aqueous solubility (Pan et al., 2001; Alsenz and Kansy, 2007; Hoelke et al. 2009). However, in practice it is not possible to experimentally determine thermodynamic solubility value in HTS approaches. This is because of large number of compounds which might be more than 1000 compounds in each HTS experiment or little amount of synthesized compounds which is around a few milligrams and is another limiting factor (Pan et al., 2001; Alsenz and Kansy, 2007; Hoelke et al. 2009).

Kinetic solubility determination methods were used for covering this problem. The advantages of the kinetics solubility determination in comparison with thermodynamic solubility determination methods are capability to being easily automated, accuracy, rapidity and requiring less amount of the solute (Pan et al., 2001; Alsenz and Kansy, 2007; Hoelke et al. 2009). Its disadvantages might include not assessing the crystal effect on the solubility, the cosolvent action of the dimethyl sulfoxide (DMSO), and its applicability is good for compounds which have solubility more than 10^{-6} molar. Some of the well established approaches include: nephelometric, UV-Spectroscopic, and HPLC methods which are discussed in the following.

2.2.1 Nephelometric method

The nephelometry is based on turbidimetry. Figure 2 shows a schematic view of the mechanism of turbidimetry. For sample preparation in this method, a 10 millimolar concentration of a solute was prepared by dissolving suitable amounts of the solute in DMSO. Then, this stock solution is used to prepare sample solutions in the range of 5×10^{-7} to 5×10^{-4} molar. For concentrations above the 10^{-4} molar, the solutions prepared by direct dilution of the stock solution and for the lower concentrations, serial dilutions were used where the dilutant is a buffer. These dilutions are directly take place in a 96-well plate with the total 5% concentration of DMSO and the final volume of $\approx$200 µL (Pan et al., 2001; Hoelke et al. 2009). This optimum volume is based on the fact that light scattering (for a specific condition) is nearly constant for a range of particle sizes (Pan et al., 2001) which make the process reproducible and accurate.

For sample analyzing after the preparation section, the 96-well plate is placed in a nephelometer apparatus for measurement of the light scattering. It uses a laser beam (with a fixed wavelength in the range of 550-750 nm) as the light source, and a detector which is placed with a specific angle to the light source. Based on plotting turbidity against prepared concentrations, and drawing its asymptotes and finding their meeting point x coordination, gives the kinetic solubility (see Figure 3) (Pan et al., 2001; Hoelke et al. 2009).

With this method, the kinetic solubility for a plate of 96 samples can be measured in a few minutes.

2.2.2 UV/Vis-spectroscopic method

There are two methods using UV/Vis-spectroscopy for kinetic solubility determination: Method 1 is based on turbidimetry and the other is based on light absorbance intensity as a function of concentration (Pan et al., 2001).

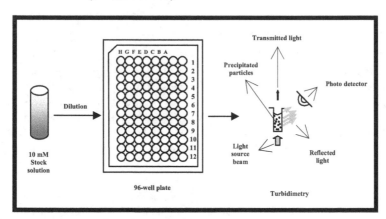

Fig. 2. Schematic representation of turbidimetry.

2.2.2.1 UV/Vis-spectroscopic method 1

The sample preparation is like nephelometry method, but the analyzing is with a 96-well plate UV/Vis-spectroscopy apparatus. This provides a wider range of wavelength to choose for reading the samples turbidity (190-1000 nm) (Pan et al., 2001). The lower the wavelength, the smaller particle is detected. However, in practice, wavelengths greater than 500 nm is used. This is because of the fact that most of organic compounds which have UV absorbance (e.g. contain a benzene ring) also have fluorescence property and might interfere with turbidimetry which reads the amount of reflected light (or fluorescence emission light) (Pan et al., 2001). An example of this is phenol red which has light absorption in 430 and 560 nm and is exited by these wavelengths which results in fluorescence emission (Pan et al., 2001). Another limitation is the UV absorbance of the most plates which are made of plastics (Pan et al., 2001).

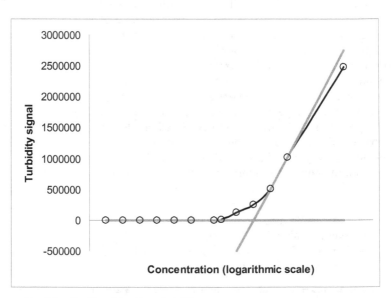

Fig. 3. The method for finding kinetic solubility.

2.2.2.2 UV/Vis-spectroscopic method 2

In this method, sample dilution in range of 7×10^{-9} to 5×10^{-4} molar is performed. But after precipitation of the stock solution by the aqueous solution, the samples are filtered to another plate. And in this part, 20% acetonitrile is added to the filtered samples for prevention of solute precipitation during analysis. Then the plate is read with a 96-well plate UV/Vis-spectroscopy apparatus and the recorded data changed to molar concentration (determined by calibration curve obtained by standard solutions using another plate) (Pan et al., 2001; Hoelke et al. 2009).

2.2.3 HPLC method

The sample preparation for this method is the same as UV/Vis-spectroscopic method 2 and the transferring of samples to the 96-well plate is not required. However, filtration of samples is done prior to injection to the HPLC or online filtration is applied. A calibration curve is required for the determination of the concentrations of the prepared samples. This method is the most accurate one in comparison with other mentioned methods (limit of detection $< 10^{-8}$ molar). But it must be considered that it consumes much more time (around 6 hours for 96 samples) (Pan et al., 2001; Hoelke et al. 2009). A comparison between the mentioned methods is given in Table 1.

Method	Calibration	Specificity	Easy	Cut off	LOD	Rapidity
Nephelometric	Not required	Low	Yes	No	Low	High
UV/Vis 1	Not required	Low	Yes	<500 nm	Low	High
UV/Vis 2	Required	Medium	No	<250 nm	Medium	Medium
HPLC	Required	High	No	No	High	Low

Table 1. The comparison between four kinetic solubility determination methods

Kinetic solubility values are valuable source in early stage of drug discovery in place of thermodynamic solubility values where there is good correlation between trends of these two values for a set of compounds (Hoelke et al. 2009). However, because of the amorphic nature of the solutes, in most of the cases the kinetic solubility is higher than thermodynamic solubility values. The effect of 5% DMSO as a cosolvent on the solubility value in kinetic solubility determination methods also should be considered. This is very important where most of the drugs have very low aqueous solubility and very small amounts of solubilizing agents such as cosolvents (e.g. DMSO) enhance their solubility largely.

Also the effect of time after dilution is important, especially in turbidimetry methods. Hoelke et al. have shown that by increasing the time after dilution and precipitation, the determined solubility become smaller (Hoelke et al. 2009).

2.3 Data validation

The collected data could be compared with the previously reported data in order to ensure the accuracy of the experimental procedure employed. Any mistake in the dilution steps, and miscalculations, or using un-calibrated instruments, such as un-calibrated balances, temperature variation and some other factors could be resulted in different solubility values for a given drug dissolved in a solvent at a fixed temperature.

3. Computational methods for solubility prediction

Computational methods in recent decades have become an important part of drug design and discovery. They are classified as theoretical, semi empirical and empirical equations. Most of models used in pharmaceutical sciences are semi-empirical (which is theoretical correlation of experimentally determined values) or empirical equations (which is mathematical correlation of experimentally determined values). Examples for semi-empirical models are those correlations which use physicochemical parameters in their relationships. In other word, it is needed for them to be calculated based on experimental determinations at least for one time. For example in Noyes-Whitney equation, the diffusion coefficient must be determined at least for one time for a solute. So the Noyes-Whitney equation is a semi-empirical model. The quantitative structure property relationships (QSPR) and quantitative structure activity relationships (QSAR) are examples for empirical modelling. The pioneer for this type of equations in pharmaceutical sciences is Prof. Crowin H. Hansch. He has developed a QSPR model for solubility prediction of liquids, based on their partition coefficient (Hansch et al., 1968):

$$-\log S = 1.339 \log P - 0.978 \qquad (3)$$

where $\log P$ is the logarithm of the partition coefficient between octanol and water for a specific liquid.

In another grouping, the correlation could be developed using linear modelling or non-linear modelling. Linear modelling is the simple linear regression (or multiple linear regression) and non-linear modelling is artificial neural network, as examples. There are advantages and disadvantages for each type of modelling which is listed in the Table 2:

Modelling type	Advantages	Disadvantages
Linear	- Simple to perform - Fast - Robust - Reproducible - Easy to use - The resulted model can be analyzed theoretically - Performable with small number of cases	- It cannot analyze non-linear and complex behaviour - Most of the time the results have low accuracy
Non-linear	- Can analyze non-linear and complex behaviour - The results have high accuracy	- Easily over fitting occurs - Many iterations are required - Need almost large number of cases - Reproducibility is hard - You must have the trained model to be able to predict new cases - It gives a black box instead of a model

Table 2. Advantages and disadvantages of linear and non-linear modelling in QSPR studies

In QSPR modelling, the variables used for correlation of physicochemical properties are called descriptors. These descriptors include simple structure derived parameters (e.g. number of carbon atoms, number of single bonds), overall structural parameters (e.g. molecular weight, and molecular volume), structure residues parameters (e.g. distance between two atoms, total charge on oxygen atoms), or physicochemical properties (e.g. melting point, partition coefficient). In solubility correlation almost all kinds of descriptors have been used. Around half of the models use $\log P$ as one of descriptors in modelling (Dearden, 2006). The following categories of descriptors have been used in solubility correlation:

1. PCPs (such as melting point, molecular weight, molar refraction, …),
2. structure related descriptors (such as molecular volume, solvent accessible surface area, number of rotatable/rigid bonds, number of hydrogen bond donor/acceptor atoms, …),
3. quantum chemical descriptors (such as optimized total energy, HOMO and LUMO energies, …),
4. topological parameters,
5. molecular connectivity indices,
6. electrostatic state (E-state) descriptors,

7.   group contribution method or fragment based approach (different fragments derived rom structure, SMILIES/InChI codes),

8.   solvatochromic parameters (Dearden, 2006; Katritzky et al., 2010; Jouyban et al., 2010b). Other descriptors have been used as well, and a number of mixtures of the mentioned parameters are used, too. In the next section, the easiest and the most accurate models for solubility prediction are discussed. Also approaches like mobile order theory and differential equations of activity coefficient for the calculation of solubility have been used as semi-empirical methods (Dearden, 2006; Katritzky et al., 2010).

For modelling, multiple linear regression (MLR), partial least square (PLS), support vector machine (SVM), artificial neural network (ANN), random forest (RF), Monte Carlo simulation (MCS), and other methods are used. Mostly, correlation coefficients of the non-linear methods are better than linear methods and the related errors are smaller (Dearden, 2006; Katritzky et al., 2010). This might suggest a nature of non-linear behaviour for solubility.

3.1 Aqueous solubility

Available models and software to predict the aqueous solubility of drugs were reviewed in a recent work (Jouyban et al., 2008). Solubility of drugs in water could be predicted using different models presented in the literature. The general single equation of Yalkowsky is the simplest and the most common method in the pharmaceutical area. The model requires experimental melting point (mp) and logarithm of partition coefficient ($\log P$) as input data and is expressed as:

$$\log S_W = 0.5 - 0.01(mp - 25) - \log P \tag{4}$$

where S_w is the molar aqueous solubility of a drug at 25 °C. If the solute has a melting point less than 25 °C, the (mp-25) term is set to zero (Ran et al., 2001). The two parameters, $\log P$ and mp are good representatives of effects of hydrophobicity and crystal packing on the solubility of a certain solute. Jain et al. (2008) provided some theoretical background for general single equation from thermodynamic principles. The simplicity of the model is its main advantage and a possible disadvantage is the melting point as an experimental parameter which may not be available for some of the compounds in early stages of drug discovery. An attempt has been made to predict the melting points from chemical structure was not successful (Jain and Yalkowsky, 2010) and it is recommended to use experimental values of melting point in the computations using general single equation (Chu and Yalkowsky, 2009). Also drugs with high melting points which decompose before melting are not suitable to be predicted by this model. The $\log P$ is measured using experimental methods such as HPLC, and/or calculated by some computational methods, then applied to solubility prediction.

The linear solvation energy relationship is another model developed by Abraham and his co-workers (Stovall et al., 2005a) and is presented as:

$$\log S_W = 0.395 - 0.955E + 0.320S + 1.155A + 3.255B - 0.785A \cdot B - 3.330V \tag{5}$$

in which E is excess molar refraction of the compound, S is dipolarity/polarizability, A and B are hydrogen bond acidity and basicity, respectively, which these later three parameter (S,

A and B) determined from solubility data of a compound in water and different organic solvents, the $A \cdot B$ term is a representative of hydrogen-bond interactions between acidic and basic functional groups of the drug in its pure solid or liquid, V is one percent of the McGowan volume and simply is calculated using group contribution method (Stovall et al., 2005).

In a recent work from our group, a simple equation was proposed to predict the aqueous solubility of drugs trained by the solubility data of pharmaceuticals (220 drugs) and was validated using various validation methods (Shayanfar et al, 2010). The proposed model is:

$$\log S_W = -1.120E - 0.599C \log P \qquad (6)$$

Both parameters (E and ClogP or computed logP) employed in equation 6 are computed using Pharma-Algorithms (Pharma Algorithms, 2008), therefore, the model is an *in silico* model and no experimental data is required in the prediction procedure. In the pharmaceutical literature, an external prediction set consisting of aqueous solubility of 21 pharmaceutical and non-pharmaceutical compounds (Ran et al., 2001) usually were used to test the prediction capability of the proposed models. This data could not well represent the aqueous solubility data of pharmaceutical compounds, and another data set has been proposed consisting of the solubility of 75 official drugs collected from the literature. A list of the proposed test set and the experimental and predicted aqueous solubilities using equations 1-3 are listed in Table 3.

Drug	Experimental	Equation 4	Equation 5	Equation 6
Acetaminophen	-1.06	-1.18	-0.63	-1.39
Acetazolamide	-2.49	-1.18	0.06	-1.43
Acyclovir	-2.24	-0.37	0.91	-1.26
Allopurinol	-2.26	-2.19	0.38	-1.30
Amiloride	-3.36	-1.96	-0.07	-2.74
Amoxicilin	-2.17	-0.11	-1.90	-2.38
Antipyrine	0.39	-0.9	-1.16	-1.91
Atenolol	-1.30	-0.98	-1.85	-1.81
Atropine	-2.12	-1.77	-3.77	-2.43
Azathioprine	-3.21	-1.98	-1.95	-3.16
Baclofen	-1.67	-0.53	-1.84	-0.76
Benzocaine	-2.33	-1.98	-1.82	-2.14
Celecoxib	-3.74	-3.73	-5.38	-4.55
Chloramphenicol	-2.11	-1.57	-2.16	-2.55
Chlorpromazine	-5.27	-4.82	-5.97	-5.72
Ciprofloxacin	-3.73	-1.11	-2.78	-2.04
Colchicine	-0.96	-1.76	-3.93	-3.00
Cortisone	-3.00	-2.72	-4.43	-2.88
Dapsone	-3.19	-2.43	-2.05	-2.94
Diazepam	-3.76	-3.34	-4.58	-4.06

Diethylstilbestrol	-4.57	-5.805	-4.94	-4.82
Digoxin	-4.16	-3.12	-10.31	-4.94
Diltiazem	-2.95	-4.39	-4.64	-4.41
Ephedrine	-0.47	-0.52	-1.28	-1.65
Estradiol	-4.84	-4.95	-4.53	-4.43
Famotidine	-2.48	-0.09	-1.18	-2.53
Fluorouracil	-1.03	-1.24	0.55	-0.38
Gemfibrozil	-3.16	-4.26	-4.44	-3.54
Griseofulvin	-4.61	-3.45	-3.47	-3.28
Guaifenesin	-0.60	-0.36	-1.10	-1.45
Haloperidol	-4.43	-4.08	-5.44	-4.22
Halothane	-1.71	-1.68	-1.99	-1.56
Hydrochlorothiazide	-2.63	-1.61	-1.04	-2.18
Hydroquinone	-0.18	-1.66	-0.23	-1.56
Isoniazid	0.01	-0.154	0.97	-0.85
Ketoprofen	-3.25	-2.73	-3.95	-3.27
Labetalol	-3.45	-3.44	-4.32	-3.75
Lamotrigine	-3.14	-4.05	-3.48	-4.26
Levodopa	-1.72	-0.02	-0.35	-0.29
Lindane	-4.60	-4.08	-4.53	-3.76
Lovastatin	-6.01	-5.40	-6.42	-4.18
Manitol	0.06	1.08	0.89	-0.18
Maprotiline	-4.69	-5.28	-5.91	-5.03
Meprobamate	-1.82	-1.36	-1.62	-1.44
Mercaptopurine	-3.09	-1.84	-0.70	-1.66
Metoclopramide	-3.18	-2.99	-2.85	-3.04
Metronidazole	-1.22	-0.585	-1.14	-1.09
Minoxidil	-1.98	-2.97	-2.19	-2.46
Mitomycin C	-2.56	-2.53	-0.12	-2.46
Mycophenolic acid	-4.39	-3.30	-4.99	-3.19
Nifedipine	-4.78	-2.10	-3.71	-2.42
Nitrofurantoin	-3.24	-2.19	-0.98	-2.03
Nitroglycerin	-2.26	-1.19	-2.22	-1.66
Omeprazole	-3.62	-3.21	-3.00	-4.43
Oxytetracycline	-3.09	0.07	-4.04	-3.30
p-Aminobenzoic acid	-1.37	-1.93	-0.65	-1.65
Papaverine	-3.87	-4.43	-4.66	-4.67
Phenobarbital	-2.29	-2.39	-1.90	-2.59
Phenytoin	-3.99	-4.07	-3.20	-3.35
Progesterone	-4.40	-4.35	-5.64	-4.08
Propofol	-3.05	-3.38	-3.82	-3.28
Propoxyphene	-5.01	-4.38	-6.45	-4.14
Prostaglandin-E_2	-2.47	-2.73	-5.22	-3.16

Quinine	-2.82	-2.11	-4.01	-4.06
Riboflavin	-3.65	-0.43	-2.77	-2.21
Salicylic acid	-1.93	-2.87	-1.53	-2.24
Sertraline	-4.94	-6.59	-6.17	-4.98
Sulfacetamide	-1.23	-0.99	-0.83	-1.64
Terfenadine	-6.69	-6.63	-9.05	-6.39
Testosterone	-4.06	-4.02	-4.89	-3.66
Theophylline	-1.38	-2.09	-0.18	-1.71
Thiabendazole	-3.48	-4.68	-3.21	-3.94
Tolbutamide	-3.46	-2.93	-3.13	-2.93
Trimethoprim	-2.95	-2.22	-6.11	-2.61
Warfarin	-3.89	-3.19	-7.40	-3.61

Table 3. List of the test data set for evaluating the capability of the models for aqueous solubility prediction, the experimental ($logS_W$) and predicted values by equations 4-6

The solubility value of a drug is affected by pH which is largely depends on whether the compound has acid/base ionizable functional groups. Most of the pharmaceutical compounds are weak acids or bases which could be dissociated according to the following equlibria:

$$Acidic\ Drug:\quad HA + H_2O \xleftrightarrow{pKa} A^- + H_3O^+ \quad,\quad pK_a = \frac{\left[A^-\right]\cdot\left[H_3O^+\right]}{[HA]}$$

$$Basic\ Drug:\quad B + H_2O \xleftrightarrow{pKb} BH^+ + OH^- \quad,\quad pK_b = \frac{\left[BH^+\right]\cdot\left[OH^-\right]}{[B]}$$

where HA and B are acidic and basic drugs, respectively, pK_a is the acid dissociation constant, and pK_b is basic dissociation constant. The solubility of a weak acid or base in solutions with different pH is calculated by Henderson–Hasselbalch equation:

$$Acidic\ Drug:\quad \log S_T = \log S_0 + \log\left(10^{pH-pKa} + 1\right) \tag{7a}$$

$$Basic\ Drug:\quad \log S_T = \log S_0 + \log\left(10^{pKa-pH} + 1\right) \tag{7b}$$

where S_T and S_0 are total and intrinsic solubility, respectively. So for solubility prediction of a drug at different pH values we need to have intrinsic solubility and pK_a value for the drug (Sinko and Martin, 2006).

However, having a specific pK_a value for a compound does not mean it will have complete activity in every pH values which is the case for most of the drugs which do not have complete activity in aqueous solutions.

There are some mathematical models for calculation of the solubility and pK_a of the compounds (Dearden, 2006; Jouyban, 2009; Katritzky et al., 2010). However, complete activity will be gained in two conditions: 1- infinite dilution and 2- strong acidic condition for basic compounds (or strong basic condition for acidic compounds).

3.2 Solubility in organic solvents

Few models were presented to calculate the solubility of drugs in organic solvents. Yalkowsky et al. (1983) calculated the mole fraction solubility of weak electrolytes and non-electrolytes in n-octanol at 30 °C as:

$$\log X_{Oct} = -0.011 mp + 0.15 \tag{8}$$

$$\log X_{Oct} = -0.013 mp + 0.44 \tag{9}$$

Dearden and O'Sullivan (1988) proposed the following equation for calculating the molar solubility of drugs in cyclohexane (S_{Cyc}):

$$\log S_{Cyc} = -0.0423 mp + 1.45 \tag{10}$$

which was tested on the solubility of 12 pharmaceuticals and the mean percentage deviation was 85.1 (± 21.6) % (Jouyban, 2009).

Sepassi and Yalkowsky (2006) proposed another version of equation 8 to compute the molar solubility of drugs in octanol as:

$$\log S_{Oct} = -0.01(mp - 25) + 0.5 \tag{11}$$

The mean percentage value of equation 11 was 147 (± 247) % (Jouyban, 2009).

The Abraham solvation model provides a more comprehensive solubility prediction method for organic solvents (Abraham et al., 2010). The Abraham model written in terms of solubility is:

$$\log\left(\frac{S_S}{S_W}\right) = c + e \cdot E + s \cdot S + a \cdot A + b \cdot B + v \cdot V \tag{12}$$

where S_S and S_W are the solute solubility in the organic solvent and water (in mole/L), respectively. In equation 12, the coefficients c, e, s, a, b and v are the model constants (i.e. solvent's coefficients), which depend upon the solvent system under consideration. These coefficients were computed by regression analysis of measured $\log\left(\frac{S_S}{S_W}\right)$ values, infinite dilution activity coefficients and partition coefficients of various solutes against the corresponding solute parameters (Abraham and Acree, 2005). The Abraham solvent coefficients (c, e, s, a, b and v) and Abraham solute parameters (E, S, A, B and V) represent the extent of all known interactions between solute and solvents in the solution (Stovall et al., 2005b).

3.3 Solubility at different temperatures

Solubility of a solute in an ideal solution could be mathematically represented by van't Hoff equation:

$$\log S = \frac{a}{T} + b \tag{13}$$

where a is the slope of the linear plot of $\ln S$ against $\dfrac{1}{T}$ and b is the intercept. The a term is

equal to $\dfrac{-\Delta H_f}{2.303R}$ and b is equal to $\dfrac{\Delta H_f}{2.303RT_m}$ for ideal solutions in which R is the molar gas

constant and T_m is the melting point expressed as K. Equation 13 provides good relationship in the narrow range of temperature. For ideal solutions, the enthalpy of mixing is zero, therefore the enthalpy of solution (ΔH_s) is equal to the enthalpy of fusion (ΔH_f). The ΔH_s is always endothermic for ideal solutions, and the solute solubility will be increased by increasing the temperature. The pattern is different for gases, liquids and solids as shown in Figure 4 where the solubility of gases decreases with increased temperature. The Hildebrand equation is an alternative model and expressed as:

$$\log S = a \ln T + b \qquad (14)$$

in which a and b are the adjustable parameters. Equations 13 and 14 fail to represent the solubility-temperature relationship of most of pharmaceutical compounds in water and other pharmaceutically interested solvents especially at a wide temperature range. There are some physico-chemical reasons for this deviation from linear relationships, e.g. formation of polymorphs or solvate forms of the drug, which was discussed in details by Grant et al. (1984). To represent such data, a combined version of the van't Hoff and Hildebrand equations could be used. The equation is:

$$\log S = \frac{a}{T} + b \ln T + c \qquad (15)$$

in which a, b and c are the adjustable parameters calculated by a least square analysis (Grant et al., 1984).

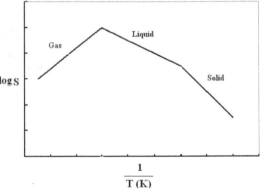

Fig. 4. The van't Hoff plot for gases, liquids and solids

3.4 Solubility in mixed solvents
The log-linear model of Yalkowsky is the simplest and famous model to calculate the solubility of pharmaceuticals in mixed solvent systems and is expressed by:

$$\log S_m = \log S_2 + \sigma \cdot f_1 \qquad (16)$$

where S_m is the solubility of the solute in the mixed solvent system, S_2 denote the aqueous solubility of drug, σ is the solubilization power of the cosolvent and theoretically is equal to $(\log(S_1 / S_2))$ in which S_1 is the solubility in the neat cosolvent (Yalkowsky and Roseman, 1981). The general form of the log-linear model for multi-component solvent systems could be written as:

$$\log S_m = \log S_2 + \sum \sigma_i f_i \qquad (17)$$

where σ_i and f_i are the solubilization power and the fractions of cosolvent i (Li, 2001).

Valvani et al. (1981) reported a linear relationship between σ and logarithm of drug's partition coefficient ($\log P$) which is a key relationship and could improve the prediction capability of the log-linear model. The relationship was expressed as:

$$\sigma = M \cdot \log P + N \qquad (18)$$

where M and N are the cosolvent constants and are not dependent on the solute's nature. The numerical values of M and N were reported for most of the common cosolvents earlier (Li and Yalkowsky, 1998) and listed in Table 4. This version of the log-linear model could be considered as a predictive model and provided the simplest solubility estimation method and requires the aqueous solubility of the drug and its experimental/calculated logP value as input data. The log-linear model was developed to predict the solubility of drugs at room temperature (22 – 27 °C) however the solubility at other temperatures are also required in the pharmaceutical industry.

Solvent system	M	N
Acetone - water	1.14	-0.10
Acetonitrile – water	1.16	-0.49
Butylamine – water	0.64	1.86
Dimethylacetamide – water	0.96	0.75
Dimethylformamide – water	0.83	0.92
Dimethylsulphoxide – water	0.79	0.95
Dioxane – water	1.08	0.40
Ethanol – water	0.93	0.40
Ethylene glycol – water	0.68	0.37
Glycerol – water	0.35	0.26
Methanol – water	0.89	0.36
Polyethylene glycol 400 – water	0.74	1.26
1-Propanol – water	1.09	0.01
2-Propanol – water	1.11	-0.50
Propylene glycol - water	0.77	0.58

Table 4. Updated Table from (Li and Yalkowsky, 1998; Millard et al., 2002.)

The Jouyban-Acree model was adopted from the combined nearly ideal binary solvent/Redlich-Kister equation proposed by Prof. Acree (1992) which was derived from a thermodynamic mixing model that includes contributions from both two-body and three-body interactions (Hwang et al., 1991). The model was presented for solubility calculations in binary solvents at a fixed temperature and expressed as:

$$\log S_m = f_1 \log S_1 + f_2 \log S_2 + f_1 f_2 \sum_{i=0}^{2} A_i \left(f_1 - f_2 \right)^i \tag{19}$$

where A_i stands for the model constants. The A_i values are calculated by regressing $\left(\log S_m - f_1 \log S_1 - f_2 \log S_2 \right)$ against $f_1 f_2$, $f_1 f_2 (f_1 - f_2)$ and $f_1 f_2 (f_1 - f_2)^2$ by a no intercept least squares analysis (Jouyban-Gharamaleki and Hanaee, 1997). The applicability of the model was extended to other physico-chemical properties in mixed solvents at various temperatures as:

$$\log S_{m,T} = f_1 \log S_{1,T} + f_2 \log S_{2,T} + \frac{f_1 f_2}{T} \sum_{i=0}^{2} J_i \left(f_1 - f_2 \right)^i \tag{20}$$

where $S_{m,T}$, $S_{1,T}$ and $S_{2,T}$ are the solubility in solvent mixture, mono-solvents 1 and 2 at temperature T (K) and J_i is the model constants. The main limitations of the Jouyban-Acree model for predicting drug solubilities in solvent mixtures are: a) it requires two data points of solubilities in mono-solvent systems, and b) numerical values of the model constants. To overcome the first limitation, the solubility prediction methods in mono-solvent system should be improved. To address the second limitation, the following solutions were examined during last couple of years:

i.   the J_i terms are obtained using solubility of structurally related drugs in a given mixed solvent system, and then predict the un-measured solubility of the related drugs where the expected mean percentage deviation was ~ 17 % (Jouyban-Gharamaleki et al., 1998).

ii.   the model constants could be calculated using a minimum number of experimental data points, i.e. three data points, and then predict the solubilities at the rest of solvent compositions where the expected prediction mean percentage deviation was < 15 % (Jouyban-Gharamaleki et al., 2001).

iii. the trained versions of the Jouyban-Acree models could be employed for solubility prediction of drugs in the aqueous mixtures of a number of organic solvents were reported. Using this version of the model, only the solubility data in mono-solvents are required. Table 5 listed the numerical values of the Jouyban-Acree model constants for the 5 cosolvents studied.

Solvent system	J₀	J₁	J₂	Prediction % error
Dioxane - water	958.44	509.45	867.44	27
Ethanol – water	724.21	485.17	194.41	48
Polyethylene glycol 400 – water	394.82	-355.28	388.89	40
Propylene glycol - water	37.03	319.49	-	24
Ethanol – ethyl acetate	382.987	125.663	214.579	13

Table 5. The constants of the Jouyban-Acree model for a number of solvent systems, data taken from (Jouyban and Acree, 2007; Jouyban, 2008)

iv.   in the trained versions of the Jouyban-Acree model, we assumed the extent of the solute-solvent interactions are the same, however, it is not the case since various solutes possess different functional groups leading to various extent of the solute-solvent interactions. To cover this point, the deviated solubilities from the trained versions of the Jouyban-Acree model were correlated using available solubility data sets in ethanol – water and dioxane – water mixtures at various temperatures and the following equations are obtained:

$$\log S_{m,T} = f_1 \log S_{1,T} + f_2 \log S_{2,T}$$

$$+ \left(\frac{f_1 f_2}{T} \right) \{ 558.45 + 358.60E + 22.01S - 352.97A + 130.48B - 297.10V \}$$

$$+ \left(\frac{f_1 f_2 (f_1 - f_2)}{T} \right) \{ 45.67 - 165.77E - 321.55S + 479.48A - 409.51B + 827.63V \} \qquad (21)$$

$$+ \left(\frac{f_1 f_2 (f_1 - f_2)^2}{T} \right) \{ -493.81 - 341.32E + 866.22S - 36.17A + 173.41B - 555.48V \}$$

and

$$\log S_{m,T} = f_1 \log S_{1,T} + f_2 \log S_{2,T}$$

$$+ \left(\frac{f_1 f_2}{T} \right) \{ 648.01 - 404.99E + 428.69 + S340.99A - 59.03B - 56.94V \}$$

$$+ \left(\frac{f_1 f_2 (f_1 - f_2)}{T} \right) \{ -135.95 - 41.11E - 192.19S + 237.81A + 363.87B + 310.30V \} \qquad (22)$$

$$+ \left(\frac{f_1 f_2 (f_1 - f_2)^2}{T} \right) \{ -1102.49 - 667.02E + 2070.16S + 421.15A - 924.73B - 271.54V \}$$

The mean percentage deviation values for ethanol and dioxane were 34 and 22 %, respectively (Jouyban et al., 2009).

v. a generalized version of the Jouyban-Acree model was proposed using its combination with the Abraham solvation parameters where the model constants of the Jouyban-Acree model were correlated with the functions of the Abraham solvent coefficients and the solute parameters as:

The mean percentage deviation of this model was 42 % for 152 data sets which was significantly less than that of the log-linear model (78 %). Figure 5 shows the relative frequency of the individual percentage deviations of the predicted solubilities using equations 23 and 16 (log-linear) in which the error distribution of equation 23 is better than that of the log-linear model. It should be noted that the Jouyban-Acree model requires two experimental data points, i.e. $S_{1,T}$ and $S_{2,T}$, whereas the log-linear model needs just aqueous solubility of the drug as input data. The main advantage of equation 23 is that it could be used to predict the solubility in mixed solvents where the Abraham solvent parameters (i.e. c, e, s, a, b and v) are available. Table 6 listed these parameters for a number of more common solvents in the pharmaceutical industry. Unfortunately these parameters are not available for a number of more common pharmaceutical cosolvents, such as propylene glycol and polyethylene glycols, and this is a disadvantage for this model.

$$\log S_{m,T} = f_1 \log S_{1,T} + f_2 \log S_{2,T}$$

$$+ \left(\frac{f_1 f_2}{T}\right) \begin{Bmatrix} 1639.07 - 561.01\left[(c_1 - c_2)^2\right] - 1344.81\left[E(e_1 - e_2)^2\right] - 18.22\left[S(s_1 - s_2)^2\right] \\ -3.65\left[A(a_1 - a_2)^2\right] + 0.86\left[B(b_1 - b_2)^2\right] + 4.40\left[V(v_1 - v_2)^2\right] \end{Bmatrix}$$

$$+ \left(\frac{f_1 f_2 (f_1 - f_2)}{T}\right) \begin{Bmatrix} -1054.03 + 1043.54\left[(c_1 - c_2)^2\right] + 359.47\left[E(e_1 - e_2)^2\right] - 1.20\left[S(s_1 - s_2)^2\right] \\ +30.26\left[A(a_1 - a_2)^2\right] - 2.66\left[B(b_1 - b_2)^2\right] - 0.16\left[V(v_1 - v_2)^2\right] \end{Bmatrix} \quad (23)$$

$$+ \left(\frac{f_1 f_2 (f_1 - f_2)^2}{T}\right) \begin{Bmatrix} 2895.07 - 1913.07\left[(c_1 - c_2)^2\right] - 901.29\left[E(e_1 - e_2)^2\right] - 10.87\left[S(s_1 - s_2)^2\right] \\ +24.62\left[A(a_1 - a_2)^2\right] + 9.79\left[B(b_1 - b_2)^2\right] - 24.38\left[V(v_1 - v_2)^2\right] \end{Bmatrix}$$

In addition to the above discussed models to predict the solubility of drugs in solvent mixtures, there are some models derived from molecular thermodynamic approaches. These models require relatively complex computations and did not attract more attention in the pharmaceutical area. These models provide comparable prediction accuracies with the above discussed models. As an example, the prediction error of a method based on statistical mechanical fluctuation solution theory varied 0.3-58 % (Ellegaard et al., 2010) whereas the corresponding value for the common models in the pharmaceutical area varied between 8 to 19 % (Jouyban-Gharamaleki et al., 1999).

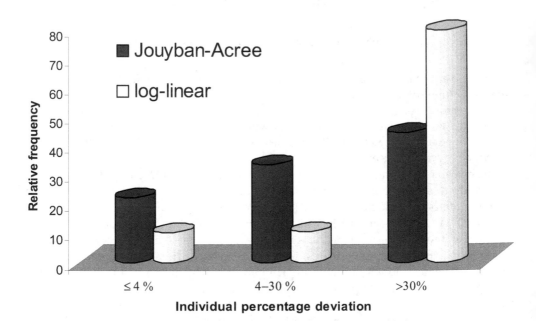

Fig. 5. The relative frequencies of the predicted solubilities in binary solvent mixtures using Jouyban-Acree and log-linear models

Solvent	c	e	s	a	b	v
Acetone	0.335	0.349	-0.231	-0.411	-4.793	3.963
Acetonitrile	0.413	0.077	0.326	-1.566	-4.391	3.364
Dimethyl formamide	-0.438	-0.099	0.670	0.878	-4.970	4.552
Dioxane	0.098	0.350	-0.083	-0.556	-4.826	4.172
Ethanol	0.208	0.409	-0.959	0.186	-3.645	3.928
Ethylene glycol	0.243	0.695	-0.670	0.726	-2.399	2.670
Methanol	0.329	0.299	-0.671	0.080	-3.389	3.512
2-Propanol	0.063	0.320	-1.024	0.445	-3.824	4.067
Water	-0.994	0.577	2.549	3.813	4.841	-0.869

Table 6. The Abraham solvent parameters of a number of common solvents (data taken from Stovall et al., 2005a; 2005b)

3.5 Solubility in the presence of surfactants

Equation 24 is one of the equations used for the solubility calculation in presence of surfactant (Rangel-Yagui et al., 2005):

$$\chi = \frac{\left(S_T - S_W\right)}{\left(C_{Surfactant} - cmc\right)} \tag{24}$$

where χ is the ratio of the concentration of the drug in micelles to the concentration of the micellar surfactant molecules, S_T is the total drug solubility in the solution, S_W is the aqueous solubility of the drug, $C_{Surfactant}$ is the molar concentration of the surfactant in the solution, and cmc is the critical micelle concentration. Another equation is (Rangel-Yagui et al., 2005):

$$K = \frac{S_T - S_W}{S_W} \tag{25}$$

where K is the micelle-water partition coefficient of the drug.

However, these equations require at least two other experimental data as input for total solubility prediction of the drug in micellar solutions.

Abraham et al. (1995) have proposed two models for prediction of K for different solutes in the presence of sodium dodecylsulfate (SDS) as:

$$\log K_x = 1.201 + 0.542E - 0.400S - 0.133A - 1.580B + 2.793V$$
$$R = 0.9849 \quad, \quad N = 132 \quad, \quad \text{standard deviation} = 0.171 \tag{26}$$

and

$$\log K_x = 1.129 + 0.504 \log P + 1.216V$$
$$R = 0.9755 \quad , \quad N = 132 \quad , \quad \text{standard deviation} = 0.215 \tag{27}$$

where K_x is the definition of K of equation 25 in mole fraction unit (Abraham et al., 1995). Ghasemi and coworkers have developed a MLR model for micellar solubility prediction in the presence of SDS for a diverse set of compounds:

$$\log K_S = -0.638 + 0.001E_b + 0.384MR - 0.112LUMO + 0.570C\log P - 0.001\,\text{Re}\,pE$$
$$R^2 = 0.9679 \quad , \quad N = 62 \quad , \quad RMSEP = 0.124 \tag{28}$$

where K_S is the micellar solubility, E_b is bending energy, MR is molar refractivity, LUMO is the lowest unoccupied molecular orbital, ClogP is logarithm of calculated partition coefficient and $RepE$ is the repulsion energy (Ghasemi et al., 2008). In other work, they have proposed a QSPR model for micellar solubility prediction for a diverse set of compounds in presence of cetyltrimethylammonium bromide (CTAB) as:

$$\log K_S = -1.1522 + 0.0070MP + 0.8089\log P - 0.1262DPLL$$
$$R^2 = 0.9624 \quad , \quad N = 40 \quad , \quad RMSEP = 0.169 \tag{29}$$

where MP is melting point of the solute, and $DPLL$ is the dipole length of the solute (Ghasemi et al., 2009).
However, as mentioned above, at least intrinsic solubility is required for total solubility prediction in the presence of a surfactant and they cannot be used as *ab initio* QSPR models for solubility prediction.

3.6 Solubility in the presence of complexing agents
In most of the cases, by adding complexing agents (e.g. cyclodextrins) to the solution, the solubility of a specific ligand (i.e. drug) is enhanced. But this enhancement could have different types as illustrated in Figure 6.
As has been seen, different kinds of drugs show different behaviours. But except for one condition, in the smaller amounts of complexing agent, the solubility changes are the same for other types. This common part of the curves is considered as a straight line with a slope of:

$$Slope = \frac{K_{1:1}S_0}{1 + K_{1:1}S_0}$$
$$K_{1:1} = \frac{[Host.Ligand]}{[Host]\cdot[Ligand]} \tag{30}$$

where $K_{1:1}$ is the complex formation coefficient, [*Host.Ligand*] is the concentration of the formed complex between drug and complexing agent, [*Host*] is the concentration of the complexing agent, and [*Ligand*] is the concentration of the drug (Sinko and Martin, 2006; Brewster and Loftsson, 2007). To correlate solubility value in presence of a complexing agent in this part of the solubility curve, one can use the following equation:

$$S_{Total}^{Complex} = S_0 + Slope \cdot C_{Host} \tag{31}$$

where $S_{Total}^{Complex}$ is the total solubility amount in the presence of a complexing agent, S_0 is the intrinsic solubility, *Slope* is the slope of the first part of solubility curve versus complexing agent concentrations, and C_{Host} is the concentration of the complexing agent (Sinko and Martin, 2006; Brewster and Loftsson, 2007).

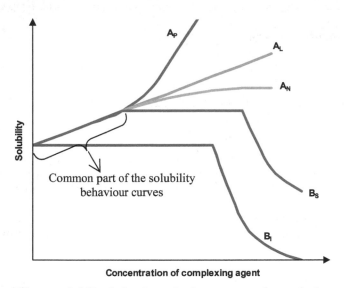

Fig. 6. Possible different solubility behaviours in the presence of complexing agent.

Again, like the pH and surfactant effects, one must have intrinsic solubility and *Slope* (or $K_{1:1}$) for solubility prediction in presence of complexing agents. However some QSPR models have been developed for prediction of *Slope* (or $K_{1:1}$). But most of them only considered the effect of complexing agent on the solubility enhancement (i.e. *Slope*). Demian (2000) has proposed equation 32 for the correlation of the *Slope* of the above mentioned equation for aromatics and terpenes with hydroxypropyl-β-cyclodextrin:

$$Slope = 2.86 - 0.11 \times SterimolL - 0.34 \times \log P$$
$$R = 0.788 \quad , \quad N = 19 \quad , \quad \text{standard error} = 0.336$$

(32)

where *SterimolL* is a steric parameter which is calculated by ChemOffice software (Demian, 2000). Choi et al. (2006) have developed a QSPR model for the correlation of the *Slope* for A_L type solubility curves between drugs and α/β/γ-cyclodextrines as following:

$$Slope = -0.012E_{h-g} + 0.102E_{np\_h-g} + 0.328E_{np\_g-g} + 0.305$$
$$R^2 = 0.913 \quad , \quad N = 63 \quad , \quad \text{standard error} = 0.028$$

(33)

where E_{h-g} is the interaction energy between host and guest, E_{np_h-g} is the difference between nonpolar components of free energy of solvation of the host–guest complex and those of individual host and guest molecules, E_{np_g-g} is the difference between nonpolar components of free energy of solvation of the guest–guest dimer and those of individual guest molecule (Choi et al., 2006). These energy values are calculated after a Monte Carlo docking simulation between each drug and related complexing agent. Trapani et al. (2005) have developed a QSPR model for the correlation of the ratio of the total versus intrinsic solubilities of 25 drugs in the presence of 2-hydroxypropyl-β-cyclodextrin as following:

$$\log \frac{S_{Total}^{Complex}}{S_0} = 3.766 + 0.182CMR - 0.150C \log P - 0.00683TPSA - 0.0844\delta_{tot}$$
(34)

$$R^2 = 0.793 \quad , \quad N = 25 \quad , \quad Q^2 = 0.711$$

and

$$\log \frac{S_{Total}^{Complex}}{S_0} = 1.827 - 0.00508MW + 0.0122MV - 0.179C \log P - 0.00547TPSA$$
(35)

$$R^2 = 0.763 \quad , \quad N = 25 \quad , \quad Q^2 = 0.605$$

where CMR is calculated molecular refractivity, $TPSA$ is total polar surface area, δ_{tot} total solubility parameter, MW is molecular weight, and MV is molecular volume. Equation 34 was derived using a MLR method and equation 35 was derived using a PLS method (Trapani et al., 2005).

However, as mentioned earlier, none of these models can be applied directly for solubility prediction in the presence of complexing agents and intrinsic solubility is required for all of them.

3.7 Available software

There is almost a large number of software for solubility prediction. A thorough review of these software was provided in an article (Jouyban et al., 2008). In this chapter, more useful solubility prediction applications and those which are newly developed or related with drug design and development is discussed.

ACD/Solubility DB predicts aqueous solubility at different pH with an accuracy of average error of 0.47±0.67 (in decimal logarithm) for solubility prediction of 1125 compounds (ACD/Labs).

ACD/DMSO Solubility predicts whether a compound is soluble (a result of 1) or insoluble (a result of 0) in DMSO. Using a hybrid model of logistic regression with PLS method, its predictive model was trained with solubility related physicochemical parameters, and considering the effects of charged groups, atom chains, and ring scaffolds. It provides 30% high reliability, 70% moderate reliability and <1% low reliability in prediction, with an overall accuracy of 82% in correct prediction (Japertas et al.).

Simulations plus' ADMET predictor™, predicts aqueous solubility using 2D and 3D descriptors as input data with average error of 0.432 and 0.423 in logarithm scale for 2817 and 711 number of compounds in train and test sets, respectively (ADMET Predictor™). It can also predict the solubility in biorelevant medium of the fasted state simulated gastric fluid (FaSSGF), the fasted state simulated intestinal fluid (FaSSIF), and the fed state simulated intestinal fluid (FeSSIF). Its average errors in logarithm scale for FaSSGF are 0.510 and 0.470 for 137 and 20 compounds, respectively. Its average errors in logarithm scale for FaSSIF are 0.469 and 0.417 for 141 and 16 compounds, respectively. Its average errors in logarithm scale for FeSSIF are 0.424 and 0.409 for 136 and 21 compounds, respectively. These predictive tools are designed using 2D descriptors as inputs and ADMET Modeler's ANNE methodology for modelling (ADMET Predictor™). This package also can predict possibility of supersaturation in water. It calculates ratio of kinetic solubility versus intrinsic solubility and if the result is higher than 1.3, then the answer to possibility of supersaturation is true. It classified 95 and 23 out of 97 and 24 compounds correctly as train and test sets (ADMET Predictor™).

Finally, Solvomix is a recently developed free software available via Handbook of Solubility Data for Pharmaceuticals as a tool for prediction of solubility in monosolvents and mixtures of solvents. It uses GSE and Abraham models for the prediction of solubility in monosolvents and trained versions of log-linear model of Yalkowsky and Jouyban-Acree model for solubility prediction in mixtures of solvents (Jouyban, 2009).

4. Conclusion

Although preparation of a drug solution is a simple procedure, the associated problems are still a challenging subject in the pharmaceutical area. Brief review of its importance, various experimental and computational methods to determine the solubility and a number of more common methods to alter the solubility are discussed in this chapter. A comprehensive compilation of aqueous solubility data of chemical/pharmaceutical compounds is available from a reference work of Yalkowsky et al. 2010. The solubility data of pharmaceuticals in organic mono-solvents and also aqueous and non-aqueous solvent mixtures are compiled in a recent work (Jouyban, 2009).

5. Acknowledgment

This work is dedicated to Professor S.A. Mahboob, Tabriz University of Medical Sciences, Tabriz, Iran, for his life long efforts in training pharmacy students in Tabriz.

6. References

Abraham, M.H.; Chadha, H.S.; Dixon, J.P.; Rafols, C. & Treiner, C. (1995). Hydrogen Bonding. Part 40. Factors That Influence the Distribution of Solutes between Water and Sodium Dodecylsulfate Micelles. *Journal of the Chemical Society, Perkin Transactions 2*, pp. 887-894, ISSN *0300-9580*

Abraham, M.H. & Acree Jr., W.E. (2005). Characterisation of the Water-Isopropyl Myristate System. *International Journal of Pharmaceutics*, Vol. 294, pp. 121-128, ISSN *0378-5173*

Abraham, M.H.; Smith, R.E.; Luchtefeld, R.; Boorem, A.J.; Luo, R. & Acree Jr., W.E. (2010). Prediction of Solubility of Drugs and Other Compounds in Organic Solvents. *Journal of Pharmaceutical Sciences*, Vol. 99, pp. 1500-1515, ISSN *0378-5173*

ACD/Labs. Advanced Chemistry Development. Available from http://207.176.233.196/products/phys_chem_lab/aqsol/

ADMET Predictor™. Simulations plus inc. available from http://www.simulations-plus.com/Products.aspx?grpID=1&cID=11&pID=13

Acree Jr., W.E. (1992). Mathematical Representation of Thermodynamic Properties. Part II. Derivation of the Combined Nearly Ideal Binary Solvent (NIBS)/Redlich-Kister Mathematical Representation from a Two-Body and Three-Body Interactional Mixing Model. *Thermochimica Acta*, Vol. 198, pp. 71-79, ISSN *0040-6031*

Allen, L.V.; Popovich, N.G. & Ansel, H.C. (2006). *Ansel's Pharmaceutical Dosage Forms and Drug Delivery Systems*, Lippincott Williams & Wilkins, ISBN 978-078-1770-17-0, Philadelphia, US

Alsenz, J. & Kansy, M. (2007). High Throughput Solubility Measurement in Drug Discovery and Development. *Advanced Drug Delivery Reviews*, Vol. 59, pp. 546-567, ISSN 0169-409X

Black, S.N.; Collier, E.A.; Davey, R.J. & Roberts, R.J. (2007). Structure, Solubility, Screening, and Synthesis of Molecular Salts. *Journal of Pharmaceutical Sciences*, Vol. 96, pp. 1053-1068, ISSN 0022-3549

Blagden, N.; de Matas, M.; Gavan, P.T. & York, P. (2007). Crystal Engineering of Active Pharmaceutical Ingredients to Improve Solubility and Dissolution Rates. *Advanced Drug Delivery Reviews*, Vol. 59, pp. 617-630, ISSN 0169-409X

Bolen, D.W. (2004). Effects of Naturally Occurring Osmolytes on Protein Stability and Solubility: Issues Important in Protein Crystallization. *Methods*, Vol. 34, pp. 312-322, ISSN 1046-2023

Brewster, M.E. & Loftsson, T. (2007). Cyclodextrins as Pharmaceutical Solubilizers. *Advanced Drug Delivery Reviews*, Vol. 59, pp. 645-666, ISSN 0169-409X

Burgess, R.R. (2009). Chapter 20 Protein Precipitation Techniques. *Methods in Enzymology*, Vol. 463, pp. 331-342, ISSN 0076-6879

Choi, Y.; Cho, K.W.; Jeong, K.; Paik, S.R. & Jung, S. (2006). Computational Prediction for the Slopes of A_L-Type Phase Solubility Curves of Organic Compounds Complexed with α-, β-, or γ-Cyclodextrins Based on Monte Carlo Docking Simulations. *Journal of Inclusion Phenomena*, Vol. 55, pp. 103-108, ISSN 1388-3127

Chu, K.A. & Yalkowsky, S.H. (2009). Predicting Aqueous Solubility: The Role of Crystalinity. *Current Drug Metabolism*, Vol. 10, pp. 1184-1191, ISSN 1389-2002

Dearden, J.C. & O'Sullivan, J.G. (1988). Solubility of Pharmaceuticals in Cyclohexane. *Journal of Pharmacy and Pharmacology*, Vol. 40, p. 77P, ISSN 0022-3573

Dearden, J.C. (2006). In Silico Prediction of Aqueous Solubility. *Expert Opinion on Drug Discovery*, Vol. 1, pp. 31-52, ISSN 1746-0441

Demian, B.A. (2000). Correlation of the Solubility of Several Aromatics and Terpenes in Aqueous Hydroxypropyl-β-cyclodextrin with Steric and Hydrophobicity Parameters. *Carbohydrate Research*, Vol. 328, pp. 635-639, ISSN 0008-6215

Ellegaard, C.; Abidsko, J. & O'Connell, P.O. (2010). Molecular Thermodynamic Modelling of Mixed Solvent Solubility. *Industrial and Engineering Chemistry Research*, Vol. 49, pp. 11620-11632, ISSN 0888-5885

Fakhree, M.A.A.; Delgado, D.R.; Martínez, F. & Jouyban, A. (2010). The Importance of Dielectric Constant for Drug Solubility Prediction in Binary Solvent Mixtures: Electrolytes and Zwitterions in Water+Ethanol. *AAPS PharmSciTech*, Vol. 11, pp. 1726-1729, ISSN 1530-9932

Galcera, J. & Molins, E. (2009). Effects of the Counterion on the Solubility of Isostructural Pharmaceutical Lamotrigine Salts. *Crystal Growth and Design*, Vol. 9, pp. 327-334, ISSN 1528-7483

Ghasemi, J.; Abdolmaleki, A.; Asadpour, S. & Shiri, F. (2008). Prediction of Solubility of Nonionic Solutes in Anionic Micelle (SDS) Using a QSPR Model. *QSAR and Combinatorial Science*, Vol. 27, pp. 338-346, ISSN 1611-020X

Ghasemi, J.B.; Abdolmaleki, A. & Mandoumi, N. (2009). A Quantitative Structure Property Relationship for Prediction of Solubilization of Hazardous Compounds Using GA-

Based MLR in CTAB Micellar Media. *Journal of Hazardous Materials*, Vol. 161, pp. 74-80, ISSN 0304-3894

Gibaldi, M.; Lee, M. & Desai, A. (2007). *Gibaldi's Drug Delivery Systems in Pharmaceutical Care*, Lea & Febiger, ISBN 978-158-5281-36-7, Philadelphia, US

Golightly, L.K.; Smolinkse, S.S.; Bennett, M.L.; Sunderland III, E.W. & Rumack, B.H. (1988). Pharmaceutical Excipients Adverse Effects Associated with Inactive Ingredients in Drug Products (Part I). *Medical Toxicology and Adverse Drug Experience*, Vol. 3, p. 128-165, ISSN 0113-5244

Grant, D.J.W. & Abougela, I.K.A (1983). A Synthetic Method for Determining the Solubility of Solids in Viscous Liquids. *International Journal of Pharmaceutics*, Vol. 16, pp. 11-21, ISSN 0378-5173

Grant, D.J.W.; Mehdizadeh, M.; Chow, A.H.L. & Fairbrother, J.E. (1984). Non-Linear van 't Hoff Solubility - Temperature Plots and Their Pharmaceutical Interpretation. *International Journal of Pharmaceutics*, Vol. 18, pp. 25-38, ISSN 0378-5173

Hankinson, R.W. & Thompson, D. (1965). Equilibria and Solubility Data for Methanol – Water -1-Nitropropane Ternary Liquid System. *Journal of Chemical and Engineering Data*, Vol. 10, pp. 18-19, ISSN 1520-5134

Hansch, C.; Quinlan, J.E. & Lawrence, G.L. (1968). The Linear Free-Energy Relationship Between Partition Coefficients and the Aqueous Solubility of Organic Liquids. *Journal of Organic Chemistry*, Vol. 33, pp. 347-350, ISSN 0022-3263

Hao, H.X.; Hou, B.H.; Wang, J.K. & Zhang, M.J. (2005). Solubility of Erythriol in Different Solvents. *Journal of Chemical and Engineering Data*, Vol. 50, pp. 1454-1456, ISSN 1520-5134

Higuchi, T. & Connors, K.A. (1965). Phase-solubility techniques. *Advances in Analytical Chemistry and Instrumentation*. Vol. 4, pp. 117-212

Hoelke, B.; Gieringer, S.; Arlt, M. & Saal, C. (2009). Comparison of Nephelometric, UV-Spectroscopic, and HPLC Methods for High-Throughput Determination of Aqueous Drug Solubility in Microtiter Plates. *Analytical Chemistry*, Vol. 81, pp. 3165-3172, ISSN 0003-2700

Hwang, C.A.; Holste, J.C.; Hall, K.R. & Mansoori, G.A. (1991). A Simple Relation to Predict or to Correlate the Excess Functions of Multicomponent Mixtures. *Fluid Phase Equilibria*, Vol. 62, pp. 173-189, ISSN 0378-3812

Jain, P.; Sepassi, K. & Yalkowsky, S.H. (2008). Comparison of Aqueous Solubility Estimation from AQUAFAC and GSE. *International Journal of Pharmaceutics*, Vol. 360, pp. 122-147, ISSN 0378-5173

Jain, P. & Yalkowsky, S.H. (2010). Prediction of Aqueous Solubility from SCRATCH. *International Journal of Pharmaceutics*, Vol. 385, pp. 1-5, ISSN 0378-5173

Japertas, P.; Maas, P. & Petrauskas, A. DMSO Solubility Prediction. Available from http://www.acdlabs.com/products/pc_admet/physchem/dmso/

Jouyban-Gharamaleki, A. & Hanaee, J. (1997). A Novel Method for Improvement of Predictability of the CNIBS/R-K Equation. *International Journal of Pharmaceutics*, Vol. 154, pp. 245-247, ISSN 0378-5173

Jouyban-Gharamaleki, A.; Barzegar-Jalali, M. & Acree Jr., W.E. (1998). Solubility correlation of structurally related drugs in binary solvent mixtures. *International Journal of Pharmaceutics*, Vol. 166, pp. 205-209, ISSN 0378-5173

Jouyban-Gharamaleki, A.; Valaee, L.; Barzegar-Jalali, M.; Clark, B.J. & Acree Jr., W.E. (1999). Comparison of Various Cosolvency Models for Calculating Solute Solubility in

Water-Cosolvent Mixtures. *International Journal of Pharmaceutics*, Vol. 177, pp. 93-101, ISSN 0378-5173

Jouyban-Gharamaleki, A.; York, P.; Hanna, M. & Clark, B.J. (2001) Solubility Prediction of Salmeterol Xinafoate in Water-Dioxane Mixtures. *International Journal of Pharmaceutics*, Vol. 216, pp. 33-41, ISSN 0378-5173

Jouyban, A. & Acree Jr., W.E. (2007). Prediction of Drug Solubility in Ethanol-Ethyl Acetate Mixtures at Various Temperatures Using the Jouyban-Acree Model. *Journal of Drug Delivery Science and Technology*, Vol. 17, pp. 159-160, ISSN 1773-2247

Jouyban, A.; Fakhree, M.A.A. & Shayanfar, A. (2008). Solubility prediction methods for drug/drug like molecules. *Recent Patent on Chemical Engineering*, Vol. 1, pp. 220-231, ISSN 1874-4788

Jouyban, A.; Soltanpour, Sh.; Soltani, S.; Tamizi, E.; Fakhree, M.A.A. & Acree Jr., W.E. (2009). Prediction of Drug Solubility in Mixed Solvents Using Computed Abraham Parameters. *Journal of Molecular Liquids*, Vol. 146, 82-88, ISSN 0167-7322

Jouyban, A. (2009) *Handbook of Solubility Data for Pharmaceuticals*, CRC Press, ISBN 978-143-9804-85-8, Boca Raton, USA.

Jouyban, A. & Soltanpour, Sh. (2010). Solubility of Pioglitazone Hydrochloride in Binary and Ternary Mixtures of Water, Propylene Glycol, and Polyethylene Glycols 200, 400 and 600 at 298.2 K. *AAPS PharmSciTech*, Vol. 11, pp. 1713-1717, ISSN 1530-9932

Jouyban, A.; Fakhree, M.A.A. & Shayanfar, A. (2010a). Review of Pharmaceutical Applications of N-Methyl-2-Pyrrolidone. *Journal of Pharmacy and Pharmaceutical Sciences*, Vol. 13, pp. 524-535, ISSN 1482-1826

Jouyban, A.; Fakhree, M.A.A.; Shayanfar, A. & Ghafourian, T. (2010b). QSPR Modelling Using Catalan Solvent and Solute Parameters. *Journal of Brazilian Chemical Society*, In press, ISSN 0103-5053

Katritzky, A.R.; Kuanar, M.; Slavov, S.; Hall, C.D.; Karelson, M.; Kahn, I. & Dobchev, D.A. (2010). Quantitative Correlation of Physical and Chemical Properties with Chemical Structure: Utility for Prediction. *Chemical Reviews*, Vol. 110, pp. 5714-5789, ISSN 0009-2665

Kawakami, A.; Miyoshi, K. & Ida, Y. (2005). Impact of the Amount of Excess Solids on Apparent Solubility. *Pharmaceutical Research*, Vol. 22, pp. 1537-1543, ISSN 0724-8741

Li, A. & Yalkowsky, S.H. (1998) .Predicting Cosolvency. 1. Solubility Ratio and Solute logKow. *Industrial and Engineering Chemistry Research*, Vol. 37, pp. 4470-4475, ISSN 0888-5885

Li, A. (2001). Predicting Cosolvency. 3. Evaluation of the Extended Log-Linear. *Industrial and Engineering Chemistry Research*, Vol. 40, pp. 5029-5035, ISSN 0888-5885

Li, X.; Yin, Q.; Chen, W. & Wang, J. (2006). Solubility of Hydroquinone in Different Solvents from 276.65 to 345.10 K. *Journal of Chemical and Engineering Data*, Vol. 51, pp. 127-129, ISSN 1520-5134

Lim, L.-Y. & Go, M.-L. (2000). Caffeine and Nicotinamide Enhances the Aqueous Solubility of the Antimalarial Agent Halofantrine. *European Journal of Pharmaceutical Sciences*, Vol. 10, pp. 17–28, ISSN 0928-0987

Millard, J.F.; Alvarez-Nunez, F.A. & Yalkowsky, S.H. (2002). Solubilization by Cosolvents. Establishment Useful Constants for the Log-Linear Model. *International Journal of Pharmaceutics*, Vol. 245, 153-166, ISSN 0378-5173

Mizuuchi, H.; Jaitely, V.; Murdan, S. & Florence, A.T. (2008). Room Temperature Ionic Liquids and Their Mixtures: Potential Pharmaceutical Solvents. *European Journal of Pharmaceutical Sciences*, Vol. 33, pp. 326-331, ISSN *0928-0987*

Myrdal, P.B. & Yalkowsky, S.H. (1998). Solubilization of Drugs, In: *Encyclopedia of Pharmaceutical Technology*, Swarbrick, J. & Boylan, J.C. (Eds.), 161-217, Marcel Dekker, ISBN 978-082-4728-19-9, New York, US

Pan, L.; Ho, Q.; Tsutsui, K. & Takahashi, L. (2001). Comparison of Chromatographic and Spectroscopic Methods Used to Rank Compounds for Aqueous Solubility. *Journal of Pharmaceutical Sciences*, Vol. 90, pp. 521-529, ISSN *0022-3549*

Patel, D.M.; Bernardo, P.; Cooper, J. & Forrester, R.B. (1986). Glycerine. In: *Handbook of Pharmaceutical Excipients*, 203-213, America and Great Britain Pharmaceutical Societies, London, UK

Peisheng, M.A. & Qing, X. (2001). Determination and Correlation for Solubility of Aromatic Acids in Solvents. *Chinese Journal of Chemical Engineering*, Vol. 9, pp. 39-44, ISSN *1004-9541*

Pharma-Algorithms (2008). ADME Boxes, Version 4.0, PharmaAlgorithms Inc., Toronto, Canada

Ran, Y.; Jain, N. & Yalkowsky S.H. (2001). Prediction of Aqueous Solubility of Organic Compounds by the General Solubility Equation (GSE). *Journal of Chemical Information and Computer Science*, Vol. 41, pp. 1208-1217, ISSN *0095-2338*

Rangel-Yagui, C.deO.; Pessoa Jr., A. & Tavares, L.C. (2005). Micellar Solubilization of Drugs. *Journal of Pharmacy and Pharmaceutical Sciences*, Vol. 8, pp. 147-163, ISSN *1482-1826*

Ren, B.Z.; Chong, H.G.; Li, W.R. & Wang F.A. (2005). Solubility of Potassium p-Chlorophenoxyacetate in Ethanol + Water from (295.61 to 358.16) K. *Journal of Chemical and Engineering Data*, Vol. 50, pp. 907-909, ISSN *1520-5134*

Rubino, J.T. (1990). Cosolvents and Cosolvency, In: *Encyclopedia of Pharmaceutical Technology*, Swarbrick, J. & Boylan, J.C. (Eds.), 375-398, Marcel Dekker, ISBN 978-082-4728-19-9, New York, US

Sepassi, K. & Yalkowsky, S.H. (2006). Solubility Prediction in Octanol: A Technical Note. *AAPS PharmSciTechnol*, Vol. 7: p. E1-E8, ISSN *1530-9932*

Shayanfar, A.; Fakhree, M.A.A. & Jouyban, A. (2010). A Simple QSPR Model to Predict Aqueous Solubility of Drugs. *Journal of Drug Delivery Science and Technology*, Vol. 20, pp. 467-476, ISSN *1773-2247*

Sinko, P.J. & Martin, A.N. (2006). *Martin's Physical Pharmacy and Pharmaceutical Sciences*, Lippincott Williams & Wilkins, ISBN 978-078-1750-27-1, Philadelphia, US

Spiegel, A.J. & Noseworthy, M.M. (1963). Use of Nonaqueous Solvents in Parenteral Products. *Journal of Pharmaceutical Sciences*, Vol. 52 pp. 917-927, ISSN *0022 -3549*

Stovall, D.M.; Acree Jr., W.E. & Abraham M.H. (2005a) Solubility of 9-Fluorenone, Thianthrene and Xanthene in Organic Solvents. *Fluid Phase Equilibria*, Vol. 232, pp. 113-121, ISSN *0378-3812*

Stovall, D.M.; Givens, C.; Keown, S.; Hoover, K.R.; Barnes, R.; Harris, C.; Lozano, J.; Nguyen, M.; Rodriguez, E.; Acree Jr., W.E. & Abraham, M.H. (2005b). Solubility of Crystalline Nonelectrolyte Solutes in Organic Solvents: Mathematical Correlation of 4-Chloro-3-Nitrobenzoic Acid and 2-Chloro-5-Nitrobenzoic Acid Solubilities with the Abraham Solvation Parameter Model. *Physics and Chemistry of Liquids*, Vol. 43, pp. 351-360, ISSN *0031-9104*

Strickley, R.G. (2004). Solubilizing Excipients in Oral and Injectable Formulations. *Pharmaceutical Research*, Vol. 21, pp. 201-230, ISSN 0724-8741

Trapani, A.; Lopedota, A.; Denora, N.; Laquintana, V.; Franco, M.; Latrofa, A.; Trapani, G. & Liso, G. (2005). A Rapid Screening Tool for Estimating the Potential of 2-Hydroxypropyl-β-Cyclodextrin Complexation for Solubilization Purposes. *International Journal of Pharmaceutics*, Vol. 295, pp. 163-175, ISSN 0378-5173

Trevino, S.R.; Scholtz, J.M. & Pace, C.N. (2008). Measuring and Increasing Protein Solubility. *Journal of Pharmaceutical Sciences*, Vol. 97, pp. 4155-4166, ISSN 0022-3549

Tsai, P.S.; Lipper, R.A. & Worthington, H.C. (1986). Propylene Glycol, In: *Handbook of Pharmaceutical Excipients*, 241-242, America and Great Britain Pharmaceutical Societies, London, UK

Valvani, S.C.; Yalkowsky, S.H. & Roseman, T.J. (1981). Solubility and Partitioning IV: Aqueous Solubility and Octanol-Water Partition Coefficients of Liquid Nonelectrolytes. *Journal of Pharmaceutical Sciences*, Vol. 70, pp. 502-507, ISSN 0022-3549

Waldo, G.S. (2003). Genetic Screens and Directed Evolution for Protein Solubility. *Current Opinion in Chemical Biology*, Vol. 7, pp. 33-38, ISSN 1367-5931

Wang, L.C.; Ding, H.; Zhao, J.H.; Song C.Y. & Wang J.S. (2008). Solubility of Isonicotinic Acid in 4-Methylpyridine + Water from (287.65 to 361.15) K. *Journal of Chemical and Engineering Data*, Vol. 53, pp. 2544-2546, ISSN 1520-5134

Wang, Z.; Burrell, L.S. & Lambert, W.J. (2002). Solubility of E2050 at Various pH: A Case in Which Apparent Solubility Is Affected by the Amount of Excess Solid. *Journal of Pharmaceutical Sciences*, Vol. 91, pp. 1445-1455, ISSN 0022-3549

Ward, H.L. (1926). The Solubility Relations of Naphthalene. *Journal of Physical Chemistry*, Vol. 30, pp. 1316-1333, ISSN 0022-3654

Weiwei, S.; Peisheng, M.A.; Lihua, F. & Zhengle X. (2007). Solubility of Glutamic Acid in Cyclohexane, Cyclohexanol, Their Five Mixtures and Acetic Acid. *Chinese Journal of Chemical Engineering*, Vol. 15, pp. 228-232, ISSN 1004-9541

Wells, J.I. (1988). *Pharmaceutical Preformulation*, ISBN 978-074-5802-76-3, Ellis Harwood Ltd., Chiester, England.

Widenski, D.J.; Abbas, A. & Romagnoli, J.A. (2009). Effect of the Solubility Model on Antisolvent Crystallization Predicted Volume Mean Size. *Chemical Engineering Transactions*, Vol. 17, pp. 639–44

Yalkowsky, S.H. & Roseman, T. (1981) Solubilization of Drugs by Cosolvents In: *Techniques of Solubilization of Drugs*, Yalkowsky, S.H. (Ed.), 91-134, Marcel Dekker, ISBN 978-082-4715-66-3, New York, US

Yalkowsky, S.H.; Valvani, S.C. & Roseman, T.J. (1983). Solubility and Partitioning. VI: Octanol Solubility and Octanol-Water Partition Coefficients. *Journal of Pharmaceutical Sciences*, Vol. 72, pp. 866-870, ISSN 0022-3549

Yalkowsky, S.H.; He, Y. & Jain, P. (2010) *Handbook of Aqueous Solubility Data*, CRC Press, ISBN 978-143-9802-46-5, Boca Raton, USA.

Yang, Z.S.; Zeng, Z.X.; Xue W.L. & Zhang Y. (2008). Solubility of Bis(benzoxaolyl-2-methyl) Sulfide in Different Pure Solvents and Ethanol + Water Binary Mixtures between (273.25 and 325.25) K. *Journal of Chemical and Engineering Data*, Vol. 53, pp. 2692-2695, ISSN 1520-5134

Yu, Q.; Black, S. & Wei H. (2009). Solubility of Butanedioic Acid in Different Solvents at Temperatures between 283 K and 333 K. *Journal of Chemical and Engineering Data*, Vol. 54, pp. 2123-2125, ISSN 1520-5134

Permissions

The contributors of this book come from diverse backgrounds, making this book a truly international effort. This book will bring forth new frontiers with its revolutionizing research information and detailed analysis of the nascent developments around the world.

We would like to thank Dr. William Acree, for lending his expertise to make the book truly unique. He has played a crucial role in the development of this book. Without his invaluable contribution this book wouldn't have been possible. He has made vital efforts to compile up to date information on the varied aspects of this subject to make this book a valuable addition to the collection of many professionals and students.

This book was conceptualized with the vision of imparting up-to-date information and advanced data in this field. To ensure the same, a matchless editorial board was set up. Every individual on the board went through rigorous rounds of assessment to prove their worth. After which they invested a large part of their time researching and compiling the most relevant data for our readers. Conferences and sessions were held from time to time between the editorial board and the contributing authors to present the data in the most comprehensible form. The editorial team has worked tirelessly to provide valuable and valid information to help people across the globe.

Every chapter published in this book has been scrutinized by our experts. Their significance has been extensively debated. The topics covered herein carry significant findings which will fuel the growth of the discipline. They may even be implemented as practical applications or may be referred to as a beginning point for another development. Chapters in this book were first published by InTech; hereby published with permission under the Creative Commons Attribution License or equivalent.

The editorial board has been involved in producing this book since its inception. They have spent rigorous hours researching and exploring the diverse topics which have resulted in the successful publishing of this book. They have passed on their knowledge of decades through this book. To expedite this challenging task, the publisher supported the team at every step. A small team of assistant editors was also appointed to further simplify the editing procedure and attain best results for the readers.

Our editorial team has been hand-picked from every corner of the world. Their multi-ethnicity adds dynamic inputs to the discussions which result in innovative outcomes. These outcomes are then further discussed with the researchers and contributors who give their valuable feedback and opinion regarding the same. The feedback is then collaborated with the researches and they are edited in a comprehensive manner to aid the understanding of the subject.

Apart from the editorial board, the designing team has also invested a significant amount of their time in understanding the subject and creating the most relevant covers. They scrutinized every image to scout for the most suitable representation of the subject and create an appropriate cover for the book.

The publishing team has been involved in this book since its early stages. They were actively engaged in every process, be it collecting the data, connecting with the contributors or procuring relevant information. The team has been an ardent support to the editorial, designing and production team. Their endless efforts to recruit the best for this project, has resulted in the accomplishment of this book. They are a veteran in the field of academics and their pool of knowledge is as vast as their experience in printing. Their expertise and guidance has proved useful at every step. Their uncompromising quality standards have made this book an exceptional effort. Their encouragement from time to time has been an inspiration for everyone.

The publisher and the editorial board hope that this book will prove to be a valuable piece of knowledge for researchers, students, practitioners and scholars across the globe.

List of Contributors

Abolghasem Jouyban
Drug Applied Research Center and Faculty of Pharmacy, Iran

Somaieh Soltani
Liver and Gastrointestinal Diseases Research Center, Tabriz University of Medical Sciences, Tabriz, Iran

Amadeo Pesce, Cameron West and Kathy Egan-City
Millennium Research Institute, USA

William Clarke
Johns Hopkins School of Medicine, USA

Alexandra Eder, Arne Hansen and Thomas Eschenhagen
Department of Experimental Pharmacology and Toxicology, University Medical Centre Hamburg-Eppendorf, Germany

Abolghasem Jouyban
Drug Applied Research Center and Faculty of Pharmacy, Tabriz University of Medical Sciences, Tabriz, Iran

Anahita Fathi-Azarbayjani
Faculty of Medicine, Urmia University of Medical Sciences, Urmia, Iran

William E. Acree, Jr. and Laura M. Grubbs
University of North Texas, United States

Michael H. Abraham
University College London, United Kingdom

Hans-Georg Breitinger
The German University in Cairo, Egypt

Nasir Mohamad
Department of Emergency Medicine, School of Medical Sciences, Health Campus, Universiti Sains Malaysia, Kubang Kerian, Kelantan, Malaysia Pharmacogenetic Research Group, Institute for Research in Molecular Medicine (INFORMM), Health Campus, Universiti Sains Malaysia, Kubang Kerian, Kelantan, Malaysia

Nor Hidayah Abu Bakar
Department of Pathology, Hospital Raja Perempuan Zainab II, Kota Bharu, Kelantan, Malaysia

Tan Soo Choon, Sim Hann Liang, NIM Nazar, Ilya Irinaz Idrus and Rusli Ismail
Pharmacogenetic Research Group, Institute for Research in Molecular Medicine (INFORMM), Health Campus, Universiti Sains Malaysia, Kubang Kerian, Kelantan, Malaysia

Anoka A. Njan
Department of Pharmacology and Toxicology, Faculty of Pharmaceutical Scinces, Usmanu Danfodiyo University, Sokoto, Nigeria

Abolghasem Jouyban
Drug Applied Research Center and Faculty of Pharmacy, Iran

Mohammad A. A. Fakhree
Liver and Gastrointestinal Diseases Research Center, Tabriz University of Medical Sciences, Tabriz, Iran

Printed in the USA
CPSIA information can be obtained
at www.ICGtesting.com
JSHW011418221024
72173JS00004B/579

9 781632 423511